AFTERWARDS,
YOU'RE A GENIUS

AFTERWARDS, YOU'RE A *Genius*

Faith, Medicine, and the Metaphysics of Healing

Chip Brown

Riverhead Books
a member of Penguin Putnam Inc.
NEW YORK   1998

Parts of this book appeared in different form in
*The New York Times Magazine, Glamour, Mademoiselle,
Vogue,* and *Travel & Leisure*

Riverhead Books
a member of
Penguin Putnam Inc.
375 Hudson Street
New York, NY 10014

Library of Congress Cataloging-in-Publication Data

Brown, Chip.
Afterwards, you're a genius: faith, medicine, and the
metaphysics of healing / by Chip Brown.
p.   cm.
ISBN 1–57322–113–9
1. Medicine—Philosophy.   2. Healing—Philosophy.
3. Medicine—Religious aspects.   4. Therapeutics, Suggestive.
5. Spiritual healing.   6. Mental healing.   7. Mind and body
therapies.   8. Faith—Health aspects.   I. Title.
R723.B695   1998   98–36015 CIP
615.5'01—dc21

Printed in the United States of America

1 3 5 7 9 10 8 6 4 2

This book is printed on acid-free paper. ∞

BOOK DESIGN BY LYNNE AMPFT

FOR KATE

CONTENTS

AFTERWARDS,
YOU'RE A 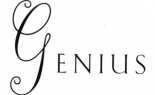ENIUS

CHAPTER ONE

The gods have become diseases.

— C. G. JUNG

1. THE FLOWER OF THE DEAD

More than a few years ago, when I was in a bad way, wallowing in a sob story about an actress who'd exchanged me for a used-car salesman in California, I went to see a psychic. It was half a lark, or so I thought at the time. The heartache that inspired the visit was real enough, but I was not able to make any sense of it until much later, when I happened on Borges's description of love as a religion organized around a fallible god. For the millions of us who press on in a secular age, under Darwin's empty heaven, love may be all we ever know of religion, and the loss of love is that much more wrenching for its likeness to a crisis of faith. What else but a confusion of divine and human realms can account for the pain of misplaced devotion? Pain made worse by the ludicrousness of it all, the ersatz savior and the preposterous church and the disillusioned parishioner, who stumbles around in the aftermath—stupefied, in my case, by the sight of his highly beloved on Channel 7 in a Fruit of the Loom commercial. There she was! Dressed as a guava or possibly a passion fruit. Something tropical. I couldn't see clearly. I was too busy gasping for air. She turned up again a few weeks later as a guest star on a cheesy detective show, but this time there was an offsetting, even therapeutic, consolation: She got shot in the head.

In those premillennial days, there were no psychic hotlines or $3.95-a-minute clairvoyants with has-been celebrities vouching for their skills, and the whiff of charlatanism that has always attended the guild of seers was not half as ripe as it seems now. There were shrinks, of course, but I wanted to look ahead to the future, where I imagined redemption was waiting, and not back, at the estrangement and misery of the recent past. A friend had given me the card of the Reverend Diane Nagorka at the National Spiritual Science Center, which was described as "an oasis of spirit in the Nation's Capital." I made an appointment, and on a mild February morning, I rode a bus up to the address in an old, middle-class neighborhood. At the end of a little path was a large house with a roomy porch. The receptionist who answered the door showed me into a living room where the walls were hung with paintings of saints. The shades were drawn, and in the Rembrandt gloom, the holy figures seemed almost luminous.

At length, Reverend Diane emerged. The mistress of the oasis was in her early sixties and resembled a scuffed-up Katharine Hepburn—a little unkempt but invincibly confident, and clearly not in the habit of suffering fools for more than three seconds. "I've been described as the no-nonsense psychic," she said as she led me up the stairs to a candlelit, book-lined consulting room where an effigy of the laughing Buddha gleamed in the corner. After many years, Reverend Diane had completed her doctorate in religious studies. She said she considered herself both a "psychic" and an "intuitive healer." She believed that universal energies unknown to science pervaded the human body; they contained information that could be read and used to promote health on any of the various tiers of a person's being.

With the laughing Buddha looking on, we settled into chairs across from each other. She fastened a small microphone to the collar of her dress and scribbled the date on a blank cassette, which she then popped into a tape recorder. She closed her eyes. She took a deep breath. And then she raised her hands as if she had just come back from a fly-fishing trip and were regaling me with the tale of the big one that got away.

"Mother-Father-God we thank thee, for thou hast said when two or three are gathered together there thou will be also." The invocation, spoken in her sandy voice, seemed to refine the air between us and impart a mood of ceremony and sacredness. You can work in Washington all your life and never hear anyone use the word "hast."

Reverend Diane's predictions can't really be of much interest all these years later. She claimed only the ability to foresee the upcoming eighteen months. She talked nonstop, mostly with her eyes closed, speaking smoothly and articulately as she presented the scenes and images appearing in her mind's eye. I later came to appreciate that she did not resort to the usual "cold reading" tactics of many so-called psychics; she did not fish for information, or pepper me with questions, or pursue themes on the strength of cues and confirmations gleaned from my responses. She said she would offer the highlights I might expect in the coming months, periods of excitement, transitions. And she stressed the provisional nature of her forecast, giving me the standard clairvoyant disclaimer that "all is chosen."

I have to say that most of what she said seemed scarcely more interesting than newspaper astrology, general enough not to be instantly refutable, but hardly profound. Of course, I wonder now if I was ready to listen to any of it, as I didn't have the foggiest idea where or how she got her information, or how anyone could envision events that hadn't happened yet. The very idea seemed crazy: an affront to the laws of the universe, at least as I presumed to understand them, which is to say an affront to the received wisdom of the culture I was trained in, a culture that had established science as the ultimate arbiter of reality. Science—or the pop distillate of it—said that what can be objectively measured is intrinsically more trustworthy, more valuable, more "real" than what can be subjectively felt. Science had lionized matter at the expense of psyche and spirit, and imagined that its preference reflected the natural order of things, not a metaphysical choice. Bones before dreams.

I was jolted out of my reverie hearing Reverend Diane say I had a sort of ethereal aide de camp, a five-thousand-year-old Chinese man who acted as a spirit guide and who stayed mostly in the background but nevertheless entered my hand whenever I wrote or played the piano. *How odd*: I hadn't told her I wrote; I hadn't mentioned having a piano.

Altogether, she spoke for half an hour, and then abruptly broke off. "It's like a movie on a screen, and when it's over, that's it," she said, opening her eyes. She asked if I had any questions. Were there people I wanted to know about? Sure, I said. She was careful to advise that she would not be invading their privacy, only reading what she could see of them in the field of my being. I tossed out the names of siblings, my parents, some old friends.

Then I threw out the name of my mop-haired heartthrob, who had inspired so many fervent journal entries and whom I could still picture in the Off-Broadway play I first saw her in, singing a song called "Tiny Lily." After the performance, when I'd recovered from my rapture in the back row, we'd gone to dinner at a fish joint in the East Village, and as we were leaving, I swiped a long-stemmed lily from a vase by the door and presented it to her. That night was the first night I stayed in her apartment. Lilies were carved on the mantel of her fireplace. Lilies in the song, lilies by the door, lilies on the mantel. It had always seemed that our affair was born under the sign of the lily, that we were wreathed in lilies, the flower of the dead.

Reverend Diane screwed up her brow for a moment—her eyes were closed again—and then shrugged, opened her eyes, and said offhandedly, as if she was sorry not to have more to tell, "Well, I see a lily."

Well, I see a lily.

You could have knocked me over with a flower. No doubt she could have said a hundred things that would have been equally true, equally disorienting. A hundred things that would have disturbed me as much for lack of knowing how she came by them. She had a lot of material to work with. My highly beloved had been ahead of her time. She had tried hard to balance the material cravings that attracted her to my American Express card with nobler, more spiritual aspirations. She meditated. She followed a guru; she quoted *pensées* about the "mystic traveler consciousness." She resolutely maintained her practice of magical thinking even though she was disappointed when the five bucks she put in a coffee can never metamorphosed into fifty or when—the harder fate—her hopes for fame and success in acting never yielded more than a few bit parts and the Fruit of the Loom spot.

I can see now that she was one of those dream-drunk seekers in the vanguard of our disenchanted age for whom the great grail is simply to feel good about themselves. She was dedicated to healing herself—but of what, exactly, it was never clear. When the emollients of fame and money weren't availing, she chased the chimera of perfect health as if it were some sort of Utopia that could be attained by effort and technique. She had her food allergies analyzed by an applied kinesiologist and steered clear of wheat. She launched juice fasts. She made appointments with a "white witch" to have her "aura brushed." She was delivered of emotional blocks in sessions with a "rebirther" and had her colon periodically flushed with coffee enemas. (She kindly warned me never to use the earthy-looking towel on the back of the bathroom door.)

So had the reverend said, "I see a beleaguered AmEx card" or "I see some coffee, not for drinking . . ." I would have been just as flabbergasted. There was an immense volume of detail my clairvoyant apparently did not perceive or find fit to report. But all the same, how had she divined the significance of *lily*? Why lily? Why not zinnia, gardenia, or furbish lousewort, which all meant nothing when lily meant the world? Many of the scoundrels who staged séances in the nineteenth century used to keep crib books of pertinent information on the prominent families who might want their services. Reverend Diane might have surmised that I worked at the local newspaper, but there were only two people in North America who could have grasped the import of lilies in the context of my love life, and, actually, at that point, given how thoroughly and rapidly I had been eclipsed, I'm pretty sure there was only one. And that was me. And yet here was some old hast-speaking wisewoman pulling it out of the ether.

All these years later, I can still recall the peculiar urgency of that hour. "Our life is not so much threatened as our perception," Emerson wrote. What was this country where science left off? Where the laws of ordinary existence seemed to be suspended and sacramentalizing crones could pinpoint the flower in a stranger's heart? Again, this time in closing, Reverend Diane raised her hands and gave thanks to her mother-father-god for that wherever-two-or-three-were-gathered place. And by then it seemed to me that we were up to our keisters in lilies, all of them glowing like that glass of poisoned milk in Hitchcock's *Notorious*. Ominous life-altering lily-light filled the room. It seemed to me my frame of reference had been broken. My assumptions had been undermined. There was a wound in my metaphysics.

Over the years, I have had but to murmur to myself "I see a lily" to bring back the depths of amazement and affliction I felt that day. Sometimes I would hear in the words a rebuke or a challenge to all the pretty categories of good sense and sound thinking that we flatter ourselves are true simply because we have established them; sometimes I would hear a summons from across the border, the siren call of uncharted territory. I began to read about psychics and their counterparts in healing circles who attempted not just to see with clairvoyant sight but to induce changes on the basis of their strange vision.

And I began to wonder about that country. In an age when the gods have become diseases, could one travel there with no qualification but curiosity, or was more required—the visa of illness, the passport of faith? Was it possible to report intelligibly about a place where facts were half dissolved in myth, and no two maps agreed, and the light, the weather, the customs, and even the substance of the inhabitants were widely held to be indescribable by the seekers and screwballs who had been there already? I wondered, because someday I meant to go.

2. SHE STARTED TO DO BETTER

Shin, the snow leopard at the San Francisco Zoo, took a turn for the worse in early May of 1995. She was a month shy of her tenth birthday, and she'd lost a third of her weight. It was clear to the veterinarians, who had her on antibiotics, that she was exhausted and dangerously ill. Their tentative diagnosis: inflammatory bowel disease. By midmonth, Shin stopped eating. She refused further medicine and would not come down from her perch. The luster of her coat was fading. She had never seen the world she was produced for, having been born in the Bronx Zoo and having spent her whole life in captivity. But her native Asian habitat was reflected in her beautiful coat: The gray of her fur was the hue of its mountain mists, the brown of her camouflage spots was the color of its ragged earth. Shin's secretive sisters were rarely seen in the wild, but their footprints were sometimes spotted as high as twenty thousand feet in the snows of Tibet.

As it happened, the third week of May, eleven Tibetan monks arrived in San Francisco from their home-in-exile in Tenzin Gang, India. They had been invited to perform their Gyuto Tantric chants by Mickey Hart, the drummer of the Grateful Dead. They asked the keepers of the San Francisco Zoo if there were any sick animals for whom they might offer a *puja*, a traditional prayer of purification, a prayer that Tibetans believe is not simply a petition for health but a way of actually strengthening the flow of life-energy in a sick creature. The sound itself rights the body.

And so the monks, dressed in their saffron robes, were shown to the Feline Conservation Center, where Shin was draped listlessly on her perch. They formed two rows in front of her cage. None of them had ever laid eyes on a snow leopard; like Shin, most of them had never even been to Tibet. But when they raised their voices in the droning overtone chant of their monastic tradition, Shin stirred. She climbed down the logs from her perch fifteen feet above the ground and came to the edge of her cage. Her whiskers poked through the wire mesh. She blinked and rubbed her face with her paws. And as the monks sang, Shin sat raptly as if she recognized some music she had never heard from a country she had never hunted. The *puja* lasted only five minutes, but it seemed much longer to the people in attendance—the keepers from the feline center, zoo staff, an Associated Press religion reporter. It seemed timeless and exquisitely beautiful. It was as if a bond had formed between the monks and the leopard, and with each minute that Shin remained at the edge of the cage, listening, some old kinship bound the wounds of exile in man and animal both.

When the chanting stopped, Shin turned and walked away. Later that day, her appetite came back, and for the first time in two weeks she showed some enthusiasm for her diet of horse meat and fortified meal. "She seemed so peaceful," said Nancy Chan, the zoo's publicist. "She started to do better."

Alas, healing and curing are not the same. On the ninth of June, her tenth birthday, the snow leopard died.

3. FRIGHTS AND MARVELS

Healing, from the Old English word *haelen*: to make whole. Whole, as in stitch the gash, reduce the fracture, bind the wound, assuage the burn, slake the fever, ice the chill, purge the poison, drain the pus, pull the bullet, excise the tumor, check the bug, dissolve the clot, uncloud the eye, allay the pain, reflate the lung, restart the heart, replace the liver, repair the mind, revive the spirit, retrieve the soul, redeem the life. Long before healing was a science, it was an art, a piece of faith, a form of magic. The catalogue of frights and marvels compiled in its name is almost beyond imagining.

In Ireland in the seventeenth century, it was said whooping cough could be cured by drinking water from the skull of a bishop. For tuberculosis (which ravaged Mozart, Goethe, Emerson, Kafka, Dostoevsky, Chekhov, Keats, and Shelley) people hung cans of dog fat over their shoulders; they swallowed monkey gallstones and slime from snails; they lingered in barns, inhaling draughts of dung-tanged air. In many parts of Europe, the odor of semen freshly ejaculated into a handkerchief was thought to cure anemia in young girls, and to improve their looks too. Flu patients sucked holy pebbles and drank urine and sprinkled the dirt of graveyards on their doorways. In the late nineteenth century, one of the members of the Brahmin Crowninshield family carried a horse chestnut in his pocket for relief from rheumatism (and at the time he was overseeing curriculum reform at Harvard's medical school).

Two years before he died in the eruption of Vesuvius, in 79 A.D., Pliny the Elder noted a Persian cure for headache: tightly bind your temples with a rope procured from the estate of someone who recently used it to commit suicide. For skin ulcers, apply goat dung kneaded with vinegar; for a chafed foot, ointment made from the ashes of an old shoe. For snakebite, apply one half of a severed mouse. (Which half? Apparently it didn't matter.) Much later, an especially elaborate cure for syphilis was tendered to Cesare Borgia, the son of Pope Alexander VI: He was to find "someone of worthless estate" to suck out his sores, then have his lesions poulticed with live frogs chopped in half, and then get some rest inside the carcass of a freshly disemboweled mule. And on and on it went. Powdered Egyptian mummy was a popular ingredient in Renaissance prescriptions. People drank a purée of old shoe soles for dysentery. They found a cure-all in moss scraped from the skulls of executed criminals.

Lest you think the twentieth century can't compete, there has been no shortage of mail-order panaceas available C.O.D. In 1928, after your morning coffee enema, you could hook up the "Vitalizer," which consisted of two "Vitality" batteries, a long wire cord, and a six-inch bar of metal, which was to be carefully inserted in the rectum, where it could then distribute one and a half volts of life-affirming electricity and quickly cure diabetes, cancer, and TB. The perfect gift for the new graduate contemplating a career in the secret police. A few decades later, people bought "Z ray" generators at fifty dollars each, which were supposedly able to expand the space between their body's atoms and thus relieve the pain of arthritis. In the 1950s, patients paid money to sit in old mine tunnels for some uncertain benefit. Seawater was advertised all over the U.S. in the 1960s for the treatment of pimples, gray hair, baldness, diabetes, and cancer. Those were the good old days of robust government intervention. Federal marshals fanned out across six states, seized two thousand bottles of Florida-packed seawater, and broke up a scam the Food and Drug Commissioner denounced as a "nationwide seawater swindle."

If the desperation weren't so pitiable, you could almost admire the inventiveness of the minds that saw healing remedies in chopped frogs and old-shoe ashes. "The history of medicine," the medical novelist Richard Gordon once wrote, "is largely the substitution of ignorance by fallacies." If Americans want to choke down unpasteurized seawater and possibly jeopardize their kidneys, why should they be restrained by their public officials? The real danger has always been the remedies that are worse than worthless, that wreak havoc in the name of healing. The American doctor Benjamin Rush, who had enormous influence on Revolutionary War–era medicine in America, thought the human body contained twice as much blood as it actually does and advocated draining four-fifths of that exaggerated quantity from sick patients. Given the treatment the English king Charles II got after toppling over backwards while being shaved one morning in February 1685—the victim of what may have been a stroke or a heart attack—he might have preferred a weekend in a gutted mule. As the king went into convulsions—his mouth foaming, his eyes rolling back—fourteen doctors rushed to his aid. They were all disciples of the medical approach that came to be known with thanks-but-no-thanks irony as "heroic medicine." One, a Dr. Scarburgh, kept a record of their unmerciful assistance. (The often-cited account I'm indebted to was first published in 1929 in a book called *Devils, Drugs and Doctors* by the physician and Yale physiology professor W. Haggard.)

First a pint of blood was taken from His Majesty's right arm. Then his shoulder was cut open and another eight ounces of blood were "cupped" out. He was given an emetic to make him vomit, two purgatives, an enema, another purgative, and two hours later, still another purgative. His head was shaved; his scalp was blistered. He was dosed with powdered hellebore root to make him sneeze and powdered cowslip flowers to fortify his brain. To soothe his system after the cathartics, he was given barley water flavored with licorice, and almonds; cups of absinthe and white wine also were provided. His feet were plastered with a mix of Burgundy pitch and pigeon dung. Again he was bled, and purged with a variety of medicaments prepared from flowers, spices, various barks, even dissolved pearls. "Later came gentian root, nutmeg, quinine, and cloves." The king rallied the next morning, and bells were rung across London, but he again went into convulsions. Forty drops of extract of human skull were administered. Then, a "rallying dose of Raleigh's antidote" was forced down his throat. It contained "an enormous number of herbs and animal extracts." The king was given bezoar stone—probably not the bezoar stone which legend held to be the crystallized tears of a deer that had been bitten by a snake, but gallstones harvested from a goat's stomach. "Alas," Dr. Scarburgh noted. "After [another] ill-fated night his serene majesty's strength seemed exhausted to such a degree that the whole assembly of physicians lost all hope and became despondent; still, so as not to appear to fail in doing their duty in any detail, they brought into play the most active cordial." And, Haggard concludes, "As a sort of grand summary to this pharmaceutical debauch, a mixture of Raleigh's antidote, pearl julep, and ammonia was forced down the throat of the dying king."

A woodcut from the time depicts Charles on the throne—in better days—laying his hands on the head of a tubercular subject. Priests and courtesans look on; the king smiles serenely. It's more than a little ironic that Charles was a practitioner of this much gentler form of healing, which was known as the "royal touch." Certainly it might have served him better than his doctors, but then, as king, he had a monopoly on the practice and, short of abdicating and quickly crowning his successor, he would have been in the strange position of having to treat himself. In between fishing and hunting and playing tennis and riding horses out in the morning to watch hawks, and roughhousing with his King Charles spaniels and his pet monkey, and reigning over "one of the most tumultuous periods of English history," not to mention attending to some thirty-nine mistresses—he left behind at least fourteen illegitimate children and was of the opinion that "God will never damn a man for allowing himself a little pleasure"— Charles II was an especially busy healer. Between 1667 and 1684, more than 68,000 people put themselves in His Majesty's hands. The crowds were so large in 1684 that half a dozen people were trampled to death. The presenting complaint was mainly scrofula, or facial tuberculosis. (People with epilepsy went to see executioners, who strangely enough supplemented their income with a little hands-on healing.) "As far as the records go, [Charles] appeared to believe in his own powers," writes the English osteopath Harry Clements in his 1952 book *Magic, Myth and Medicine*. Clements noted that the effort may well have been in vain as "mortality rates of the period showed no real diminution." And when William III came to the throne, he made no secret of his dubious view of the royal touch, saying to patients, "God give you better health and more sense."

Whatever the efficacy of royal touch—Sir Richard Blackmore, writing in 1726, said the credit for its success belonged to the "wonderful Power of Imagination"—a dose of hands-on healing would not have mauled the principle of First Do No Harm as badly as the official physicians did. Alas, as Scarburgh said; alas. There may be reasons to prefer life in the seventeenth century, but royal doctoring isn't one of them. Before he died, in what may reign forever as the sovereign example of English civility, Charles II apologized to his medical team.

4. A DEPLORABLE STORY

M odern Western doctors don't learn much history of medicine, the medical essayist Lewis Thomas once observed, because it "is so unrelievedly a deplorable story." We might ask: Would it make any difference if they did? Would familiarity with medicine's confounding history do anything but reinforce the conviction that only the most modern ideas have merit? Life in industrial countries is buoyed by the myth of medical progress, the long inspirational march from the darkness of ignorant dogma and superstition to the truths of science. At first blush, and maybe second, the case is compelling. Look at the trephined skulls dug up from ancient Incan burial sites; look at the eighteenth-century lithographs depicting French surgical attendants restraining some poor wretch on the brink of a septic and unanesthetized amputation; look at the twentieth-century photographs of medical helplessness, the swollen-faced boys in insulin comas, the polio wards littered with paralyzed kids. Survey the fallacies promoted not by quacks and witch doctors but by distinguished physicians, the best and brightest.

For thousands of years, medicine was practiced with no understanding of bacteria, viruses, genes, vitamins, hormones, neurotransmitters, antibodies, sodium channels, blood clotting factors, and a welter of other discoveries that now glut libraries and MEDLINE, the computerized medical information bank. The treatment of sickness rested with spell-casting, god-appeasing shamans and medicine men who saw the hand of the supernatural manifest in the diseases of the body. They were part chief, part priest, part counselor, part magician, part herbalist. Their medicine relied on the not-to-be-underestimated power of ritual to stimulate the body's innate healing ability: that's to say, the healing power of nature, *vis medicatrix naturae*. They depended on the power of authority, symbolic associations, and the magic embedded in what has been called the "doctrine of similarities." To treat the eye they found plants like eye-bright that resembled an eye. Walnuts looked like little brains, ergo the Rx for some head ailments. A wound in an enemy could be inflamed if the spear that had caused the cut was heated in a fire. Disease often was considered to be a malignant spirit that the shaman could suck out of the body with his mouth.

But the traditional healers were also shrewd enough to acquire over centuries a subtle empirical understanding of therapeutic plants and preparations, and healing techniques. Magic was balanced with keen reasoning. Native North Americans sewed up wounds with sutures of human hair, deer tendons, and basswood. They treated scurvy before science understood the role of vitamin C. For malaria, they peeled the bark of the cinchona tree, from which quinine was eventually derived. Willow bark gave them the essence of aspirin. The heart medicine later known as digitalis came from foxglove. Some estimates say the botanical knowledge generated largely by native people has contributed about one-third of the number of drugs in the modern pharmacy. "There can be no doubt that by trial and error they arrived at an understanding of the properties and effects of many useful botanical medicines," wrote Virgil J. Vogel in his 1970 classic, *American Indian Medicine*.

With the civilizations of the ancient world, the principles that underlay medicine shifted from magic to philosophy. The great innovation of Hippocrates in ancient Greece was the theory that disease was natural, not a supernatural affliction caused by gods. (The word "physician" comes from the Greek word *physis*, meaning "nature.") Hippocratic methods were empirical—empiricism being from the Greek *empeirikos* for "a doctor relying on experience alone." Hippocratic physicians stressed observation and experience, not the appeasement of religious deities. Epilepsy, for instance, "the sacred disease," had been considered a scourge from the gods, but a Hippocratic author writing in late fifth or early fourth century B.C. argued it was a natural phenomenon. As G. E. R. Lloyd notes in his book, *Magic, Reason and Experience*, that was an enormous conceptual shift. Of course, to attribute a natural cause is not necessarily to attribute a "correct" explanation, or one with scientific basis. In the view of the ancient doctor, epilepsy could be explained by an inundation of phlegm in the brain during a southerly wind. Not content to interpret omens, a Hippocratic investigator sawed open the head of a goat—goats were thought to be particularly susceptible to epilepsy—and observed the brain, "wet, full of fluid, and foul smelling," which to him provided "convincing proof that disease and not the deity is harming the body."

Reasoning of this ilk is akin to the logic that still persuades sailors in Micronesia that the morning sun is cool because it has come up from an overnight dip in the ocean. Empiricism as a method, especially when pressed into service of Greek philosophy, is no more immune to unfounded conclusions than medicine based on magic. Despite the impulse to query nature, the early physicians diagnosed and treated on the basis of what they thought the body should be like, not on the study of what it actually was like. "It took seventy generations to find how the body worked," says Dr. Guido Majno in his magnificent book *The Healing Hand: Man and Wound in the Ancient World.* The Greeks believed the left half of the heart was blood-free because it was reserved for man's intelligence. They thought disease was governed by the stars and the seasons, and that good health meant finding the proper balance among the four humors. They passed along the regimen of bleeding, purging, and starving that was to dominate medicine for the next two millennia. Their fixation with enemas, which has haunted medicine for centuries, may have come from the Egyptians, who, according to Herodotus, set aside three days every month for the cleansing of their bowels. There was even a court official assigned to the (unhappy?) job of irrigating the Pharaoh's colon; he was known as the Shepherd of the Royal Anus. (This piece of trivia comes from the insanely interesting *Encyclopedia of Metaphysical Medicine* by Benjamin Walker.) The Egyptians were also early pioneers of bleeding, apparently having gotten the idea from watching hippopotamuses—creatures that seemed to deliberately draw their own blood by thrashing around on sharp river rocks. Deliberately is what the people watching them thought, but I'm going to go out on a limb and say that the mind of a hippopotamus is probably not something Homo sapiens can know.

Trial and error established remedies that seemed to work. Trial and error produced invaluable discoveries all over the ancient world. Eighth-century-B.C. Assyrian stone carvings show a physician clutching poppies, recognition of the gift of pain relief. The ancient Greeks grasped the importance of draining wounds and practiced auscultation, the diagnostic art of listening to the body. Roman doctors lacking knowledge of infection observed that sword wounds healed better when plasters included myrrh, which now is known to have antibacterial properties. Chinese healers established an enormous pharmacopeia, and a successful preventive medicine, and the theory of energy flow in the body, on which acupuncture is based and which still confounds modern science. Ancient Hindu surgeons were highly skilled, and clever enough to suture wounds with the pincers of beheaded ants, a practice also known to native healers in Africa and to South American Indian tribes.

The apparent success of empirically derived methods often gave credence to baseless measures when credit properly belonged to *vis medicatrix naturae*. The body, then as now, is the great healer. Healings may occur for reasons other than those the empiricist believes. In fact, cures may happen despite treatments. One can imagine how the royal doctors would have swelled with pride had Charles II recovered, how they would have touted the proven efficacy of their murderous therapy. Even today, much of a doctor's success can be attributed to the power of suggestion, or the "placebo effect." Sometimes an empirically derived treatment would have what we narrowly and at times misleadingly think of as a "real" effect—that is to say, it would cause an organic, physiological change. Other times, it stimulated the body's latent healing ability by working on the patient's emotions or imagination. Thomas Sydenham, the English Hippocrates and the recognized founder of clinical medicine and epidemiology, was no enemy of medication. He introduced the use of opium, treated anemia patients with iron, and gave quinine to people suffering from malaria. But, as a former cavalry officer, he also recognized the therapeutic value of long horseback rides, and according to one famous story, he ordered a patient suffering from bad headaches to horse it all the way to Edinburgh, or Inverness (the sources disagree), where a brilliant headache doctor would cure what ailed the man. There was no doctor of the sort in Edinburgh or Inverness. The patient was ticked off by Sydenham's deception, but by the time he returned from his wild goose chase, he was no longer complaining about his head. One of Sydenham's more winsome, not to say insightful, observations was that "the arrival of a good clown exercises more beneficial influence upon the health of a town than twenty asses laden with drugs."

Most of the medicine in the world today—the traditional medicine that serves eighty percent of the earth's people—is practiced under the banner of empiricism. Empiricism cares more that healing happens than why. The empirical approach gives more weight to the question "Does the medicine work?" than "Why does it work?" or "Does the way it works make sense according to the principles of science as we understand them?" Practical experience will eventually assay the worth of dog fat and halved frogs, but the empiricist's position is simple: If a patient improves after a nap in a disemboweled mule, and naps in a disemboweled mule don't exacerbate the condition, then bring on the mules. As the osteopath Harry Clements wrote: "In the long history of medicine, this fact stands out more clearly than any other: reduce the violence of the treatment and the patient's chance of recovery is increased."

Medicine's long march out of magic and philosophy began with the ascendancy of science in the seventeenth century, but it took three hundred years to make the revolutionary match that allied the art of healing with the experimental study of anatomy, physiology, and biochemistry. The union was considerably delayed by Galen, the prolific physician who revived the Hippocratic texts, finished three books of his own by the time he was thirteen, and wrote more than five hundred works altogether, twenty volumes of which survive. Throughout the Middle Ages, Galen attained such cult authority that his views on anatomy were received as gospel, even though he reached them without the benefit of ever dissecting a human corpse. For epilepsy, he recommended a nine-times-a-day dose of liver from a gutted gladiator. Galen's endorsement of bleeding, starving, and purging secured that ghastly regimen's franchise for nearly fifteen hundred years. Even up until 1910, the landmark textbook of William Osler, one of the American champions of the Viennese less-is-more school known as "therapeutic nihilism," recommended bleeding for patients with pneumonia.

Locating the wellsprings of modern medicine is like finding the headwaters of the Amazon: perhaps it is the iatrochemistry of the great Swiss physician and alchemist Paracelsus, who overthrew the doctrine of the four humors; perhaps the anatomy of Vesalius, who defied Galenic dogma and took a closer look at the human corpse. Osler himself, during the Harveian Lecture at the Royal College of Physicians in London in 1906, cited the epoch-making contribution of William Harvey, whose monograph "Motions of the Heart and Blood in Animals" was published in 1628: "But at last came the age of the hand," Osler noted. "The thinking, devising, planning hand; the hand as an instrument of the mind, now reintroduced to the world in a modest little monograph of seventy-two pages from which we may date the beginning of experimental medicine." The pantheon was enlarged for Edward Jenner, who devised the smallpox vaccine, and James Lind, who worked out a cure for scurvy. Lind enlisted a dozen scurvy patients in an experiment aboard a ship in 1747. He gave two a daily quart of cider; two others received "twenty-five guts of elixir vitriol," which was apparently the only thing that King Charles II didn't get; another pair got a couple of spoonfuls of vinegar; a third pair received "a course of seawater"; two others were given "the bigness of a nutmeg"; and the final two subjects got two oranges and a lemon. The improvement was most dramatic in the citrus-eating limeys.

And so they came, little moments of enlightenment. In Paris, in 1835, the French clinician Pierre Charles Alexandre Louis discovered by means of statistical analysis the inefficacy of the lance and started the seventy-year process of stopping the bleeding. In his studies of yeast fermentation, the great Louis Pasteur founded the science of bacteriology. Claude Bernard developed the still underappreciated concept of host resistance. Joseph Lister pioneered asepsis, his genius bathetically commemorated today in the mouthwash Listerine.

To most of us, the supremacy of modern medicine seems incontestable, and we compliment ourselves when we mock the fallacies of the ignorant past. What Luddite half-wit thinks he's not fortunate to live in the time of anesthesia and penicillin? Who can quarrel with a system of medicine based on rationally justifiable treatments that promise results without having to summon gods or appease spirits? The science of medicine has come so far so fast we scarcely remember how young it is, how little could be done for a sick person even fifty years ago. (In the 1950s, Christian Scientist practitioners, who treat all disease with prayer, were nearly as numerous as M.D.s.) Before 1923, nothing could be done to resurrect people in diabetic comas. Sulfa drugs, which gave doctors the first effective means of treating infectious diseases in history, were not introduced until 1937, and the serendipitously discovered bacteria-inhibiting mold penicillin was not clinically available before 1941. The randomized double-blind controlled clinical trial—the so-called gold standard of medical research, which purports to prove that a medicine will work whether you believe in it or not—wasn't established until after the Second World War. Over the course of the twentieth century, life spans have increased in Western industrialized countries. The mean life span in ancient Rome was twenty-two years; in medieval England, thirty-three years. In the United States, by 1900, it had risen to forty-seven years, and in 1990, it was seventy-three years. Chauvinists of scientific medicine often claim the credit for the increase in life spans, but the averages were held down in ancient times by high childhood mortality—if you got past your early youth and stayed clear of snakebites, wars, and accidents, you could expect to reach a ripe-enough age. And longevity gains in modern times are due mainly to soap, sewers, better housing, and improvements in economic standards. "The major improvement in health conditions," wrote Albert Sabin, one of the pioneers of the polio vaccine, "occurred before the advent of the miracle drugs and other important therapeutic measures." But inarguably medicine contributed to the decline of infant mortality. Today, vaccines exempt children once condemned to death by infectious diseases. Smallpox has been eradicated; polio may well be gone by the end of the century.

The proud partisans of modern medicine can fling statistics out like tickertape. Heart disease has dropped by half in America since 1963. Cancer survival rates have doubled since 1930. Complex operations like coronary artery bypasses and liver transplants are almost routine. Doctors can operate on prenatal hearts the size of chickpeas. Magnetic resonance imaging can produce pictures of the body never before available—or maybe available only to clairvoyants and shamans. The wealth of knowledge is incalculable. Textbooks fifty years ago were half as thick. The number of medical journals at the Academy of Medicine library in New York exceeds 3,700. Discoveries crowd the news. We are living in the golden age of molecular biology and brain science. Researchers can deposit snippets of human genetic code into bacteria, inject the bacteria into hamster ovaries, and so cultivate synthetic hormones such as epoetin alfa that can treat anemia in people suffering from chronic kidney disease. Perennial mysteries of consciousness like depression and schizophrenia have been correlated with structural and chemical abnormalities in the brain. Scientists have even found a gene related to anxiety.

Yesterday's miracles, such as the suppression of tuberculosis or the restoration of sight by the removal of cataracts, are today's routine cures. In short, the conjunction of the clinic and the lab has produced more knowledge of human disease in the last hundred years than was amassed in all the other centuries. In this, the century of scientific medicine, what could possibly be amiss that would cause anyone to question the virtue of that revolutionary partnership, the alliance of science and medicine? What could resurrect old questions of philosophy and cast doubt on the direction the art of making whole has taken in the last thirty years? To find out, you have to look to the countercurrent of dissent and heresy that has been running against the tide of scientific medicine in the United States since the sectarian wars of the nineteenth century, and to a kind of report card issued in the first decade of the twentieth century, which in some ways partitioned what would be known as mainstream in medicine from what would be known as fringe.

5. THE DOLPHIN ENERGY

It is the nature of the fringe—the alternative medicine outlands—that when you come back from a trip there, people ask with raised eyebrows, or a pained smile, or a dismissive upturn of the voice: "Are you a believer now?" As if the question were the key, and once it was answered, all the discomfiting ambiguities of medical heresy and dissent would be resolved. It irritated me at first, mostly for the note of condescension and doubt. Doubt about my competence as a witness; doubt about my commitment to the unquestioned virtues of reason and the self-righteous principles of objectivity. Invariably, the person would say, "Well I'm very skeptical of this sort of thing, you know." And I'd have to bite my tongue to keep from snapping back that there is a difference between being a skeptic (from the Greek *skeptesthui*, meaning "one who looks around") and a narrow-minded know-nothing.

It wasn't just that the question of belief was broached with the insinuation that I had abandoned critical thinking and had become some credulous faith-hungry screwball who sowed money in coffee cans and dialed psychics after derailed love affairs. It was the implication that there is only one kind of truth, and one way of understanding it. It is certainly not hard to make the ideas and therapies of the medical outlands sound outlandish, not to say cliché, stupid, ridiculous, venal. Not to say, even—where people of antilibertarian sentiment favor the idea that the government should police what they can put in their bodies—dangerously misguided, subversive, criminal. The truth is, it *was* hard to know what to believe when you had come back from a trip to the fringe—from, say, a session with a Chinese acupuncturist who pinned a dozen needles in your face and then shook open the paper to read the race results from Aqueduct; or from a "journey to the boundless," where you spent the weekend doing chair yoga and listening to weirdly seductive quantum mush in a New Jersey hotel room; or from a consultation at an ayurvedic spa where you had your *doshas* analyzed and underwent the genuine transports of having warm sesame oil dripped onto your forehead.

The question of belief was there whenever I plunged into the postmodern madness of the great American alternative-medicine shows. Every year, health expos set up camp in hotel ballrooms in major American cities. The first of these carnivals I stumbled into was in Manhattan's Roosevelt Hotel. Thousands of people were milling around display tables laden with mineral supplements, six-packs of blue-green algae, boxes of copper bracelets, vitamin sprays, super-juicers, foot-massage dowels, water revitalizers, colloidal silver generators, nonsurgical face-lift contraptions, and trove upon trove of health books never seen in regular bookstores. There were aromatherapy displays reeking of sage and sandalwood, and crystal kingdoms that had been hacked out of Arkansas caves, and amazing magnets that promised to dissolve unwanted calcium and cholesterol. There were gems configured to balance the body "at the

Nuclear Cell level." There were wristwatches embedded with copper induction coils that supposedly could neutralize the effects of harmful electromagnetic radiation and strengthen "the harmonically resonating frequencies of the body's natural bioenergy field."

You could have your aura photographed by an "Innervision" camera. (Mine looked oddly like the out-of-focus, light-slashed snapshots my mother was always sending out for review after Thanksgiving.) If you didn't like the Innervision picture, you could try the Aura Spectrophotometer from Korona Enterprises; the Oakley, California, company says their system "detects and measures the human energy field," but that claim is not half as candid as the one in their ad copy, which brags that "the system is a commercial gold mine." You could spend twenty minutes in a machine that resembles the Orgasmatron in Woody Allen's movie *Sleeper*. It was supposed to heal by simulating six-thousand-year-old Tibetan chants. Or something. I tried it. Very nice. Probably no more effective for inflammatory bowel disease than a *puja* from an actual chorus of Tibetan monks. Weirdly, and to his credit, the operator told me that if I sang the A above middle C, I could open the energy center in my throat and heal myself, and would have no need for the Orgasmatron.

Around another corner, I fell into conversation with a macrobiotic advocate who ticked off a horrifying list of food-additive hazards. He looked terrible—sick and pale. From the looks of him, thinking about all the additives on the list was worse than ingesting them. After a couple of hours at the expo, I began to think I had wandered into some upside-down universe, where people who looked healthy were sick and people who looked sick were healthy; the situation was analogous to health-food-store produce sections, where the dull, shriveled apples are the good organic ones and the preternaturally plump, shiny, Revlon-red standbys are the supermarket Frankensteins that have been adulterated with every pesticide, preservative, and color enhancer known to science.

Truth to tell, it was starting to seem as if there was something sick about the American obsession with health, and that Flaubert was onto something when he noted in his *Dictionary of Accepted Ideas*, "Too much health, the cause of illness." How, amid the greatest medical progress in history, could such levels of dissent and paranoia and disgust with the system of medicine thrive? How could millions of people have been persuaded that medicine does not hold them in good hands? Had the enlightenment of science only deepened their anxieties?

As the day wore on, my suspicions grew. There were lectures and talks and seminars from a staggering variety of fringe advocates with books to hawk, testaments to post, confessions to divulge, doctrines to unfold, conspiracies to unmask, truths to proclaim. And, as ever, livings to make. Acupuncturists, body workers, colonic irrigators, aromatherapists, makers of angel key chains . . . A soft-voiced, doe-eyed woman in her late twenties was representing an energy-healing school in Santa Fe. She stood in front of one audience swaying slowly and gently entreating the crowd to "connect to the dolphin energy." It is probably harder to connect to the dolphin energy in midtown Manhattan than it was for the bleeding Egyptians of the ancient world to connect to the hippopotamus energy. Or at least it was that day, thanks in part to a bunch of bumptious octogenarians who were unhappy with the airy-fairy fare of the seminar and decided to make a conspicuous departure.

By contrast, the rage of Charlotte Gerson down the hall was almost refreshing. A severe and autocratic woman, well known as a fixture of the fringe, Gerson had become deeply embittered over the years by the laws that prevent her Mexican-based clinic from operating in the United States. Here she was hammering on the virtues of the carrot juice and five-coffee-enemas-a-day cancer treatment pioneered by her late father, physician Max Gerson. "Cancer is totally preventable; nobody needs to get it," she said, shouting at the crowd as if it were full of FDA bureaucrats and pompous physicians. "You can't heal cancer with poison. Cancer is impossible in a healthy body. A normal body has healthy defenses."

Maybe so. Maybe many thousands of deluded war-on-cancer researchers have been barking up the wrong tree for thirty years, unable to see the genius of enhancing the body's natural defenses with antioxidant-rich carrot juice, and too enamored of "magic bullets" and militaristic metaphors to comprehend the benefits of a back-assward cup of coffee. Maybe, as Gerson says, nothing untoward is possible in a healthy body. But even the most ardent idealist has to be suspicious of Gerson's claims, if only because they jibe so neatly with how we wish things were. What a wonderful world where nothing untoward can happen in a healthy body!

Gerson's claims, of course, were infused with the same myth of perfect health that dazzled my former mop-haired heartthrob. It was lurking everywhere at the expo, in every feel-good tip and revitalizing gizmo, and indeed it had been running through healing ideology for centuries. It is the chimera that beguiled the exponents of the "mind cure" in nineteenth-century America. It is the pot of gold at the end of the rainbow that best-selling physician-authors like Deepak Chopra cash handsome checks against. The myth of perfect health is flourishing now in our millennial climate, which is marked by nostalgia and anxiety, by the erosion of scientific authority and the rise of pluralism. When postmodernists in the medical counterculture are arguing that facts about disease are not solid, objective determinations but subjective constructions that reflect hidden social forces and metaphysical assumptions, how you assess the question of whether "cancer is totally preventable" has less to do with the weight of evidence than with the angle of your beliefs.

So you can see why it was so easy to waffle when someone asked, "Are you a believer?" and why sometimes I was tempted to ask right back, "What's it to you?" Most of the secular academic world equates faith with naive self-delusion and holds that to entertain the fairy tales of a higher power is to affront the only real higher power, which is reason. I suppose I was especially nettled because I didn't really know what I believed, and the question often was posed by fellow journalists or magazine editors who seemed to have made up their minds and who, with a cynicism that was second nature to them, were quick to mock the dolphin energy, as quick as I. I suppose they all reminded me that I was drifting out of step, restless in the complacencies of my old identity but with nothing available yet to hang a new one on, nothing except a clutch of Flipper-come-home platitudes and a batch of dopey speculations that flew in the face of good sense. I can't downplay the lure of convention, the powerful longing to be part of your community, even one as half-baked and hypocritical as the news media. Past a certain age, we do not yield our identities lightly. By the same token, we come to see that the line between communing and conforming is very thin. Like beliefs about any social activity, beliefs about the self, the body, the mind, about the nature of healing, are shaped by the pressures of consensus. This the Swiss

medical historian Henri Ellenberger knew well. As he wrote in his classic book *The Discovery of the Unconscious*: "Curing the sick is not enough;
one must cure them with methods accepted by the community."

But what community? And whither did you come by it? And
whereof your alienation? Maybe the point I want to make is that when
you are having a hard time reconciling your contradictions, it's tempting
to try reconciling somebody else's. I was a house divided, equivocation
personified; I shuttled between points of view like a frazzled birdie in a
badminton match, always eager to shift my doubts and ambiguities onto
someone else. I didn't care what side of the argument I had to take. I was
as ready to challenge a curmudgeonly know-it-all who dismissed any
treatment not sanctioned by the American Medical Association as I was
to shoulder the burden of dissuading a rapt New Age pilgrim who
insisted that it was only the program of culturally instilled beliefs that kept
her from sinking through the molecular interstices of the Earth.

How do we decide what to believe? In this century, the age of the
"half-believer," as it has been called, how do we critically evaluate ideas
of mind and body that address the limitations of the critical mind? Some
therapies are not meant to be analyzed or measured or quantified, but are
meant, as perhaps was the case with the infernal dolphin energy, to be felt
and acknowledged and lived. Much of what exists on the fringe of medicine challenges the divide between the observer and the participant, and
underscores the one paradoxically absolute truth of postmodern discourse, which is that there is no absolute truth, truth being something
that is "made," not "found." If making some key discovery is predicated
on believing, is it rational to refuse to at least gesture in the direction of
belief? Why would we refuse to experiment with going at a problem dif-
ferently if the attempt promised to teach us something we wouldn't learn
otherwise? If blind faith was too hard, could we at least suspend or tamp
down the reflex of militant disbelief?

Here was the no-win gambit that only a trial lawyer could love:
Confess belief and you disqualify yourself as an impartial witness. Declare
your opposing conviction and you undermine the relevancy of your
researches. Why even bother with the fringe if it was all bunk and fraud?
Fresh proof that the outlands were full of rot would only deepen the com-
placency of closed minds. And fresh proof that the outlands were rife with

marvels hardly mattered to people already disposed to the truths of faith. It was clear to me early on that I would have to learn to balance between these two poles; I would have to develop a knack for hovering in that awkward position between faith and disbelief. And it was then that I understood why the question of faith had always been raised with such priority and haste. The reason everybody asked whether I believed was not to belittle my experiences; it was to avoid the intricate trouble of having to reach a verdict for themselves.

6. SUCH A RATTLING OF BONES

When he bid his wife and two children good-bye in New York and boarded a train bound for New Orleans in January 1909, Abraham Flexner was forty-three years old, a balding, energetic man with the mien of an owl and a passion for Shakespeare and Keats. He had just been hired by the Carnegie Foundation, and as he recalled many years later in his autobiography, he was relieved to be heading far out of town, because he was "keenly conscious of my ignorance and inexperience." By training, Flexner was an educator; while obviously a quick study— he'd graduated from Johns Hopkins University in two years, and had earned a couple of master's degrees—his professional life had been spent far from medical politics, so far, in fact, that when he was first approached about the Carnegie job he thought the foundation officials had mixed him up with his older brother Simon, a noted bacteriologist who isolated the bug that causes dysentery (*Shigella flexneri*). Flexner the Obscure had made his career in Louisville, where he'd been raised, the sixth of nine children of Czech and German immigrants. He taught Greek at the local high school and then established his own college-prep classrooms under the name "Mr. Flexner's School." Now he was pointed south, bound for the medical school at Tulane University, the first stop on a mission that would take him to 155 medical schools around Canada and the United States, and would in the years to follow change the character of medicine.

Prompted by the American Medical Association (the AMA)—hardly a disinterested party—the Carnegie Foundation had commissioned Flexner to report on the education of doctors. It was clear some serious muckraking was in order. New medical schools were springing up like mushrooms—moneymaking operations formed without a second thought by any ragtag group of doctors who had an extra box of bones, some empty offices, and an eye for profits. Getting a medical degree in the United States had more to do with the ability to pay tuition than with achievements in medicine. Doctoring was an overcrowded, cutthroat free-for-all, marked by fierce disputes over medical ideology. The country had more than four times the number of doctors per capita as Germany, and practitioners of radically different medical sects were obliged to vie not just for social and professional legitimacy but for economic footholds too. Hydropaths were treating illness with applications of water. Osteopaths were manipulating joints. Chiropractors, who got started with Daniel David Palmer in 1895, were cracking spines and aligning subluxated vertebrae. When they weren't haggling with one another over doctrine, homeopaths were practicing the "like cures like" therapy pioneered by the formidable German physician Samuel Hahnemann. Eclectics were writing botanical prescriptions. So-called regular doctors, dubbed "allopaths" by Hahnemann because they tried to fight the symptoms of disease head-on, were practicing their heroic brand of medicine, using highly concentrated drugs and, of course, lots of bleeding and purging.

In the latter half of the century, the Viennese school of therapeutic nihilism was beginning to spread the gospel that in treatment less is more. Oliver Wendell Holmes, addressing the Massachusetts Medical Society in 1860, had made the now famous remark that if all drugs could be sent to the bottom of the sea, "it would be better for mankind and all the worse for the fishes." The real changes filtering through medicine came from the influence of the biological sciences and the late-century bid to link the clinic with the lab and with a new breed of "laboratory men." The movement had influential supporters; Flexner was one.

Before commencing his grand tour, Flexner read everything he could find on medical training in America. He made a preliminary trip to Chicago to consult with the AMA, which had been pushing for reform in medical education. (The fact that an AMA representative traveled with him on many of his trips is something Flexner didn't think worth mentioning in his autobiography.) He also called on the medical deans and professors at his alma mater, Johns Hopkins University; the medical department there had been established in 1893 and was reputed to be the best in the country. Flexner later called Johns Hopkins the "one bright spot" among the medical schools of America. It "possessed ideals and men who embodied them," he wrote, "and from it have emanated the influences that in a half century have lifted American medical education from the lowest status to the highest in the civilized world. All honor to Gilm Welch, Mall Halsted and their colleagues and students who hitched their wagon to a star and never flinched!"

Once under way, Flexner followed a simple plan. He arranged interviews with medical-school deans. He asked about the entrance exams; he asked about the size of the faculty and the school's endowment, if any. He asked about hospital affiliations, if any. He asked to see the classrooms, and the laboratories, if any. Impressions were fast in coming. He took encouragement from the advice given to him by the chairman of the General Education Board, the Rockefeller-financed foundation that in years to come would, largely on Flexner's say-so, channel $600 million into medical education reform: "You don't need to eat a whole sheep to know it's tainted."

In Salem, Washington, when Flexner asked about the physiology lab, the dean brought out a small sphygmograph, an instrument to register the pulse: that was the physiology lab. At an osteopathic school in Des Moines, Flexner found all the classroom doors locked. Later, unknown to the dean, he returned, slipped a janitor five dollars, and looked at the equipment in the rooms marked anatomy, physiology, pathology. It was all the same: a desk, a blackboard, some chairs. Flexner leaned on a dean in Raleigh: He photographed "filthy" medical buildings and told the man the pictures would be published. At the Georgia College of Eclectic Medicine and Surgery he reached the conclusion that "nothing more disgraceful calling itself a medical school can be found anywhere."

In November, he hit fourteen cities in sixteen days. At the Missionary Medical College in Battle Creek, Michigan, he found "a combination of business, religion, and pseudo-science that was very revolting." In Kirksville, Missouri, the "fountainhead of osteopathy," he wrote, "I have seen much of gullibility in the last ten months, but commend me to the father of osteopathy and his sons as past masters of therein. Here are almost six hundred students 'taught' in a building that might accommodate seventy-five, each student paying $150. The teaching is mainly done by upperclass students and young osteopaths receiving a bare pittance. The net profits of the two owners must be upward of $60,000 a year."

When asked by some officials what changes he would recommend, he replied, form new faculties, reorganize clinical facilities, raise an endowment. Medical schools had to "answer to modern requirements." Where he saw no hope of their doing so, he told them they just ought to close their doors for good. The conditions of medical education almost everywhere, in his view, were "sordid, hideous, unintelligent even where honest." And there is so little "that is even honest," he said.

When Flexner was finished traveling, he repaired to a house in the Berkshires to write his report. Within six months, he produced a 180-page monograph entitled *Medical Education in the United States and Canada*. It has since become a landmark.

Years later in his autobiography he allowed himself to crow: "Such a rattling of dead bones has never been heard in this country before or since. The medical profession and the faculties of the medical schools, as well as the state boards of examiners, were absolutely flabbergasted by the pitiless exposure." Flexner's fame surpassed his brother's. He received anonymous letters warning him he would be shot if he set foot in Chicago ("the plague spot of the country in respect to medical education"). He was threatened with lawsuits, and actually sued for libel for $150,000. He didn't trouble to report the outcome in his autobiography, so perhaps it wasn't worth mentioning.

What shocked the country were his unminced descriptions of tattered labs and stinking anatomy rooms. The Great Quack-buster was particularly severe with the country's thirty-two sectarian schools. The eclectics were "drug mad," he said. The osteopathic schools "reeked of commercialism." The osteopathic school in Des Moines "is a disgrace to the state and should be summarily suppressed. In the absence of police power to terminate its career in this way, its graduates, undertaking as they do to treat all sorts of diseases, should be compelled to meet whatever standards are applied to other practitioners."

Almost immediately, medical schools began to collapse. Fifteen medical schools in the plague spot of Chicago were consolidated into three. Within two decades, the number of medical schools in America had been sliced in half. The seven black schools Flexner reviewed were eventually reduced to two. The number of women graduating from medical schools fell by a third, and doctors were much harder to find in poor and rural communities. The Flexner report, noted physician Leo Galland in his 1997 book *The Four Pillars of Healing*, "succeeded in increasing the social and intellectual homogeneity of the medical profession, driving out the lower classes and the immigrants, reducing the number of blacks and women, and, initially, of Jews."

The sectarian schools had the roughest going. Flexner professed not to question their tenets; indeed, their laboratories were so wretched, their commercialism so rank, their dissembling so pathetic that you get the feeling he thought it would have been almost unsporting to tackle their theories of illness. Homeopathic schools shrank in number from twenty-two at the outset of the century to two in 1923. The number of practitioners dwindled from fifteen thousand to a handful. Such was his scorn for chiropractic that Flexner did not bother with actual visits and inspections but contented himself with noting that chiropractors (along with "mechano-therapists") were "unconscionable quacks" best dealt with by "the public prosecutor and the grand jury."

If the tightening of standards was a boon to the public, the loss of rival medical ideas redounded to benefit allopathic doctors, who did not mourn the decline of their competitors. They had allied themselves with the scientific method; a number of their own more slovenly institutions were gored, but the recommendations and prestige of the Carnegie Report helped secure their franchise. Decades later, following the path Flexner blazed, the AMA's Committee on Quackery launched a secret campaign to destroy the chiropractic profession, an effort that was eventually stopped when they were sued by the chiropractors in a case resolved by the U.S. Supreme Court.

It would be an overstatement to say Flexner single-handedly lifted allopathy above its rivals; he makes a point of asserting that scientific medicine cares nothing for the dogma of homeopathy and allopathy, only for facts. In his seigniorial book *The Social Transformation of American Medicine,* Paul Starr writes: "The triumph of the regular profession depended on belief rather than force, on its growing cultural authority rather than sheer power, on the success of its claims to competence and understanding rather than the strong arm of the police. To see the rise of the profession as coercive is to underestimate how deeply its authority penetrated the beliefs of ordinary people and how firmly it had seized the imagination even of its rivals."

But Starr's point has been contested by Marxist scholars such as Richard Brown who see the Flexner Report aimed not just at the issue of public health but also at industrial capitalist society's preference for a convenient, standardized health-care machine. Whatever the case, the enmity the Flexner report arouses in present-day homeopaths and other descendants of medical sectarianism is mirrored by the gratitude of the allopathic community. At a dinner in Flexner's honor nearly half a century after his findings rocked the country, a representative of the AMA told a distinguished assembly of medical school deans and faculty that Abraham Flexner had made "the greatest single contribution" in the history of medical education.

What seems easier to see today, eighty years after the Flexner report, are the author's turn-of-the-century assumptions—his idealization of progress and technology, his confidence in facts, and his unquestioning faith in science—science not just as a superior method for learning about nature but science as a privileged body of knowledge before which all other modes of knowing and interpretation must bow.

This is not to pick on a guy who worked hard, spoke Greek, and recited Shakespeare; who was married to a successful playwright; who subsequently reviewed medical education in Europe, and then did another Carnegie report on prostitution in Europe, which one somehow senses was not a hands-on roustabout like his first medical opus. As secretary to the Rockefeller Foundation's General Education Board, Flexner shunted $500 million in philanthropic contributions to major university medical schools. He championed a new figure in medicine, the doctor as research scientist. In 1930, he set up the Institute for Advanced Study at Princeton.

But it's worth trying to dig out the assumptions in his point of view, because they typify the attitudes and philosophy on which scientific medicine rests. In fact, Dr. Galland and others have argued that the Flexner report's most profound and lasting effect was not its economic impact but the way the new science-based technocentric medicine would alter the relationship of patient and physician, turning a suffering subject into a diseased object. Flexner had a pure, and, we can say now in hindsight, naive faith in science itself, which to him was exempt from dogma and apparently immune to politics, social pressure, and ethical perversion as well. Flexner was a proud, reform-minded modern, a champion of logic and rationality, but he stood blissfully unaware on the threshold of the most genocidally "rational and logical" century in history. A patronizing note crept into his view of people who did not see health care and illness as he did; particularly where sectarian ideas persisted against all good sense, he counseled a strong paternalistic hand to safeguard against irrational excesses. "In dealing with the medical sectary, society can employ no special device," he noted sadly. "Certain profound characteristics in one way or another support the medical dissenter: now, the primitive belief in magic crops up in his credulous respect for an impotent drug; again, all other procedure having failed, what is there to lose by flinging one's self upon the mercy of chance? Instincts so profound cannot be abolished by statute. But the limits within which they can play may be so regulated as to forbid alike their commercial and crudely ignorant exploitation."

That might have sounded all very reasonable and protective in a Father-knows-best sort of way in 1910. Flexner didn't leave open the possibility that the institutions which regulate and protect the public might also abuse the public, that doctors at the behest of the government might, for example, inject sick patients with plutonium. He didn't leave open the possibility that there were other ways of interpreting and healing illness, or that even within "scientific" cultures there might be widely divergent points of view. All physicians, he wrote, "are confronted with the same crisis: a body out of order. No matter to what remedial procedure they incline—medical, surgical, or manipulative—they must first ascertain what is the trouble. There is only one way to do that." Of course, there is not just one way to do that, any more than the crisis of a sick person is simply or strictly that of a body out of order. Flexner was a medical materialist, and he helped pave the way for the triumph of medical materialism, and the eclipse of the patient.

His paeans to the virtues of the scientific physician now resonate with some painful ironies:

> The scientific physician still keeps his advantage over the empiric [physician]. He studies the actual situation with keener attention; he is freer of prejudiced prepossession; he is more conscious of liability to error. Whatever the patient may have to endure from a baffling disease, he is not further handicapped by reckless medication. In the end the scientist alone draws the line accurately between the known, the partly known and the unknown. The empiricist fares forth with an indiscriminate confidence which sharp lines do not disturb.

You can't help but mark the naive optimism in that passage, given the reality behind the myth that everything done in the name of scientific medicine rests on scientific evidence. (In 1983, the U.S. Office of Technology concluded that of all the medical techniques and therapies on the market, only about one in five was actually backed by scientific evidence. The percentage of evidence-based treatment is much higher within many specialties where the practical range of therapies tends to be narrower than what's generally available.) And there is something egregiously naive in the line "not further handicapped by reckless medication" given the abuse of penicillin and prescription drugs and the catastrophes caused by medications like thalidomide and diethylstilbestrol. One recent study published in the *Journal of the American Medical Association* (*JAMA*) found that more than 100,000 Americans die annually in hospitals from adverse reactions to medication; "side effects" of prescription drugs are the nation's sixth leading cause of death and one of the main complaints in the case against modern medicine. The medical mainstream's over-reliance on drugs has reinvigorated the unorthodox medical theories Flexner helped to scotch.

Science, it turns out, is no more free of dogmas than any other cultural activity. The dogmas of biomedicine have been evolving since the time of Descartes, Galileo, and Newton, whose philosophy and experimentation and mathematics created the great scientific awakening in the seventeenth century. The principles that defined science and shaped its explorations also shaped medicine, the youngest science—with magnificent benefits and still-unfolding costs. In Flexner's day, the accent was on the benefits; the costs were scarcely imaginable.

Taking its cue from Newtonian physics, modern scientific medicine starts with the idea that the body is a machine whose systems operate deterministically, like the gearing of a clock. And, indeed, the body does behave very much like a machine at times, maybe most of the time. As the example of an atheist might demonstrate, the body seems able to function without any conscious spiritual programming or creed. Cuts are healed, food is digested, molecules of oxygen are distributed to famished cells.

Next, biomedicine incorporates the principle of reductionism into its machine metaphor: To see how the body works, you must reduce it to its constituent elements. As with a clock, nothing about the whole can't be known from studying the sum of the parts. Reduction, it is assumed, provides the real story. Water can be reduced to hydrogen and oxygen. Corybantic religious ecstasy can be reduced to a spritz of neuropeptides in the brain. And finally, biomedicine relies on two stalwart principles of modern scientific epistemology—objectivism and positivism—which, in essence, assign pride of place to the material aspects of the body and dismiss mind, emotion, belief, even consciousness itself as so much "noise." The axioms of positivism and objectivism insist that the only things that are "real" are the things that can be counted, weighed, or in some way quantified; the only significant propositions are the ones that can be verified. An especially severe exponent of this view once said there were two kinds of people, "logical positivists and goddamn English professors." There's no mistaking who were the softheaded knaves in his opinion.

But science is more perspicaciously viewed as a method for proposing theories than extracting truths. The revolution of Isaac Newton, which prevailed as scientific gospel for three hundred years, was itself overthrown. Not overthrown so much as quietly and subtly usurped by a new generation of theoreticians and experimentalists who subscribed to a new, more nuanced understanding of the behavior of matter. The physics of quantum mechanics that emerged in 1925, fifteen years after the Flexner Report, did not repeal the Newtonian laws that explained the movement of the planets or the vectors of falling apples, but it did collapse the idea that nature was a great deterministic clockwork that could be observed objectively without affecting the phenomena under observation.

Dissident doctors poetically raise the metaphor of quantum mechanics to support a new approach to the body, but mainstream medicine has hardly begun to grapple with the provisional, uncertain status of matter implicit in twentieth-century physics. The youngest science is still based on the dogmas of nineteenth-century science. Its job is much harder than the job of the other sciences. It is not strictly concerned with a pancreas, or a cell in the pancreas, or a protein in that cell, or a molecule in that protein, or a carbon atom in that molecule, or a proton in that carbon atom, or a quark in that proton. It is concerned with the whole system of a human being, an aggregate of some three trillion cells, growing and energizing and interacting and dying amid an even larger number of bacteria. Gazillions of proteins. A googolplex of uniquely bundled atoms. There is no reckoning with the complexity of such an organism.

"Abandonment of the deterministic worldview in physics has made it more difficult to regard the existing state of science as legislative of what is and what is not possible in nature," writes Cambridge University mathematician Mary Hesse. "We are by no means sure, even in physics, that existing theories will last many decades. Moreover, we have no guarantee that existing theories will prove adequate in sciences other than physics, and in the sciences of complex systems such as the human psyche and human social groups we have only the bare beginnings of any theories at all."

A new view of the body may require a new intellectual framework. As physician Elliot Dacher, one of the leading voices of contemporary holism, argues in his book *Whole Healing*, the determinism and positivism of science have given medical science a somewhat distorted picture of how the body actually operates, precisely because the axioms belittle the role of the mind. In his view, the principles of "dynamism, holism, and

purposefulness" may be more useful in making models of the way wholeness is actually restored.

From the patients' point of view, if an incantation works, if—go figure—syphilis clears up after a night in a disemboweled mule, why should
scientific medicine have a greater claim? Why should patients be
offended—as rationalists sometimes want them to be—by empirical
treatments that work but lack scientific evidence or a suitably "rational"
explanation? Empiricism isn't a philosophy contrary to Flexner's suggestion. It's a method, widely employed by witch doctors and scientists alike.
It's a process of trial and error that can yield results, and those results can
either yield new theories or confirm old ones. They can buttress the cosmology that binds any community, no matter how sophisticated. The
models of disease that guide scientific medical research and treatment are
ultimately dogmas—a set of beliefs sanctioned by society. True, the dogmas that empower the shaman who capers around in a Big Bird costume
are not the dogmas that underlie the scientific experiment. The shaman
and the doctor may have an explanation for why a remedy works, and
the explanation may be "rational" within each healer's system of belief.
Outcomes in both cases may even be reliably predicted. The key difference in science is that the measurements and assessments of illness do not
depend—or depend as much—on the vagaries of human interpretation.
The diagnostic tools are not the shaman's dreaming ability but laboratory
cultures, blood tests, and X rays. As much as possible, for better or for
worse, the human element has been stripped out. And we believe that no
special beliefs are required to understand our illnesses—that is to say, no
special beliefs other than those beliefs on which science itself rests.

What might really confound the early modernists of Flexner's time
is the postmodern view of science inspired by quantum indeterminacy.
How strange it would have seemed to them that even solidly "scientific"
evidence cannot produce an authoritative conclusion, that even further
research served not to resolve the gray areas but only to illustrate the contradictions and ambiguity inherent in our attempt to know nature.
Historians of science are much more attuned than they were in Flexner's
time to the role of consensus and politics (German scientists denounced
Einstein's "Jewish physics"). They discern economic and philosophical
biases embedded in the structure of research. As current controversies

over everything from the health hazards of high-tension lines to artificial sweeteners illustrate, more studies sometimes compound the confusion, as if science were not a system for producing Flexnerian facts and self-evident truths but subtler pictures of paradox and uncertainty, increasingly nuanced insights into the limits of what we can know. (An example is the artificial sweetener debate: The TV show *60 Minutes* reported in December 1996 that good studies paid for by the company that produces the sweetener aspartame are less likely to find health-related dangers than good studies funded by independent groups.) Faced with the spectacle of hypercredentialed academics bashing each other with contradictory research, some historians of science venture to argue that it is impossible to separate "good" science from "bad," or even to distinguish "real" science from "pseudoscience." These are, the argument goes, cultural judgments.

By definition, all scientific conclusions are provisional, open to a new and "truer" vision. But as they follow their passions, scientists get attached to their ideas. They treat their current theories as incontrovertible truths—truths of nature, truths of the body, truths of disease—not truths of the perceiving and designing minds that formulated them. It's understandable that they do, for the degree to which perceptions correspond to realities is an old conundrum of philosophy. Some observations seem like inviolable laws. Gravity exists, cats fall out of windows. It matters not whether Newton or some other math whiz is at the chalkboard defining the phenomenon. But the business of science is drawing and revising theories on the basis of evidence, not asserting "proofs" of the way things "really" are or excommunicating those who disagree: History makes fools of people who ignore the distinction.

If you want to see the folly of confusing the method of science with a body of beliefs, you have only to open an old "scientific" medical textbook, a book that Flexner would have pointed to proudly as a paragon of proper "scientific" medicine. New insights into medical problems make old textbooks seem like mockable compendiums of error. A study in 1975 by physician and editor Paul Beeson concluded that sixty percent of treatments recommended in a major textbook published in 1927 were worthless, and many of them actually harmful. Did people in 1927 think they were any less sophisticated than people think themselves today? To cite one more example, were scientific chauvinists shaken when it was later discovered that a species of nematode larva did not cause cancer in rat stomachs as had been claimed by Johannes Fibiger, the Danish physician whose mistake won the 1926 Nobel Prize in medicine?

Time and again, the strength of medical science, its impulse to correct its own errors, is translated into faith in the inerrancy of science. The privileged place of science in society is under attack. Its social and political pretensions have been exposed, its mythology and hubris laid bare. Science tilts into "scientism" when scientists proclaim their church to be the one true church and their version of reality to be the way things really are. The hazards of such presumption are especially evident in the youngest science, where objective claims of knowledge encounter the mysterium of human subjectivity, that frontier where healers and physicians confront the consciousness that can posit its own existence and then dream up methods—science among them—to probe it.

As a piece of muckraking journalism, a breakthrough in the crusade for quality, Abraham Flexner's report was a vital progressive document. As a polemic, it seems suffused with the spirit of the old headmaster. Visions of Utopia, he wrote at the end of his autobiography, are achieved only by "trench warfare." Flexner took the healing professions to Mr. Flexner's school. He graded them on his curve. His opinions were embraced by medical boards that set the requirements for physicians' licenses; his opinions guided foundations that funded the schools that shaped American doctors in this century. And maybe they had consequences he didn't intend. As the physician Leo Galland has pointed out, Flexner's report changed the relation of patients and doctors: "The eclipse of the patient is the most profound, lasting, and unfortunate effect of the Flexner report." Flexner himself began to have some qualms, not about the merits of scientific medicine but about its dehumanizing side effects, which were apparent to him as early as 1925, when he wrote, "Scientific medicine in America—young, vigorous, and positivistic—is today sadly deficient in culture and philosophic background." But the point remains that after the Flexner report there were just two brands of medicine in America, "regular" and everything else. It was by way of Flexner that the mainstream was separated from the fringe. More than anyone, he put the "alternative" in front of "medicine."

7. THE MANTRA OF NO

A nd then, where modern medicine was concerned, people began to say no. Some naysayers had been saying no for years but were brushed aside as "health nuts" or "cancer charlatans," selling panaceas in Tijuana, beyond the reach of the Food and Drug Administration. Or they were religious refuseniks whose dissent attested not to their criticism of modern medicine but to the strictures of quixotic doctrine—Jehovah's Witnesses saying no to blood transfusions, Christian Scientists saying no to doctors altogether lest they compromise the therapeutics of fervent prayer. Homeopaths had been saying no for decades, but in their dwindling numbers they resembled their highly diluted medications that contain almost no molecules of the active ingredient. Naturally, naturopaths were saying no. And so were chiropractors. Tired of being persecuted by the AMA—the chairman of the AMA Committee on Quackery had compared chiropractors to "rabid dogs"—the dogs sued the archagency of biomedicine in 1976, and won a restraint-of-trade case against their bête noire, greatly helped by leaked AMA documents from an anonymous source known in the inevitable Watergate parlance as Sore Throat.

Biomedicine barely blinked. The National Institutes of Health were organized after World War II, and academic medicine boomed as millions of federal dollars flowed in. But here and there, new protestants picked up the mantra of no. The cancer patients of Harry Hoxsey, who claimed they'd been saved by the Hoxsey-family salves and formulas, surrounded the jail where the naturopath was imprisoned during one of his celebrated legal battles in the early 1950s. He anticipated the chiropractic success, winning a libel suit against the Hearst newspapers and Morris Fishbein, the editor of the AMA journal. Fishbein had called him the boldest of a breed of "wicked medical fakes" and went on to say of the species that he believed Hoxsey epitomized: "They look like men, they

speak like men, but in them, pervading them, resides a quality so malevolent that it sets them apart from others of the human race. Even in this
time of scientific progress, they, brazen, dare the daylight. With Stone Age
lures, they call. The credulous believe. They slay their patients as guiltily
as if they knifed them in the heart."

Hoxsey won but collected only a dollar and court costs.

The dissent did not always come from the outlands. One of the most
distinguished and surprising voices of demurral was the microbiologist
René Dubos. In his prescient 1959 book *The Mirage of Health* he
observed:

> Modern man, probably no wiser but certainly more con-
> ceited, now claims that the royal avenue to the control of dis-
> ease is through scientific knowledge and medical technology.
> "Health is purchasable," proclaimed one of the leaders of
> American medicine. Yet, while the modern American boasts
> of the scientific management of his body and soul, his
> expectancy of life past the age of forty-five is hardly greater
> today than it was several decades ago and is shorter than that
> of many European people of the present generation. He claims
> the highest standard of living in the world, but ten percent of
> his income must go for medical care and he cannot build hos-
> pitals fast enough to accommodate the sick. He is encouraged
> to believe that money can create drugs for the cure of heart
> disease, cancer, and mental disease, but he makes no worth-
> while effort to recognize, let alone correct, the mismanage-
> ments of his everyday life that contribute to the high incidence
> of these conditions. . . . One may wonder indeed whether the
> pretense of superior health is not itself rapidly becoming a
> mental aberration. Is it not a delusion to proclaim the present
> state of health as the best in the world, at a time when increas-
> ing numbers of persons in our society depend on drugs and
> on doctors for meeting the ordinary problems of everyday life?

When the newly created federal programs Medicare and Medicaid
began to change the practice and drive up the cost of medicine, even

some mainstream doctors began to wonder about the direction of medicine. The word "holism," which had been coined in 1926, revived the vague but deeply appealing idea of treating the "whole" person, not simply the diseased part. This idea went back to Plato, and, as Anne Harrington notes in her book *Reenchanted Science*, it enjoyed a special vogue in nineteenth-century Germany, where holistic thinking was "a vehicle for both political anxiety and social reformist zeal." Holistic ideas emerged in opposition to the pervasive metaphor of the "machine." By the early 1960s the "wellness" movement gathered adherents around the idea that health was not simply the absence of disease but a condition that could be actively cultivated. This movement marked the first wave of contemporary alternative medicine, and it seems clear today that it drew on the rebellion of the times, the energy of the alienated counterculture that was attacking establishment authority on a dozen fronts.

Defenders of the mainstream didn't take the criticism all that well. A medical economics professor at Columbia University named Harry Schwartz wrote in the January 1975 *Ohio State Medical Journal*: "If one took literally all the nonsense about the supposed 'health crisis' which is ladled out by the ton over the major communications media, one might think that the health of the American people had seriously deteriorated this past half century."

But that was the very year that sociologist Ivan Illich published *Medical Nemesis*, the most formidable piece of medical dissent this century. Marshaling the thunder of Jeremiah, Illich said no not just to one bad drug or one superfluous tonsillectomy but to the whole institutional structure of modern medicine itself. There had never been a polemic of its power. Starting with the opening salvo ("The medical establishment has become a major threat to health") Illich poured down condemnation on a system of health care that he argued was perversely causing more disease than it was curing, subjecting people to a pandemic of iatrogenic illness—illness engendered by doctors. (Medical critics noted, for instance, that the death rate in Los Angeles had declined during a doctor's strike in 1976, and had gone back up again when the doctors returned to work.) Biomedicine and the professional class of physicians, in Illich's view, prescribed too many dangerous drugs and did too many dangerous, unnecessary surgeries. A million people a year had to be hospitalized for adverse reactions to prescription drugs. While medication for high blood pressure was valuable for a small percentage of people, it was unnecessary for most and represented in Illich's view "a considerable risk of serious harm, far outweighing any proven benefit, for the 10 to 20 million Americans on whom rash artery-plumbers are trying to foist it." Modern medicine traded on the prestige of controlling infectious diseases that were in steep decline before the application of its "wonder drugs" and "magic bullets." Despite some victories, the war against cancer was essentially a stalemate, and in Illich's view the Pollyanna updates from the American Cancer Society were reminiscent of "General Westmoreland's proclamations from Vietnam." Instead of mobilizing the self-healing power of the patient, modern medical procedures transformed "the sick man into a limp and mystified voyeur of his own treatment"; the professional physician monopoly robbed people of "control over medical perception, classification and decision-making."

Medical Nemesis was an impassioned and ruthlessly well documented attack. Illich hoped it would help effect the "laicization of the Aesculapian temple" and the "delegitimizing of the basic religious tenets of modern medicine." The two decades since have only aggravated the trends and conditions that aroused his wrath. But the Jeremiahs proclaiming a crisis in the healing arts today are often M.D.s. Many of them have traced their disenchantment in bestselling books, and some have set up 800 numbers to sell herbal supplements and are sought for star turns at healing seminars and retreats. Their argument is the same. Modern medicine is sick—economically, politically, morally, therapeutically, philosophically. One need only update Illich's statistics. We've already noted the death toll exacted annually in hospitals by prescription drugs. In 1994, there were 2.2 million nonfatal adverse reactions to medications, up from 1.5 million in 1983. Coronary bypasses are seven times more frequent in the United States than in Europe, with no clear benefit to patients. In some communities, the number and kinds of surgeries have less to do with what patients need than with what local doctors are capable of supplying. Brain cancer rates have increased dramatically in the 1990s. Chronic disease is epidemic. The great victories won against microbial plagues like tuberculosis and cholera are unraveling as the gross overuse of antibiotics (and, say some epidemiologists, the mutation-accelerating effects of radioactive environmental pollution) bring virulently infectious bugs back in new drug-resistant guises.

Modern biomedicine today is even more industrial, more high tech, more specialized, more litigious, more impersonal, more riddled with economic inequities. And more expensive. From 1990 to 1994, health-care spending in the United States doubled as a percentage of gross domestic product. And yet the country ranks twentieth in the world in infant mortality, and only sixteenth in female life expectancy; it is seventeenth in male life expectancy. Each year the nation pays more and more for diminishing returns. Modern medicine's emphasis remains on patching and fixing problems, not preventing them. It turns doctors into harried technicians pitching pills at symptoms and hoping that the pills don't cause new symptoms for which more pills will have to be prescribed. The oft-repeated argument is that making medicine a science sacrificed the art. The bedside manner of modern doctors is so notorious that somebody actually devised an experiment which found that male physicians who asked patients a question would interrupt the answer after twenty-two seconds or so, while female doctors were more indulgent, giving patients approximately forty-five seconds. (I can't remember the exact numbers in these Patient Interruptus studies, but I have to wonder if the mindset that extracted the data isn't part of the problem. The fact that somebody actually went to the trouble of quantifying what one would think would be the quintessential qualitative experience of listening and being listened to seems perilously close to Experimental Science as Monty Python parody.)

Much criticism is directed at modern medicine's attachment to the bacteriological model of disease that made dramatic inroads against infectious plagues but has bogged down trying to solve the riddle of the chronic diseases that beset modern patients. The rise of immune disorders has revived the "seed or soil" debates that pitted Claude Bernard against Louis Pasteur in the nineteenth century. (On his deathbed, Pasteur confessed that Bernard was right: It was not the "bug" that mattered most but the "terrain" in which it flourished. There are, for example, TB lesions in many adults who have never had the symptoms of tuberculosis.) Modern medicine still emphasizes fighting the pathogens that presumably are the causes of disease rather than accenting the body's reaction to the bugs, or the host-pathogen relationship. Medical scientists now track causes down to the level of pathogen molecules, a development that for all of its exciting discoveries about physiology and disease still draws criticism as a medical model for treating illness. Homeopathy historian Harris Coulter writes in *Divided Legacy*, his epic four-volume account of medical orthodoxy and heresy: "The unending twistings and turnings of allopathic thought, its renunciations of concepts held with dogmatic tenacity a few years earlier, are presented by professional apologists as evidence of medical 'progress' but actually reveal scientific hollowness and inconsistency, the absence of any understanding of how the body functions as an integrated whole, and consequent inability to avoid being carried along by new externally generated scientific paradigms such as molecular biology or genetic manipulation which promise final answers to perennial medical puzzles."

The reductive, mechanistic view of the body grants no privilege to the "integrated whole." Modern medical science has evolved for most of this century as if the mind played no part in disease. Indeed, until the late 1970s and the onset of psychoneuroimmunology, many doctors refused to accept that the mind had any role in the body's immune response. Even now, the mind is seen mostly as a kind of nuisance that can cause a placebo effect that has to be factored out of studies before the "real" impact of a drug or surgical technique can be determined.

Dissent may be inevitable in a field that has enshrined the Second Opinion. After Illich and the wellness movement, a second and much larger wave of dissent began to crest in the early 1990s. Mainstream medicine protested, but prodded by Rep. Berkley Bedell, an Iowa Democrat who claimed alternative treatments for his Lyme disease and prostate cancer worked where mainstream medical treatments had failed, the U.S. Congress established the Office of Alternative Medicine at the National Institutes of Health in 1993. That same year, an AMA poll found that seventy percent of respondents said they thought people were losing faith in their doctors, and the *New England Journal of Medicine* published Harvard professor David Eisenberg's landmark survey of alternative and complementary therapies. Among other achievements, the paper demolished the shibboleth that only poor, uneducated people used "unproven" medical treatments. Eisenberg estimated that an astounding $13 billion was being spent on everything from acupuncture to yoga, more out-of-pocket money than people were spending on conventional health care.

The rebellious spirit that drove that initial wave of dissent has morphed into some powerful sort of longing now: a longing for meaning. A longing to see illness in the context of the now painfully clichéd idea of a "healing journey." A longing for a new metaphor of the body that rejects the figure of the machine and resurrects a figure from medicine's long-gone and hitherto-unlamented past. Which is to say, the romantic, neovitalist metaphor of the body as a dynamic, self-regulating, purposefully striving, mannequin-shaped opus of pulsation and light that was jump-started by the Gnostic spark, and by its nature seeks balance and harmony, and strangest of all, when sick or afflicted, can be changed, succored, affirmed, confounded, or made whole by whatever it is that animates our hands.

CHAPTER TWO

If I aspire to a metaphysical career, I cannot, at any price, retain my identity: whatever residue I retain must be liquidated; if, on the contrary, I assume a historical role, it is my responsibility to exasperate my faculties until I explode along with them. One always perishes by the self one assumes: to bear a name is to claim an exact mode of collapse.

—E. M. CIORAN

1. BLUDGEONING THE INEFFABLE

One morning in Los Angeles in the spring of 1993, while we were having some extravagantly foamed latte in cups the size of dog bowls, my friend Linda said I must go see a healer she'd just been to. I thought that in the movie-maddened spirit of Hollywood with its mix of insider buzz, personal-growth gurus, and action-hero coffee, she was just sharing her latest enthusiasm, not diagnosing some illness she had perceived in my personal domain, which, by the way—and thank you for asking—seemed okay enough at the time, apart from the usual low-grade romantic troubles. (It had been years since L.A. loomed as an orgiastic abyss of used-car dealers and colonic actresses; now it was just an abyss.)

A journalist and aspiring screenwriter, Linda was fearlessly immersed in astrology and could always be counted on to reframe writer's block so that it was not a failure of will or a testament to sloth but the only response of a sensitive mind to impossible celestial conditions. So you'd spent a feckless week staring at *All My Children*? You were lucky to get that much done with Mercury in retrograde.

The healer's name was Joel B. Wallach. "He's really powerful," Linda said, giving me his card:

TRANSFORMATIONAL AURA BALANCING
SINCE 1980

Experience deep inner peace
Clear your past & present patterns
Activate your light body • Release your potential

What all that entailed, I really had no idea, but for some reason that at the time seemed no more than the curiosity that lures house cats into shopping bags, I called the number. I would have bet back then that such a whim would have had fewer repercussions than ordering another cup of the latte. But now I can see that it marked one of those mysterious openings when a long dormancy is shaken off, and the ice starts to move in the frozen river. We review our days, Joseph Campbell once wrote, and we notice "how encounters and events that appeared at the time to be accidental became the crucial structuring features of an unintended life story."

The address brought me to a small apartment complex off Santa Monica Boulevard, not far from the freeway, in one of those bloodless L.A. neighborhoods where people keep from going quietly mad in the afternoon by imposing martial law on their lawns. The grass along the street was golf-green trim, and the prima donna scent of hyacinth weighed heavily on the air. I parked my rental car and walked through an open gate and up a flight of stairs.

Joel B. Wallach was in his late thirties, tall and lanky with long brown hair gathered in a ponytail. We shook hands. In a soft baritone, he asked me to take off my shoes. The floor of his apartment was covered with a carpet that looked as pristine as a field of new snow. The walls were a pale lavender; muted light filtered through the blinds. He showed me to a chair, and took a seat on the couch. He was dressed in loose white pants and a flowing white shirt.

I asked about the weird array of objects under his healing table—metal disks, a wire pyramid, and what looked to be a set of Pan pipes made of transparent plastic.

"I designed those," Joel said. "They collect and focus subtle energies."

Subtle energies? Joel explained they were the manifestations of the subtle bodies, the bodies of emotion, of thought, of spirit, whose energy was pitched at finer and higher frequencies than the energy of physical life.

Uh, okay. I mentioned Bill Moyers's landmark television program *Healing and the Mind*, which had recently aired—in particular the episode in which a half dozen Chinese martial arts students tried to knock their aged instructor off his stance. Like a sheriff rebuffing protestors with a water cannon, the master repelled them all, a feat disciples attributed to his command of *chi*, or vital energy, but which skeptics had glibly dismissed as demonstrating only the power of suggestion. Joel had seen the episode.

"I tuned in to what the guy was doing," he confided. "He was supplanting their energy with his own—that's why they looked like puppets."

"How do you mean you 'tuned in'?"

"I connected with what the guy was doing."

"Off the television set?"

"Yes."

I thought of a time once when I was a newspaper reporter and a guy who said his name was Cab Man telephoned and insisted that his friend Pisa had a story for me. Pisa would only talk in person, and only with Cab Man as go-between. Cab Man sounded a little squirrelly, but on the theory that you never know where the next Deep Throat is coming from, I arranged to meet him and Pisa in the lobby of the *Washington Post*, in full view of the security guard. Cab Man was well dressed, maybe too well dressed given that it was 10:30 in the morning and he was outfitted in top hat and tails. "Where's Pisa?" I said. "Pisa's in here," he said, popping the latches of his briefcase. The lid came up and inside, where you would expect to see memoranda or some such stuff from the paper world, there was a big brown snake. I leapt back. Michael Jordan should move so fast. No, no, no, Cab Man, no snakes, no thank you, see you later, not too soon, I hope.

Now here in the guise of Joel B. Wallach, maestro of the subtle world who could read living human energy in the pixels of a Bill Moyers special, was another radically disjunct reality. Would a smarter cookie have scrambled to his feet and bid Joel and his high-definition TV adieu? I guess I always wished I'd heard Pisa's story. Or maybe my five-thousand-year-old Chinese guide had locked up my legs. In any case, I stayed put. However alien and possibly demented Joel's personal cosmos might be, at least he hadn't produced a snake. And Emerson was whispering again: *Our life is not threatened so much as our perception.* And there was also the pivotal issue of Joel's eyes, which were immensely kind and suffused with a spacious, starry light, as if some patch of the Milky Way had gotten tangled in them. I had hardly been able to meet them at first, and as we talked I was struck by the fact that he wasn't meeting my eyes either. He was gazing above my head or down at my stomach, moving his hands around as if he were trying to shoo away a swarm of gnats. He was sighing under his breath, and clucking, and smiling furtively as if he couldn't get his mind off a joke he'd heard down at the barber shop from Jack Nicholson.

When I managed to stop monitoring myself for a moment, I wondered if maybe I was as unnerving to Joel as he was to me, but that idiotic conceit was quickly dashed when Joel went to work. So much was I affected by my first Transformational Aura Balancing that whenever I had an excuse to be in L.A. over the next couple of years, I called Joel, and it was during those subsequent visits that I began to understand that what made him sigh and cluck, and apostrophize under his breath, and smile with bemused irony was not his self-consciousness in my presence but his self-consciousness in his own. He spent many hours in meditation, dissolved in what mystics call the Realm of the One, where the dynamics of undifferentiated reality make it hard to talk, do business, or defend your pristine carpet. Meeting a new client meant returning to the Realm of the Many, the socially constructed I-thou duality that presented itself to him as an amusing hoax, a chronic illusion complete with the curious artifact of "personality." Was it G. K. Chesterton who said we can acquire everything in solitude except character? In the throes of small talk, Joel seemed to get reacquainted with his own particularity; Joel the trackless ocean met Joel the drop of water. There was no vanity or self-centeredness in this. He assumed the burdens of a practical self with an innocence that was poignant and a little comic: the plight of the transcendent man with his earthly head in the stars and his heavenly carpet on earth.

After what was at most ten or fifteen minutes of high-strung chitchat, I lay down on the healing table like some fluttery debutante about to be introduced to the High Society of the Subtle World. How can I describe my initiation—not just the enchantment of it, the sense of eternity and, yes, as advertised, of peace, but also the sense of the poverty of language? Few things are as exasperating as sublimity proclaimed but not conveyed. The refrain of almost every correspondent conversant with unitive states is that moments in the realm-of-the-one defy description, and almost every mystical text contains a passage begging the reader to understand how poorly language approximates the glory of the subtle world. Whatever happened to Transformational Word Balancing? And yet now I find myself wanting to post the same miserable apology and wondering whether I should have new cards printed up: BLUDGEONING THE INEFFABLE SINCE 1993 . . .

I lay on my back. Joel stayed mostly on my right side. For several minutes he settled his hands on my legs, then relocated them at various places on my torso and head. Sometimes he held his hands over me or swept them through the air. He made curious whistling and huffing sounds. He said he was clearing away bands of stagnant energy and filling holes in the energy field. He rendered the images that came to him, dazzling speculations and impressions premised on the theory that each person's life was one in a series of incarnations, a drama of energy that happened to be playing in his or her particular tissues at the moment but which existed independently, like a flame that didn't need the candle. Joel ventured to say he could see where I had been run through by a sword, a while ago this was, the seventeenth century maybe, a subtle trace of the sword still existed, he was going to pull it out . . . okay he was pulling it out . . . It was out. I had to take his word for it; in, out, I couldn't tell. He thought I had lost my left arm once; possibly it had been hacked off in a battle. *Oh that's just ducky. You lost an arm in the seventeenth century, and now in the twentieth you're losing your mind. . . .*

Had I overstayed my time in California? Though it made no sense, not then at least, not to me in the baffled drag-ass incarnation I had hauled up the stairs that morning, the whole business was bizarrely engrossing. If asked how long I had been on the table, I would have said forty-five minutes, but it was twice that when Joel finally stepped back and went to fetch a glass of water.

I lay on the threshold of a new world. I was aware of the old one outside the apartment where my rental car was parked and a lawn mower droned faintly under the silky notes of cooing doves, but I could not remember when I had last felt so centered, so serene, so devoid of latte anxiety. Or had had such rapture and room inside myself. The question is not do we live in our bodies, but how much of our bodies do we actually inhabit? The denizen of a shoe box had suddenly been given the run of Versailles! The exaltation of breadth! The visceral feeling of vastness! Even as I lay there on the table with Joel's work technically done, the sensation kept building and building, as if the scripture in the Upanishads that claimed the existence of a space within the body that was the home of the Spirit, was not just some press release or demiurgic claptrap that had to be taken on faith, but a true and accurate account of an actual phenomenon. There *was* a space, and the most highly placed of sources was confirming it with everything but footage. Here it was, whatever it was, just as the sacred texts had said: *What lies in that space does not decay when the body decays, nor does it fall when the body falls. . . .*

But now I am left wanting to address not the gift of a revelation but the forfeitures it brought about, the loss of bearings, the shipwreck of old perceptions, the way the Realm of the One ebbed away and left me back with the doves and the mowers. Because we live as if we *know* what we *see*, nothing shocks us as much as the crisis that turns that deluded proposition inside out and drives home the truth of its converse, which is that we *see* what we *know*. It's hard to do justice to the disorientation you feel when you realize your eyes are not taking pictures but making them, your mind is not reading stories but constructing them. You understand how thoroughly preconceptions are embedded in the most innocent point of view, how the eye is shaped and blinded by the mind's expectations. "As a man is, so he sees," wrote William Blake. It is precisely to clear the lifeless way we look without seeing—to disrupt the trance of rote connection—that Zen masters pose logic-busting koans and improvisation teachers make their students walk around calling mundane objects by the wrong name until every over-familiar peppermill, teapot, trumpet, and truck is blazing with a new virginity.

On a larger scale, I think Transformational Aura Balancing effected a similar disruption of my status quo; my senses had been soothed, but my intellect was up in arms. In retrospect, it was during that spring in Los Angeles that my years of sleepy, intrapsychic peace began to unravel. I awoke to find myself caught in the old quarrel between the heart and the head, where the heart signifies the hunger for faith and the head expresses the compulsion to doubt. And as it happened, by one of those accidents that become the structuring features of one's biography, I rediscovered a pair of small wooden figurines whose symbolic opposition framed the very nature of this schism and yet also posed a way of mending it.

Decades ago, my maternal great-grandfather, who was a sculptor and a painter and an opera singer and an author of children's books, but who never made any money (probably because he couldn't settle on one vocation), constructed a tableau of an Italian street scene. In a wooden box about the size of a wine crate, he painted the backdrop of a sky, a curving street, and the facades of village shops, and then he populated the foreground with two dozen figurines, which he had carved from soft wood and carefully finished with painted clothes and facial expressions—shopkeepers, an organ grinder, a peg-legged lamplighter, a woman knitting, another one churning butter, even a dog and a chipmunk. When he died in 1965, the tableau passed to my mother, who said the crowd could stand some thinning and that I should take a couple of the carvings as keepsakes. I was about twelve, and for some reason I chose the commedia dell'arte clown, who wore a white cone hat and a red ruffle around his neck, and the portly Benedictine monk, who was taller by a head and clasped his hands over his belly in prayer. I put them in a box and forgot about them.

After my trip to Los Angeles in the spring of 1993, when I was coming to grips with the costs and benefits of having a transformationally balanced aura, I found the monk and clown again, buried in the back of a closet. As I dusted them off, I was struck by their respective stances, and I began to think of them as the emblems of my conflicted psyche, the polar sensibilities of its endless point and counterpoint. On one hand I had half a mind to dismiss the whole business in Joel Wallach's office as a New Age pratfall. Auras, amputated arms, and subtle-energy amplifiers were ingredients for clown satire, weren't they? And who could want "inner peace" if the price was psychological disintegration?

On the other hand, in the spirit of the monk, I knew that no amount of rationalization could banish the conviction that I had been in some actual place that people had sought and prized since the beginning of time. Whatever wholeness meant for others, for me in the wake of that inaugural healing it seemed to entail the necessity of reconciling the rival forces of faith and doubt. It seemed to require an accord between my monk and clown. They were expediently standing together above my desk, and while it was unlikely they would ever resolve their intrinsic differences, maybe they could help me contend with mine.

As for Joel, he certainly had lived up to his end of the bargain. I wrote him a check for seventy-five dollars and went to find my shoes. As I stood unsteadily in the doorway, assembling my subtle bodies for the plunge back into what now seemed the sunstruck dream of Los Angeles, Joel said, "When you're back in New York, you might see if you can track down some of Barbara Brennan's students—if you want to keep doing this work."

2. ILLIMITABLE WHIRLWINDS, ETC.

F orce, Force, everywhere Force," Thomas Carlyle once wrote, "this huge illimitable whirlwind of Force, which envelops us here; never-resting whirlwind, high as Immensity, old as Eternity." And eternally enigmatic, the historian might have added. No mystery is more basic to medicine, religion or philosophy than this distinction between living and nonliving. What is the force or energy that from a single zygote can manifest, among other marvels, the wonder of the human hand with its complement of twenty-seven bones, its miles of nerves and blood vessels, its sensitivity calibrated acutely enough to detect a ridge of glass raised one-ten-thousandth of an inch above a smooth surface? What energy repairs its wounds and replenishes its muscles and lubricates its joints for a lifetime of executing memos and curveballs and demisemiquavers? What enables us to squeeze the hand of someone who is dying? What lets him in turn register the touch and comprehend its meaning and squeeze back until the illimitable whirlwind moves on, leaving yet a deeper enigma in its wake?

Medical dictionaries are no help. The editors of Dorland's 1994 edition tautologically define the animation of living tissue as "a certain peculiar stimulated condition of organized matter." Life according to these distinguished shatterpates is "that obscure principle whereby organized beings are peculiarly endowed with certain powers and functions not associated with inorganic matter." Thanks, fellas . . .

The obscure principle travels under many names. Idealists and religious believers call it "soul" or "spirit." The Hindus refer to it as *prana* or "breath." In ancient Greece it was known as *pneuma* (meaning "breath" as well), though given Aristotle's view that all of creation was alive, the presence of *pneuma* did not clearly delineate animate philosophers from inanimate minerals. Pacific islanders called it *mana*; Kabbalists, *astral light*; Paracelsus termed it the *archaeus*. In China, vital energy was conceptualized as *chi*, which still serves the basis of acupuncture. Like *pneuma*, *chi* pervades the inanimate world, and thus may not be the clearest indication of what makes a rat different from a rock.

And this is the problem: in the infinitesimally small realm of atoms it seems impossible to distinguish between animate and inanimate. Matter in rocks is no less animate than matter in rats. Matter is frisky, pulsatile, vibratory; matter is endlessly in contest with itself, scoured day and night by illimitable whirlwinds. Neutrinos crash through. Electrons are strong-armed into new alliances. Something like a riotous twenty-four-hour house party is raging in there. Rocks just *appear* to be slow-witted wall-flowers. Atomically speaking, they're happening. As the physicist Freeman Dyson writes:

> I judge matter to be an imprecise and rather old-fashioned concept. Roughly speaking, matter is the way particles behave when a large number of them are lumped together. When we examine matter in the finest detail in the experiments of particle physics, we see it behaving as an active agent rather than as an inert substance. Its actions are in the strict sense unpredictable. It makes what appear to be arbitrary choices between alternative possibilities. Between matter as we observe it in the laboratory and mind as we observe it in our own consciousness, there seems to be only a difference in degree but not in kind.

The idea that matter is inanimate can be traced to René Descartes, the father of modern philosophy and the godfather of modern science. Descartes, who made his break with scholastic philosophy after a series of dreams, famously split psyche and soma, and construed matter as an inert substance that had to be moved, or acted upon, or in some way animated by external forces. The human body, in Cartesian philosophy, was a machine.

The reaction against the physio-mechanical view of the body fostered by Descartes emerged as the doctrine of vitalism. Drawing on the philosophy of Aristotle, vitalists argued that something must be present in "mere matter" to account for the ways in which rats are unlike rocks. Rats could react to their environment. They pursued goals and had purposes. They acted with intent and intelligence; they could learn. More complex species possessed feelings and consciousness. The eighteenth-century chemist-physician George Ernest Stahl proposed to call the source of these qualities the *anima*. One of Napoleon's physicians, Paul Joseph Barthez, offered the phrase *principe vitale*, and the French philosopher Henri Bergson, who won the Nobel Prize for literature in 1927, proposed what he called *élan vital*. All these concepts were basically glosses on the Aristotelian idea that living beings unfolded under the guidance of an immaterial psyche.

In the sixteenth century, the great anatomist Vesalius made charts of the human body that included a *rete mirabile*, or "marvelous net," at the base of the brain. But then he began to make his own observations of dissected criminals (whose executions were sometimes scheduled at his convenience by an interested Padua judge). When he separated himself from the dogma of Galen, who had inferred human anatomy from the configuration of goat and pig innards, the fanciful nexus supposedly able to transform "animal spirit" into "human spirit" failed to show up. Before long, many discoveries in chemistry and biology were eroding distinctions between living and nonliving matter, and vitalism was forced to retreat. The German chemist Friedrich Woehler struck a famous blow in 1828 when he synthesized the organic compound urea from inorganic ammonium cyanate. What is often considered the coup de grace to vitalism was administered a century later, when the mechanism of self-replication in proteins was unraveled. Science was now satisfied that the laws of chemistry and physics applied equally to rats and rocks, and that life could be reduced to the known and measurable properties of matter. No vital extras were necessary. Indeed, the concept of *anima*, or soul, which dignifies a human, looks silly pinned on a virus.

Darwin had demolished the Aristotelian idea that the growth of an organism was guided by a final cause or purpose. Under natural selection, organisms were the products of random events and had no purpose other than to maximize their number. Even Descartes—who had reserved within his mechanistic view of the body a spot in the brain for the human soul—was trampled under the medical materialism he had helped establish. By 1949 the philosopher Gilbert Ryle could ridicule Cartesian dualism for its suggestion of a "ghost in the machine." The view of the illimitable force that prevails in scientific circles today was summed up by George Schmid in his 1982 book *The Chemical Basis of Life*: "Life is a series of complex chemical reactions. To understand the process of life you must understand the principles of chemistry."

Practitioners of alternative medicine could hardly disagree more. Encompassing as the principles of chemistry are, they seem not to account for some aspects of biological phenomena, aspects which are crucial in the realm of medicine. "The Empiric tradition," writes the homeopathy historian Harris Coulter, "has taken [vitalism] to signify recognition that the *laws* governing the living organism differ from those of lifeless matter. The organism is *reactive*, at all times coping with and attempting to overcome the stresses which impinge upon it from the outside. It behaves purposively, the nature and form of its reaction being determined by the specific environmental stress encountered. It responds to challenge, which no aggregate or assembly of nonliving substances can ever do."

So the mystery is not in the matter but in the way it's organized. Which is to say what, exactly? Are we back at the beginning, with illimitable whirlwinds, etc.? Homeopathy doesn't even bother to dress up the notion; it calls the vital force "the vital force." Chiropractic even more vaguely refers to "the innate." Naturopathy looks simply to awesome curative abilities of *medicatrix naturea*, the body's inherent ability to right itself. Even within medical science, something vitalistic lingers in the body's immunity genius. In the nineteenth century, Claude Bernard emphasized that the crucial trait of living things was their ability to maintain and defend an internal milieu. In the twentieth, the power of self-regulation was called "homeostasis" by the influential Harvard physiologist Walter B. Cannon. These ideas were extended by the Montreal-based physiologist Hans Selye, who coined the term "stress" and grappled with a property he called "adaptation energy" that seems suspiciously vitalistic. In his 1956 book, *The Stress of Life*, he wrote:

> People can get used to a number of things (cold, heavy muscular work, worries) which at first had very alarming effect; yet, upon prolonged exposure, sooner or later all resistance breaks down and exhaustion sets in. It is as though something were lost, or used up, during the work of adaptation; but what this is we do not know. The term adaptation energy has been coined for that which is consumed during continued adaptive work, to indicate that it is something different from the caloric energy we receive from food; but this is only a name, and we still have no precise concept of what this energy might be.

In the hands of hands-on healers the vitalist principle is finessed in the catch-all "energy." Energy is a synonym and metaphor for desire, libido, spirit, psyche, consciousness, soul—for life itself. When healers describe energy they sound like the Inupiat hunters of the arctic cataloguing the varieties of snow.

The variety of pulses in the Nei Ching, the ancient Chinese medical book, speaks to both the subtleties of energy and the power of the hand to differentiate among them. (And perhaps to the power of the imagination as well, imagination itself being in some minds another vitalist attribute.) The pulse can be sharp as a hook or a bird's beak, fine as a hair, and (more slander on our brothers the rocks) dead as a rock. It can be smooth as a flowing stream. It can be continuous like a string of pearls; it can be slightly indented in the middle, or crooked in the front and delayed in the back. It can be soft and fluttering like floating feathers blown by the wind, or elastic like a bending pole. Or taut as a bow when first bent. It can follow up delicately like a rooster treading ground or lifting a foot; it can be like water dripping through the roof, or resonant like striking a stone, or rapid as the edge of a knife in cutting, or vibrating as when one stops the strings of a musical instrument. Light as flicking the skin with a plume; multiple as the seeds of the flower blossom. It can arrive like a suspended hook, or be like firewood burning or scattering leaves. It can, in ways that Westerners may never comprehend, be like visiting strangers or dry mud balls, or mixing lacquer, or sparse earth, or springwater welling up. It can be like being stopped by a horizontal partition, or like a suspended curtain, or a sword lying flat ready to be used, or a smooth pill, or like glory, or like colors, like red, green, white, yellow, black.

Of course, under this unrestrictive license the pulse can also just as easily be like a Shirley MacLaine parody. What's the difference between pulse energy that is "like being stopped by a horizontal partition" and pulse energy that is like being stopped by a state trooper? "Like visiting strangers" seems to have ascended into the canon of fabulist poetry, far from any scientific comprehension of energy. While not overtly metaphorical, even the scientific definition of energy—"the capacity to do work"—only gestures at its mystery, focusing on the function of energy, on *how* it works, not *why*, not what it is in itself. In the end, the scientific definition of energy seems as nebulous as Dorland's definition of life, and lacks even the poetical appeal of the Nei Ching.

In the healer's hands the vital force is the essence of a person's subjectivity, the compelling, if scientifically elusive, stuff that pervades the living and is ipso facto absent in the dead. It follows thought; it reflects emotions. It leaps and streams and swirls. It can be braided into a curse; martial artists insist it provides the real wallop in the karate punch, and who is going to argue with them? Tell-tale traces of it are alleged to cling to objects—the killer's dropped knife, the no-good boyfriend's keys. It can be blended into an atmosphere of sacredness around altars and healing tables in otherwise secular Holiday Inn conference rooms. It can be pulled and pushed and directed through the tissue of the physical body.

In many esoteric traditions it also constitutes a body of its own, the energy body, the subtle body, the light body, some sort of quasicorporeality more rarefied than the physical being, but palpable all the same. It is refracted into colors, which healers sometimes call frequencies, or vibrations. Some aspects of it can be catalogued according to therapeutic function: there's "matrix" energy; "blue goop"; the chaotic energy of a "virus scramble"; the spine-juicing rumble of red energy, which can wake up a stagnant body and may be compared to the sound of an unmuffled motorcycle; high-pitched gold energy, which is often offered as a treatment for disorders of the nervous system, and registers—inasmuch as it's useful to describe a color as a sound—as an ultrasonic whine, like a mosquito in your ear. Given these synesthesia-type paradoxes, where light makes sounds and sounds have color, perhaps even the idea of a dolphin energy is not beyond the pale, though there remains the problem of how to distinguish the energy of an actual bottle-nosed *Delphinus delphis* happily sculling through the Coral Sea from a simulacrum of dolphin energy generated by watching old episodes of *Flipper*.

If you continue the work, it's said you can learn to feel the energy with your hands. Guidebooks recommend holding your palms six inches apart and waiting for the sensation of a spongy presence, a cushiony feeling akin to the influence of a magnetic field. Try it, write John Mann and Lar Short in their book *The Body of Light*: "If something seems to have occurred you might wish to take a further step." Further steps can include attempting to sense the vital force in tree trunks, in petting zoos, perhaps even at Sea World. You might try interacting with the energy around the body, curry-combing it as if it were the tangled coat of an Old English sheepdog. You might mold it into a shield to protect your solar plexus. Or dispose of its negative forms in basins of neutralizing saltwater and pyres of imaginary green fire. The skill in a healer's hand mixes technique and native talent, and it can be honed as tailors and card sharks and pianists hone their handicraft. In some osteopathic schools where energy diagnosis was emphasized, students were expected to refine their sense of touch until they could identify bones wrapped in blankets and detect a strand of hair beneath a piece of paper.

What some hands feel, some eyes see—which in a culture that prizes the visual opens the possibility of substantiating subtle energy phenomena not just by way of the comparatively obscure means of touch and blind intuition but by way of the seemingly more credible and cinematic medium of eyewitness description. Nascent seers may only glimpse the flow of energy as a rushing translucency in the air around the body, movement akin to the heat-distortion at the mouth of an active kiln. But adept clairvoyants behold a nimbus of light engulfing the body. Sometimes it includes the luminous lymph-like net of acupuncture meridians. Sometimes it includes the kundalini energy, which is said to be that aspect of the life force coiled in the sacrum, like Pisa in the Cab Man's briefcase, and which, when awakened, wreathes its way up the spine as two intertwining snakes. And sometimes clairvoyants see those most venerable features of the subtle world called the chakras or the lotuses— the subtle energy centers whose size and color and spin are said to reflect a pilgrim's progress toward Enlightenment. Chakra means "wheel" in Sanskrit. "In those who have reached a certain degree of development, the chakras start to rotate," writes Werner Bohm in his book *Chakras: Roots of Power*. "Whereas in those who have not undergone this development, the petals droop inactively and look dark and colorless."

So you go, up the body from crotch to crown, through storms of petals and spinning light: Muladhara, Svadishthana, Manipura, Anahata, Vishuddha, Ajna, and Sahasrara. Which is to say the red light of the tail-bone chakra, where Pisa & Company sleep; the orange light of the chakra at the belly; the yellow light at the solar plexus; the green light at the heart; the blue light at the throat; the violet light of the third eye at the brow; and finally the white light of the terminus at the crown, where the scholars of the subtle world say the vital principle breaks into the thousand-petaled lotus of the godhead. If you continue this work.

3. THE DEPARTMENT OF SUBTLE ENERGY

W ell, I did continue, though not without some static from the clown. His main qualm, apart from resenting that the chaos-loving spirit of comedy should have to defend the orderly principle of objective evidence, was that there were few, if any, bombproof scientific studies attesting to the reality of subtle-energy phenomena. Kundalini snakes, auric light bodies, and the whirlaway chakras were virtually unknown to scientific literature. On a number of points, even nonscientific reports were unhelpfully riddled with laughable contradictions: For instance, there were seven major chakras in the Hindu tradition, but six in the Tibetan and only four mentioned in Buddhist tantras. The color associated with each chakra varied across cultures. For those exotic Sanskrit names, one could just as easily substitute the days of the week and speak portentously about grounding the Monday chakra, and sexing up the Tuesday chakra, and kneeling prayerfully in the unitive transports of the Sunday chakra . . .

Chakras seemed more like metaphysical speculations with the same relation to the human body that the signs of the zodiac had to the night sky—yet another poetically beguiling set of patterns traced out by the human mind, which never met a set of dots it could resist connecting or a sequence of events it wasn't tempted to round into a story. Factual only as anecdotes of personal experience, the chakras comprised one more mythic narrative about the divine organization of the human body. Without science, was there any way to evaluate critically the claim that the chakras represented the stages of awareness or states of consciousness? It seemed fiendishly difficult to assess the idea that the chakras comprised an ingenious energy system with each lotus processing a specific kind of energy: the first, or root, chakra spinning with the energy of one's tribe; the second chakra with the energy of one's personal passions; the third with the energy of one's mental capacities; the fourth, or heart, chakra with the energy of relationships; the fifth, or throat, chakra with the energy of the will and self-expression; the sixth, or third-eye, chakra with the energy of deep insight; and the seventh, or crown, chakra with the boundless energy of being consciously engulfed in the enigma that made you.

On the other hand, to dismiss phenomena that had been accepted and harnessed for millennia because scientific evidence was lacking was to practice a ludicrously arrogant form of absolutism. And a highly selective one. Clown fire could be drawn by the pieties of scientism too. We've already noted that many standard medical practices are not anchored in conclusively demonstrated scientific results, and if you squint hard at some of the staple features of everyday life—I'm thinking of notions such as "the self," "intention," and "personal responsibility"—they will appear as scientifically doubtful constructs too. But, of course, they are no less essential for being difficult to prove or anatomize. As someone once said, not everything that counts can be counted.

So I was determined to continue. And as it happened, about six months after my trip to Los Angeles, I got a call from an assistant to the editor of *The New Yorker* who wanted to know if I would hold for Tina Brown; I said sure, and then Tina Brown came on the line and asked if I was interested in writing a story about kids who did drugs with their parents, and I said, oh yes, as if it were a subject that had been burning a hole in my files for years and finally somebody with a checkbook had twigged on it, and Tina Brown said, good, why don't you come by the office, we'll talk about it, and then she switched me back to her assistant, who set up the meeting. As I say, this was about six months after my visit to Joel Wallach, who had mentioned that I might track down some of Barbara Brennan's students if I wanted to continue the work that it seemed I had unknowingly started with him. Per his suggestion, I had gotten a copy of Barbara Brennan's book *Hands of Light: A Guide to Healing Through the Human Energy Field*. I studied it with the sort of zeal Sumerian priests reserved for the divinatory entrails of butchered goats. The day of the big meeting came. I wore a blue wool suit, but it was really hot out and my shirt was soaked through. A nice assistant gave me some paper towels and a can of diet Coke and told me to sit at the table in Tina's office; Tina would be there in a minute; I looked around at the walls, which were lined with *New Yorker* covers just like my sister Cam's bathroom; I continued to sweat. Then Tina came in, very cool and crisp in an Armani suit, and we agreed that kids who do drugs with their parents was a terrific piece. We chitchatted about one thing or another, and just as the meeting was about to end, I said, hey, you know there's another subject I think might make a good story, this woman Barbara Brennan, she's a very well-known hands-on healer, and now she has a school with around five hundred people in it; she mortgaged her house to self-publish her first book, and then it was picked up by a commercial publisher, and now it's sold more than six hundred thousand copies, and she's got another book coming out soon. I didn't know at the time that Tina took a dim view of anything "New Age" and couldn't understand why Americans were so gaga for gurus, psychics, and kooky spiritual movements, but it was obvious my pitch wasn't cutting ice. I mopped my forehead with the paper towel and rushed to point out that Brennan didn't seem like a kook, she had a master's degree in physics from the University of Wisconsin, she had worked for five years for NASA's Goddard Space Flight Center . . . This was all stuff I'd picked up from the book bio and an article. Where was the school, Tina asked, and when I said East Hampton, her eyes lit up. East Hampton! Hmmmm. I think now that she must have envisioned I would write a stinging story about a lot of rich, socially prominent nitwits credulously gadding about Flake Land. Either that or she wanted to get me out of her office. In any case, she suddenly said, okay, sure, go ahead, do it. I was giddy; I'd hit the freelancer's trifecta: two contracts from *The New Yorker* and a diet Coke. I had an expense account and a subject I didn't even have to feign enthusiasm for. I also had what I soon came to realize was not just the entrée and the status conferred by an alpha magazine but the crucial cover of the journalistic role. Ulysses sailed past the island of the Sirens with his arms lashed to the mast and his crew's ears plugged with wax. I was proposing to entertain the siren madness of the healing world safely tied to the strictures of an assignment. I wanted to explore the flaky subject without having to own up to an unseemly personal interest in it; without appearing, in the parlance of the fourth estate, to have "crossed over" or "gone native" or "become a believer" or in some other way compromised the principle of objectivity, a principle which no matter how absurd and self-deluded it might actually be was a prized component of a professional reputation. (Or as *Washington Post* editors used to say, in a maxim that wonderfully managed to confuse the merits of objectivity with the virtues of chastity: "You can cover the zoo but don't fuck the elephants.") At all times I would be *working*. And so it seemed I was at the outset. Under the cover of that artful press-pass dodge which masks so much of the reportorial profession's intrinsic voyeurism, I dived into the healing story. Those kids who did drugs with their rascally parents could wait.

On a snappingly cold morning in early December 1993, I drove out the Long Island Expressway, headed not for the media-genic precincts of East Hampton, where even in winter, hedge-fund managers were dashing over to the Barefoot Contessa for another fourteen quarts of lobster salad, but for the Radisson Hotel just off the hellish expressway in Hauppauge. It was about a ninety-minute drive from Manhattan. When she started teaching, in 1982, Barbara Brennan had six students and held classes in her office on Manhattan's Upper East Side. But by that fall of 1993, the school she had named after herself was the largest hands-on healing training center in the country. There were 470 students enrolled in the four-year program; a faculty that included sixty-five part-time teachers and graduate trainees; a full-time staff of ten; an annual budget of around $2 million. (Four years later, there were more than seven hundred students and nearly a hundred faculty members.) Success had obliged Brennan to stage the operation in two rented ballrooms at the Radisson Hotel. I hadn't gotten my assignment under completely false pretenses: The main offices of the school were located in a clapboard house in an unpretentious East Hampton neighborhood.

I parked in front of the Radisson Hotel and made my way across the icy lot. The lobby was crowded with people who, even to an untutored eye, didn't look the part—they seemed too ashen to be healers or students of the subtle world. They weren't. They were the heavily caffeinated, tobacco-smoke-wreathed members of the Firearms Safety Committee of the U.S. Department of Energy. The Department of Subtle Energy was meeting on a higher plane, one floor up.

It was another world entirely. Under the skylights, dozens of vibrant-looking people were fixing cups of herbal tea, and pinning oversized name tags on their lapels, and hugging each other with such heartfelt joy that it seemed they were reuniting after forty years of exile in Egypt, when actually they'd been in class together just the day before.

I had been assigned a guide for the day, Alix Harnden, a brown-haired woman with dark, solicitous eyes. She was in her late thirties, the daughter of a Canadian newspaperman. She had three children of her own. When she was young, she had been obsessed with hands and had spent years photographing them. She had graduated from the Barbara Brennan School of Healing in 1991 and now was training to be a teacher, commuting from her home in Ottawa to the Radisson five times a year.

As the morning program was about to begin, Alix and I found seats in one of the ballrooms, where a makeshift stage was backed by a blue drop cloth. Brennan's lectures all were audiotaped; video recordings were made of some special presentations. The stage was set with two white candles, fresh flowers, and a magnificent harp. Down in front on a long bench was a rush-hour menagerie of stuffed animals, which Alix told me had been assembled by the students as part of an "inner child" exercise. Suddenly a reverent hush fell over the room, and from the side door, Barbara Brennan came gliding in.

She was wearing white flats, a burgundy velvet jacket, and a crinkly white dress that whisked about her ankles. Her lips were done up in bright red lipstick, and blond curls trailed over her shoulders. You would not have guessed she was fifty-five years old. The lights went down. Brennan blew into a radio mike.

"Good morning," she said in a girlish voice. She had a bit of a lisp, and an abstracted, wondering air. She clicked the slide projector. Nothing happened; an assistant scrambled to check the carousel. Alix told me that Barbara—everyone called her Barbara—was extremely shy, but as a triple Pisces she could be temperamental too. She kept the exact date of her birthday secret, Alix said, because she didn't want her astrology-crazed students jumping to conclusions about her mood.

While the projector was being fixed, Brennan sat in a chair on the stage, sipping from a bottle of Evian water and swinging her legs like a schoolgirl waiting for a bus. She did not look like someone who kept ninety-hour workweeks and traveled half the year teaching workshops around the country. And but for the reading I'd done, I would never have guessed that her curriculum vitae included such resolutely un-New-Age-like publications as "Simultaneous Cloud Albedo Measurements Taken with Airborne Medium Resolution Infrared Radiometer." In *Hands of Light* she had summarized the three things healers had to offer patients and the medical profession: "A different and broadened view of the causes and cures of disease; access to information about any given life or medical situation that may not be available through other means; and working directly with the patient to enhance the patient's healing abilities."

"Are we ready now?" Brennan said. A slide popped into the projector. "Okay."

The topic that morning was "high sense perception" (HSP), a general term for all psychic faculties, including feats of clairvoyance. High sense perception was the foundation of Brennan's healing work, the means by which different and broadened views of disease and cures could be offered. Many nuances apparently distinguished psychic healing, mental healing, spiritual healing, and energy healing, but at the time I wasn't familiar with them. As I understood "healing" that morning, it was mostly as a word that spoke to the nebulous concept of "wholeness." I had gathered that healings could be performed without any special perceptual ability. A mother holding her child's hurt arm, for instance, was acting instinctively as a healer. But then a horseback ride or a shopping expedition could also constitute a healing. Some of Brennan's views as described in *Hands of Light* and the book she had just published, *Light Emerging*, drew on the long God-friendly tradition of spiritual healing, where faith was the fountain of miraculous cures and no special skills, no clairvoyant eyes, clairaudient ears or clairsentient hands were necessary. Healers in that specialty presented themselves as conduits who had only to let Providence flow through them. Higher powers happily handled the messy details.

But evidently once you started trying to deepen healing beyond the sphere of Mommy's Kiss and Thy Will Be Done, once you tried, as Brennan wanted to do, to make hands-on healing into a "science," you were bound to address the dynamics of energy, and to put forth a therapeutics based on the corporeal dance of *chi* or whatever vitalist principle seemed most congenial. Brennan's healing work was premised on the existence of a "human energy field," or aura, which surrounded the body and drew on the nourishment of a "universal energy field." A person's field had physical, mental, emotional, and spiritual dimensions. It could be therapeutically manipulated. It presupposed an infinite array of subtle energies and vibrations that could be sensed and influenced by trained healers—an array which, it almost goes without saying, had been devilishly difficult to confirm scientifically.

To read a client, Brennan was saying now, a healer expands her awareness and shifts into what she called the witness state. "When you move from the active and rational perspective to the witness state, you are allowing reality to unfold in the moment," she said. "As soon as you try to use the mind the way you learned in school, you're back in the active state.

The flow of energy is very different. Being in the witness state means being willing not to know."

Being willing not to know what she was talking about put an interesting spin on the fact that I didn't know what she was talking about. I mean, sure I understood what she was saying in theory, but in practice? Was it like reporting a story, where you didn't know what you needed to know or even what was important until you had some sense of the overarching pattern and could see the significance of previously unremarkable details? Okay, it was a pathetic analogy; I reached for it for the same reason a culturally shorn American wanders into McDonald's in Shanghai and orders a hamburger.

Brennan was widely known in healing circles for having world-class psychic vision. She had elaborated on maps of the subtle-energy system that had been first sketched thousands of years ago by clairvoyant Tibetan and Indian yoga masters and Chinese acupuncturists. The trouble was that where six zoologists will look at the skeleton of a chicken and agree what's a leg bone and what's a back bone, gifted seers are hard pressed to reach an objective consensus about the features of subtle anatomy, and their personal maps, their lexicons and landmarks, vary as maddeningly as those sixteenth-century charts of the coastline of North America.

The main features on Brennan's map were the seven "subtle bodies," which she saw as surrounding and pervading the physical body, nested within one another like a Maryushka doll, each finer in substance and higher in frequency than the one below it. The preferred verb for describing the relation of these bodies was "interpenetrated." The subtle bodies comprised the sum of a person's aura. There were chakras too, seven of them, in accord with the Hindu tradition. They pulled energy into the body from a "universal energy field." In Brennan's view, the chakras projected from both the front and the back of the torso. In *Hands of Light* she described how tears and blockages in both the chakras and on the perimeters of the subtle bodies were evidence of pathology on the physical, emotional, mental, or spiritual level. Looking at the energy field of a cocaine addict, for example, she often could see that it was scummed up with "etheric mucus." The area around the heart in the field of a cardiac patient frequently showed a kind of energetic "scarring." Disease or potential problems often appeared first as energetic imbalances, blocks, or tears, or sometimes as drabness or enervation; the chakras could spin weakly or in the wrong direction. Sometimes part of a chakra would poke out like a spring from a cheap couch. High sense perception was vital because it enabled a healer to see what was going on in a person energetically and to anticipate what might eventually be manifested as gross physical illness.

"Perceiving the Human Energy Field not only takes study and practice but also requires personal growth," Brennan wrote in *Hands of Light*. "It takes internal changes that increase your sensitivity so that you can learn to differentiate between internal noise and subtle incoming information that can only be perceived by silencing the mind."

When she was first practicing, Brennan had to meditate to achieve this altered state. Over the years, the transition became automatic and rapid; she can read people instantly, and, she says, can see what other healers are seeing as the information is coming to them.

But who can verify her vision? In the spring of 1983, for example, Brennan "looked" into the chest of her best friend, a social worker named Cindy Metz. She saw a grayish-black triangular shape in Cindy's left lung and heard a voice in her head say, "She has cancer and is going to die." The bluntness of the prophecy shocked her. She said nothing to her friend but urged Cindy to get her chest checked by a doctor. Brennan was immensely relieved to learn a few days later that her diagnosis had not been confirmed. The doctors at George Washington University Hospital couldn't find anything. Well, not at first. After four months and three CAT scans, they found a blood clot. It did not respond to treatment. When they operated they discovered mesothelioma, an incurable lung cancer. Eight months later—months in which Barbara sat with Cindy, holding her friend's head for hours on end, working on her field, watching it fluctuate with the medications, seeing the effects of a camphor-based experimental French drug called 714-X and then the effects of morphine, which seemed only to undo the benefits of 714-X—Cindy died.

It's hard to know what to make of this story. When I read it I was back in the rift valley that divides the world into logical positivists and damned English professors. Set aside the point that 714-X was eventually junked as a worthless cancer therapy. If only people with good high sense perception can tell whether someone else has good high sense perception, is it simply a matter of believers believing and belief making it so? How is the testimony of clairvoyants confirming the accuracy of each other's readings more reliable than the testimony of two members of the Flat Earth Society who say they have corroborated each other's arithmetic? On the other hand, maybe the best way to verify chakras and subtle bodies is to stop whining about objectivity and science and learn to do what Brennan says she does. Sensation is a complex act; in some ways it is a performance. You don't really know how good a great violinist is until you try to play the instrument yourself.

Many healers who have not developed clairvoyant sight and can't visually read the aura are nonetheless effective, Brennan maintains. They can sense the field with their hands. Kinesthetic perception is one of several modes of HSP. Some healers receive auditory guidance. Taste and smell can convey information from the domain of the subtle bodies. So can intuition—a sense poorly understood in the West as it is not localized in an organ or a set of nerves. Emotions can be diagnostic. Alix told me that the school requires graduates be adept in at least two forms of HSP. As ever, the tricky part is learning to separate what's going on in yourself from what's actually occurring in the client.

Now a student named Martha rose to ask a question about visual HSP. Brennan said, "Why don't you read my mother—Elmyra Lydia Brennan. She's eighty-three. No, eighty-four."

Martha, who was evidently already quite good at HSP, closed her eyes and bent her legs in a martial-arts stance.

"See there," Brennan said to the class, "she went out of her crown chakra . . ." Some time passed. "She's reached my mother, who's in the north woods of Wisconsin, where we used to go deer hunting. There's a connection here she's seeing." An expression of pained sympathy crossed Martha's face. "As she brings a conscious awareness to my mother's field, she's feeling a lot of sadness. She's feeling my mother's burden. Can anybody else here see that?"

People were nodding, affirming they could see something.

"My mother's field is starting to pulsate. Now Martha's seeing the disconnection between the upper and lower levels."

The air in the room had grown still, and warmer, and the mood strangely sacrosanct. Martha held her martial-arts stance for ten minutes, while Brennan offered a desultory play-by-play of the psychic action. When Martha sat down, the students wiggled their hands over their heads as though they were trying to pantomime the word "moose" in a charades game.

"What are they doing?"

"Clapping scatters the energy," Alix whispered.

The novelty and strangeness of the morning were unrelenting: dire diseases, paranormal phenomena, metaphysical speculations, stuffed animals, the sound of moose hand clapping. On the wall, posters depicted stick figures with a line drawn from the solar plexus to the "molten core of the earth." The molten core of the earth was represented as a kind of steaming cow flop. Countless times, students were directed to "ground" themselves to the molten core of the earth, a place none of them had actually seen, of course, but which they imagined they could feel and attach themselves to. The common denominator of so many people in the crowd seemed to be a willingness to entertain fantastic scenarios with an uncritical ingenuousness. They went at their work with an open-hearted and at times naif-like demeanor, always seeking to free themselves from the temptation of passing judgment, and as a consequence they seemed to have rinsed all trace of politics out of themselves, to have denatured their personalities of irony and bitterness and various other emotional tannins. Time and again I had the feeling of being in a weird Kiwanis Club on the far side of the looking glass, where all the friendly, hearty, civic-minded Golden Retriever—loving people just happened to have five hundred milligrams of LSD freestyling through their bloodstreams.

Stranger still was when Brennan herself was talking and suddenly slipped into the first-person plural and began sculpting the air with her hands and speaking in a staccato, portentous voice.

"We are here holding you with our hearts quite safely. Is it not truly your soul's desire to clear the shadows and live with us in the light?"

I turned to Alix.

"That's Heyoan," she said. "He's Barbara's guide."

The students seemed to take this bizarre bit of theater perfectly in stride. They all had their own guides. Training in high sense perception dispels the fiction that the self speaks with one voice. Guides, I assumed that morning, were metaphors for altered states. I learned within a day or two that guides would insist that altered states were just metaphors for them. Heyoan was Brennan's old and beloved mainstay. In *Hands of Light* she had confessed to some embarrassment upon learning that his name meant "Wind That Whispers Through the Centuries." Heyoan had been giving her advice for years. He supervised healings and kibitzed at lectures; Brennan seemed almost relieved to let him handle the harder questions put to her by the students. When she channeled Heyoan, her lisp disappeared.

To my clown-cocked ear, Heyoan's stilted cadence and mannered diction sounded a lot like Robert Benchley doing his immortal parody of the treasurer's report, but then maybe the discordant note was just a matter of style—Plato reported that Socrates frequently heard and followed the voice of a semidivine being, his so-called daemon. Brennan broke back into her own voice, but she was still hearing Heyoan's. Her hands seemed to be half hers, half his, carving the air in his characteristic way. She seemed like a real-time translator at the United Nations.

"He's saying 'Do you understand what I mean?' " Many of the students were nodding. And then Heyoan released her hands and withdrew completely, and Brennan was back on her own, speaking in her voice. She was saying that students could move the screen of their mind anywhere, outside the head, inside the bodies. They could see the auric field with their eyes, but they could also perceive it through the sixth chakra—the third eye. "That's where I get most of my information," she said. "It's more like remembering what your house looks like than seeing it in front of you. When Martha was reading my mother, I could see her sixth chakra open, and light enter through the third eye."

Each chakra had a seal on it to keep unwanted energy out. The idea was that you should see only what you were ready to see or what you could handle. What you could handle was determined in large part by the quantity of energy in your system. So there was an interesting reciprocity between the quantity of energy in your system and the quality of it. If your seals were opened but your energy levels were low, you might well be vulnerable to lower frequencies, which apparently could produce hallucinations. You might well find yourself oscillating at a rate of vibration associated with purgatorial states of consciousness. You could end up wandering around Broadway ranting about the CIA. You had to open your chakras to sharpen your high sense perception, Brennan said, but it was essential to have enough power in your field first.

"How do you get more power?" she asked. "Make your field more coherent. Make it more coherent by synchronizing the pulses. You can do this by grounding yourself down to the earth and synchronizing yourself with fluctuations in the earth's magnetic field. The harder way to make your field more coherent is the way gurus do it, which is to make all your chakras the same size at the same level, and synchronize them with each wave in the vertical power current so there are no beats and nothing is impeded."

"Vertical power current?" I said to Alix.

"It's the flow of energy that runs up and down the spine."

"There aren't many human beings that can do this," Brennan was saying. "I'm telling you this because it's what our potential is. It's part of our evolutionary process. Where we're going as a species is undreamable, provided we make it through the next several years . . ."

She closed her eyes. Here was Heyoan, butting in again. A resourceful fellow, never at a loss for answers, the sort of discarnate friend you'd like to have around as you were paging through the stock tables. Never mind whether humanity would survive the millennial turbulence. Was it time to short Microsoft? But millennial turbulence was the topic of the moment. Were we all going to make it through the next several years? But really, what was he going to say, here at the Barbara Brennan School of Healing? Was he going to tell the students "No, don't bother with your homework, *you're all going to die in a lake of fire!*" That probably wasn't his style.

To the extent that the healing school had many of the elements of a religious organization, it proposed a remarkably democratic idea of divinity and nurtured prophets with little appetite for Adventist apocalypse or Old Testament harangue. *Provided we make it through the next several years . . .* Well, would we? Brennan opened her eyes. "He says we all will," she said with a laugh. Phew! Everyone raised their arms and wiggled their hands. Alix was right about subtle applause. Some closure had been brought to the morning's lecture, but the spell of the room was still intact.

4. PUSH PULL
STOP ALLOW

After Barbara Brennan's lecture on high sense perception, everyone went out for water; the energies of healing class instill desertlike thirsts. Alix, who as a guide was beginning to seem mercifully concrete, emptied a vitamin-and-mineral powder into a water glass that was unmistakably part of the physical plane, and talked about the school. Brennan's version of hands-on healing was a good deal more elaborate—and now at $5,200 a year a lot more expensive—than other programs'. But, like many, it assumed that healing was a skill that could be taught, like, say, household wiring, and did not require a special endowment of talent beyond the gifts already latent in most people.

To qualify, prospective students had to take a four-day introductory seminar, which Brennan offered six times a year at venues around the country. Applicants also had to have two credits of anatomy and physiology, and be engaged in some kind of psychotherapy. Eighty percent of the students were women, mostly in their thirties and forties. They had come from as far away as Japan, Brazil, Italy, Alaska. Many already had experience in healing professions as nurses, psychotherapists, acupuncturists; there were several medical doctors enrolled during the term I visited the school.

The students met five times a year for week-long sessions. They worked their way up the levels of the human energy field as they advanced in grade. They had homework during and between classes. They practiced the HSP-enhancing and chakra-opening exercises from *Hands of Light*. Brennan incorporated the neo-Reichian body-psychology she had absorbed during her years at the Pathwork Center in Phoenicia, New York: Students learned to categorize people by one of five "characterologies" said to denote a person's energetic defense system and habitual style of relating to others. The students started with the pre-liminary healing technique misleadingly referred to as "chelation," which was not a chemical process but a way of clearing, balancing, and charg-ing the energy field. It had been developed by the noted healer Rosalyn Bruyere to mitigate the side effects of chemotherapy. The students went on to the more subtle elements of field work, learning how to "restruc-ture" lines of light in subtle bodies, how to "sew" tears in the auric field, how to keep their hands immobile and their energy pitched at specific frequencies. There was an aspect of play in the training—once you develop an ability to see or sense an energy field around the body, it's tempting to explore what affects it. Brennan and Jason Shulman, who at the time was one of the school's main teachers but who eventually left to start his own healing group, The Society of Souls, used to take homeo-pathic remedies and antidepressants to see if they could track the drugs' effects on each other's fields. "Xanax made the chakras spin backwards," Shulman told me. "Prozac looked very good."

It was precisely this sort of shared empirical experience that allowed healers to build up confidence in their perceptual abilities and gave Brennan the confidence to claim that what she was teaching was "heal-ing science." She hoped to make energy treatments a standard part of the medical system. But subjective agreements between two healers did not constitute the kind of scientific evidence that could persuade die-hard skeptics or even people willing to keep an open mind. You had to be chary of the term "healing science" if only because its chief instruments were human beings with their flat-Earth history of error and self-deception. In *Hands of Light*, for instance, there were significant names misspelled; there was a bibliography but no list of references; and Brennan had enthusiastically quoted experimental work supporting the human energy field hypothesis that had, in fact, been discredited.

It was conceivable you could make an empirical science of the tech-nical skills that were taught. Undergraduates had to pass dozens of tests. They had to learn how to push and pull energy with their hands, how to allow it to run, how to stop it. Push. Pull. Stop. Allow. It was basic ABC stuff but still very important, and you could get the hang of it, as you could get the hang of the French horn or the yo-yo, and teachers could confirm and grade your abilities. At the end of their senior year, students had to pass a final exam, which consisted of a presentation and defense of a healing case. Their progress was monitored by Brennan and the rest of the faculty; students were evaluated constantly, starting with their work in the required four-day introductory seminar.

But where was the "science" in learning how to summon one of the spirit guides that apparently mob the wards of the subtle realm and keep longer hours than first-year interns? Learning to get "guidance" was considered a crucial part of healing science. That alone would seem to disqualify the training as a "science." Sure, there were little-acknowledged metaphysical assumptions in science, but they still did not require a leap of faith, or at least not as screamingly large a leap of faith. "Healing science" at the Brennan School seemed to have more in common with the pseudosciences of the alternative medical realm, where procedures and theories were shaped less by data than by religious and spiritual convictions.

And given Brennan's own contention that anyone could learn to heal, was there even a need for a "science" of healing? By one measure, even the most tender greenhorns in the freshman class were already astonishing healers. Their bodies were patching cuts and consuming cancers and suppressing bugs and regulating blood pressure and churning out leukocytes and balancing sodium and potassium salts, and automatically doing a hundred million other things with no training or conscious assistance. The school's mission was to make students conscious of the healing process so that they might enhance what people already do naturally, heedlessly, while they eat or sleep or practice the French horn or toy with yo-yos. The main assumption of the school was that people *could* become conscious of the healing process; the operation of the healing process was intimated in the flow of energy. Healing ability, then, was not simply a question of technical expertise. As Brennan had written in *Light Emerging*: "The hard part about healing training is not the techniques but the personal growth one must go through to become ready to learn the techniques. The heart of healing is . . . the states of being out of which those techniques arise."

So the training inevitably deepened students' awareness and understanding of themselves, and therein lay the real drama and the true focus of the work. Alix explained to me it wasn't until junior year that the students realized the degree of personal commitment it took to become a healer. "This work is about bringing yourself forward," she said. "In the course of it, you'll be in really vulnerable states." It was her belief, and a central tenet of the school's curriculum, that people created their own reality—the reality of the body, the reality of illness or health, the reality, at some level, of fate itself. "From the viewpoint of the healer," Brennan had written in *Light Emerging,* "all disease is psychosomatic."

I was bristling with questions on this point, for it was one of the most conspicuous and controversial ideas from the medical fringe. Certainly, the extent to which the mind dictates the terms of its existence has become more of a health issue. And certainly it is now well established that some illnesses are exacerbated and even caused by the mind, and that many aspects of health and disease are influenced by attitudes and emotions. But how far can the domain of mental factors be extended? How much "control" do we have over our ailments, our bodies, our histories? In the face of the disasters that confront millions of people every day—from epidemics to birth defects to earthquakes and civil wars and genocides—the idea that individuals generate their own reality seemed awfully naive, not to say astonishingly narcissistic. In the spirit of the open-minded curriculum, I was determined to squelch the urge to make snap judgments, but it was difficult not to wonder about the millions of people who would never have the benefit of a day in healing school and the luxury of entertaining questions about whether human beings were the pawns of fate or fate's masters. Alix said that vacillating between the way the Western scientific mind had been conditioned to think and this other, take-charge view of destiny was a normal phase of the training. It was hard not to pester her with questions that would seem to refute the prevailing metaphysics of the place: Didn't healers live at the mercy of stray bullets and breaking cornices like the rest of us? Hell, if you took the logic of reincarnation at face value, which apparently most students did, how could your life follow the script you devised when your choices were predetermined by the metastory of your karma?

Still, I had to grant that the idea of writing your own script was, for lack of a better word, weirdly empowering. And the healers' point in taking responsibility for creating their own reality—bad luck and genetic misfortune notwithstanding—seemed to be that they enriched their existence by enhancing their sense of ownership. They owned even their negative aspects. They owned the body's pain. Pain was not to be fled, ignored, or stifled, but to be consulted, worked with, embraced even— and so digested for the lessons it offered, such as they were, and the changes it could produce, if any. The ultimate end of healing—of the personal growth healing entailed—was to achieve a conscious death and to overcome in life the haunting sense of the separation from the greater world, a sense of separation that seems to have its origins in the mythic story of the fall of man. "All suffering is caused by the illusion of separateness, which generates fear and self-hatred, which eventually causes illness," Brennan had written in the prologue to *Hands of Light*. When no aspect of life is separate from the totality, the power to influence outcomes and heal diseases is unlimited. Or so the theory goes. Nothing I had read or heard so far explained what fear and self-hatred had to do with a chlamydia infection, or any infectious disease, except in the very roundabout sense that fear and self-hatred might weaken the immune system. Alix's definition of health was boundless: "Health," she said, "is being as much of who you are as you possibly can be." But strictly speaking, weren't there times when a perfectly adequate definition of health could be a prescription of penicillin?

While we were talking, Brennan came up and introduced herself. She was brimming with goodwill. Her eyes were liquid and deep and shone like moonlit water in a rain barrel; as with the eyes of Joel Wallach, I found them hard to hold for very long. Partly it was her reputation for clairvoyance, the eerie sense of being seen into, of wondering if she was divining stuff not normally available on making someone's acquaintance. I'd met a number of the students, and many of them had that same scoping eye when you shook their hands. Is what makes their gaze at times uncomfortable that they want so much? Or that they offer so much?

Brennan reached around my hip and held her hand in the air.

"You seem pretty healthy," she said, meaning specifically what, I wasn't sure. "A little bit of a leak back here."

She left her hand there behind my hip a moment and then turned away to attend to some business the school's dean had just approached her with.

Since Brennan was so focused on running the school, people she'd done healings on were hard to come by, and she'd made a point of telling me I ought to talk to a middle-aged Alaska schoolteacher named Barbara Ann Nelson. Nelson was in her junior year at the school, and when I hooked up with her later, she credited Brennan with reversing her degenerative eye disease. She had gone to the eye doctor for a new pair of contact lenses in the spring of 1993 only to be told that she had an idiopathic macular hole in her left retina and an incipient hole in her right retina— a condition that her doctor said was all but certain to lead to blindness and that could be treated only by a risky surgery. She saw three more doctors who confirmed the diagnosis and made photographs. The night before her surgery, she bought a copy of *Hands of Light*, and what she read made her decide to cancel the operation. She wanted to give energy work a chance. She told me how Brennan put her on a table and said she could see that the lines of light feeding Barbara Ann's eyes were weak and in some cases broken, and needed to be restructured—restructuring being one of the most common therapeutic actions at the school. (Even now I'm not sure I know what it entails, but have imagined it to be like reaching into a pot and straightening strands of spaghetti.) "She totally restructured my eyes and my optic nerve," Barbara Ann said. "She created fluidity and space so my eyes had the ability to vibrate at a level the body would normally be at when it heals." As Brennan worked to reestablish something vital in the eyes, Barbara Ann was engulfed with memories of lives she had had in the past, of a time when she'd been a healer among a tribe who believed that clairvoyant vision was enhanced by blindness. A week after the healing, an eye surgeon could no longer find a hole in the right eye, and the hole in the left had diminished. During the semester, other students continued to work with Nelson, but heeding Brennan's instructions, they had not added to or tampered with the delicate work Brennan had done around her eyes. Steadily, Nelson's vision improved. Her doctors could only attribute the recovery to spontaneous remission—the catch-all for cures that cannot be explained by the conventional medical paradigm. One of them, eventually quoted in an article in *New Age Journal*, said he was "in awe" of what had taken place.

When I caught up with Alix again, she said the next day would be the final day of that week's classes, and a Goddess Healing was scheduled.

It would be the climax of the week. Brennan would expand her consciousness to the full extent of her range and convey into the room energies of surpassing fineness and power, her way of working on everyone at the school en masse. Sometimes it produced amazing results, Alix said. She had been asked to find out whether I would mind if Barbara included me in the work she would do on everyone in the room. "Do you want to get zapped?" she said. Here were the Sirens singing from the shore of their lethal island . . . But the monk had checked the ropes and snugged the knots and plugged the clown's ears with wax. Getting zapped—wasn't that the point?

5. FUSED IN SO-CALLED TIME

With my magazine license I had privileges that were the envy of Brennan's paying students: a sustained chunk of her time, and a format in which she was not the venerated figure on a stage, but a profile subject being called upon to make an account of herself for what she had to know—if only from having faced some difficult interviews on her book tour—was likely a skeptical audience.

Six weeks after my initial visit to the school, I drove out from New York again, this time all the way to Brennan's airy, plant-filled house adjacent to the school offices in East Hampton. Brennan was about to move to a new place in Montauk, which she had designed and built with her husband, Eli Wilner, a very successful picture-frame restorer and dealer. She met me at the door, dressed in white slacks and a white sweater. Her husband was upstairs in bed with the flu at the moment, she said. She could see the flu in his energy field but couldn't keep it out. Nor could she, a few days later, keep it out of her own field. Some viruses had no respect for her power to sew auric tears and reset chakras. They thrived where Perfect Health fell short.

I did my due diligence for Tina Brown that February day, interviewing Brennan for seven hours. We sat first in her living room, where the light in the half-moon windows waned and little prism-scattered rainbows faded on the floor, and then moved upstairs to her office, where we settled ourselves on the thick white rug by a small shrine filled with cards and candles and pictures of Mother Meera and the Dalai Lama. "My memory for dates is going," Brennan sighed. "Too many hours in nonlinear time." Minus the podium and the retinue of teachers and students, she seemed like any other East Hampton mortal who might drive into Manhattan for a regular mammogram, or explain to the folks at the summer arts fair that she had given up wearing nylon stockings because they blocked the flow of energy in the legs, or advise friends against cooking with aluminum pots because the metal took the *prana* out of food. I had not come with a tape recorder; Brennan helpfully dug one up, saying it would be good to have in case she channeled Heyoan. Heyoan's remarks tended to come out in a headlong rush. Truth to tell, I knew they would be more precious to her than to me.

I thought we might begin at the beginning, but when Brennan told me her earliest memory, I pitied the fact checker who would have to corroborate the information. Brennan had reached back well past her earliest childhood recollection of her older brother David scratching her eye while she was parked in a high chair. She had reached back past what neuroanatomists asserted were the hard-wired limits of memory in the infant cortex and had latched onto some occult zone of holographic reality where, she confided, she was able to recall the moment of her own conception, that Gnostic hour when she was nothing but the substance of a soul drawn down one spring evening by the reddish-rose light emanating from a particular bedroom in a particular house . . . She told me this with such guileless sincerity that I knew she believed it herself and didn't feel it was a grievous departure from common sense, which meant either she was, well, deranged, or she was right. But if she was right, how was I going to explain it to Tina Brown?

At any rate, about nine months after Brennan sailed into the rose light, she popped out in her new physical digs, slimy and blue with the umbilical cord around her neck. She was the second of three children, born in a shack on a wheat farm in Drummond, Oklahoma. She didn't make a sound for three days. This was in the shadow of the Great Depression. Her father, a restless Dutch-Irishman named George Brennan, had lost his job as a factory worker in Chicago and had moved his family in with his wife's Oklahoma relatives. George wasn't cut out for farming; he'd wanted to be an anthropologist. Elmyra Brennan, the daughter of German immigrants, also was brimming with unrealized hopes; she wanted to be a nurse. Strict Protestants, neither she nor George drank, but they did love to dance.

They drifted in poverty from Oklahoma to Kansas, Chicago, and finally to the central Wisconsin town of Loyal, where George tried dairy farming. They had no water in the house, and only a Sears catalogue for toilet paper in the outhouse. They couldn't afford gas for the car. The only book around was the Bible.

Brennan walked two and a half miles to a one-room school, often in killing weather. She did chores on the farm, picked strawberries, and baby-sat. She played the angel in the church pageant. Her mother sewed all the kids' clothes. Her father fished and hunted for food: bluegills, pike, crappies; squirrels, rabbits, deer. He taught his kids how to handle guns, how to hunt. The cardinal rule was you had to be stone quiet. Brennan's girlhood was an apprenticeship in the discipline of Wisconsin woods-manship. She learned to sit motionless at twenty below zero so as not to spook deer. She learned to row soundlessly on lakes. She got up before dawn to walk her brother David's trap line. In the woods, she had what she would later realize were her first experiences of high sense percep-tion. Psychic abilities often are attributed to children, under the theory that the talent exists until it is repressed, when kids become conscious of what convention says is possible. Brennan thought everybody could see a haze-like shroud around trees and locate animals without seeing them. She spent hours in expanded states without thinking they were anything special. Chipmunks ran across her feet. She would walk blindfolded, "feeling" the energy around maples and pine boles before she could actu-ally touch their bark.

When George found a job with a company that made fire engines, the family moved to Clintonville, a town of five thousand people some thirty miles west of Green Bay. At Clintonville High, Brennan poured herself into schoolwork. Academic success gave her an identity and, in time, a passport out of rural misery. She was interested in painting but was drawn to physics her senior year because it was harder. "I had a lot of ego tied up in being smart," she said. She was a model of bobby-sox adolescence: homemade skirts, saddleshoes, a ponytail, and pretty enough to be a homecoming queen, even though she felt like a hick with zero social graces. "I didn't even know how to eat a salad, because we never went to restaurants," she said.

Her parents wanted her to be a secretary or a nurse. She had her heart set on physics. She was the first person in her family to continue her education past high school, matriculating at the state college at Oshkosh. The male physics majors who asked her out usually wanted help with their homework; her dormmates in their angora sweaters thought she was odd because she wasn't in the market for a husband. "In those years, most women weren't interested in anything I was interested in," Brennan recalled. "I thought it was very romantic to know why the moon reflects light from the sun." She took time off to work—she sewed clothes, worked in a door factory, and toted trays as a carhop at an A&W root beer stand—and then she transferred to the University of Wisconsin at Madison, where she was the only woman among fifty or so men studying atmospheric physics. She would sit six hours a day at her desk studying, take a break for half an hour, and then sit for another six hours. She graduated with a bachelor's degree in science in 1962. She got her master's degree in physics in 1964, despite an attack of stage fright during her oral exam. Her professor Werner Soumi had a NASA grant to calibrate a weather satellite. He hired Brennan. The fellowship eventually led to her moving east to take a job at the Goddard Space Flight Center, in Maryland, where she spent hours aloft in airplanes packed with instruments, overflying the arctic ice caps, the North Sea, the Amazon.

For a naive Midwestern farm girl, twenty-three years old, NASA airplanes afforded the least of her revelations. Washington, D.C., was roiling with the cultural changes that were general in the country. Brennan had met Jac Conaway, a NASA soil expert and Maryland native who was active in the civil rights movement. They would eventually marry in 1971. Conaway got her involved in the women's movement. They did primal scream therapy and launched an encounter group. Their house on North Capitol Street turned into a commune filled with roommates.

After five years at NASA, Brennan was disillusioned with government science. She had always had a penchant for dramatic changes, and in 1970, pregnant with her daughter Celia, she quit and took off with Jac in a VW bus for Mexico. It was the worst year of her life. They stayed in a house in Progreso in the Yucatan, four blocks from the Gulf of Mexico. She didn't speak the language, the marriage was rocky, and the loss of her professional identity depressed her so badly she couldn't set plates on the dinner table. She retreated to the roof to meditate, and for the first time since her childhood, she began to have spiritual experiences.

When the couple returned to the States, Brennan started therapy. In three months her enthusiasm for life came back, but the marriage was a struggle. She began to study counseling at the Community of the Whole Person, a small personal-growth center led by Methodist minister Jim Cox. They did work on deep hypnosis, relaxation techniques, altered states of consciousness. One of her trainers was Ann Bowman, who though blinded by cataracts could nevertheless "read the aura." "Someone would walk in the door, and Ann would say, 'Your energy is going like this and is doing this,' and I could see what she was talking about," Brennan recalled. "What impressed me was that it wasn't light she was seeing." Brennan's own clairvoyant faculty was awakening. One morning she found herself staring at the back of her husband's neck in bed. "I was looking at this intersection of muscle and bones and thinking, how interesting! I could see long strips of muscle. Then I took a deep breath and didn't see it again for six months. You could say I drove it away, or you could say that I didn't know how to achieve and sustain a state of consciousness in which I could see into the body.

"I had strong negative psychic experiences—I took them out of *Hands of Light*, but I teach them in the sophomore class. There are things that are too frightening to people because of the old way of looking at them. There are spiritual beings that have negative intentions. I have been to levels of hell that are like Hieronymous Bosch paintings. It's terrible. I have been through Tibetan Bardos. Giving people healings, I've been in places where it's totally black and people are screaming."

In her second year of training at the Community of Whole Person, at the behest of a family member, she tried to contact the energy essence of a man named Bud, who had hanged himself. She got more than she bargained for. "I was followed for weeks by a black form. A meditation teacher saw it, and her interpretation was, 'You're being invaded by an evil dark force.' But it wasn't an evil force, it was Bud. And I didn't know how to interpret it. He came because I could call him. He'd hanged himself, and I was his life preserver. I was terrified. I didn't know what to do. I was going around with a cross. Jim Cox was there for me—he didn't send me to the hospital; he said, 'You're just having a psychic experience.' I learned I shouldn't mess around with 'lower beings.' I also began to understand that consciousness on the astral level, the fourth level of the field, takes the shape of what it thinks itself to be. All I had to do was send Bud unconditional love, and the thought-form was transformed and released."

One rainy night in 1974, Brennan was camped on the beach at Assateague, Maryland, with her family. She had gone to sleep in the Volkswagen bus. "Suddenly in the middle of the night, I heard my name called very loudly and distinctly, three times. I woke up, and the sky was clear, the whole sky had opened, and I could hear the stars—I literally heard the stars singing. I had been praying for some direction. When I was a teenager in high school I used to shake my fist at God because I didn't know everything about the world. Now here was the music of the stars telling me my prayers had been answered."

Two weeks later, the family moved up to New York to the Pathwork Center, a spiritual community in the Catskill mountains, where Brennan stayed nine years. To live at the center, she was required to give up the therapy practice she'd started in Washington. She washed toilets and cleaned house; she worked in the kitchen, cooking for the center's weekend guests. Jac managed the grounds. Brennan began the five-year "helper" training program at the center. She studied bioenergetics, a system of body psychology developed from the theories of Wilhelm Reich. Her unhappy marriage got better for a while, and then derailed.

Given her facility for seeing the aura, Brennan was drawn toward energy work at the Pathwork Center. She attempted to measure the human energy field in a darkroom. With New York psychiatrist John Pierrakos and researcher Richard Dobrin, she correlated observations of the energy field with emotional patterns. She began teaching courses about her findings. She studied with Rosalyn Bruyere, who had assisted

UCLA professor Valerie Hunt in a set of intriguing studies which correlated visual phenomena of the auric field with electromyographic readings of muscle energy at the chakra locations. Brennan found in Bruyere
a mentor who could confirm her observations of energy fields. Brennan
began to get a reputation as a healer; within three months of opening a
practice in New York, she had more clients than she could handle.

Toward the end of our conversation, Brennan was channeling
Heyoan, and I asked her to ask him: What did he think about the direction of her life? Did he know where she was going?

"He's saying, 'I know perfectly well where she's going,' " she said.
" 'She's coming to me and will be fused with me—in so-called time.' "

"And do you know when that will be?"

"Do you mean when will death occur?"

"Yes."

"I don't think she wishes to know that yet. We would be glad to take
off the veil if she so desires. But at this point in time it would not be the
best for her process. There needs to be more ego letting-go here before
that matters. When it no longer matters to her personality whether she
lives in the physical or spiritual world—in other words, when that veil is
dissolved, and she knows she will be able to communicate with her dear
Eli and her daughter and many dear friends—then perhaps she will let
go of that thought-form, and do what you call 'drop the body.' There
will be no break in conscious awareness."

I was struck by how serene the texture of the room had grown; it was
as if what had been gravel was now a fine soft sand. And the strange feeling of being steadied, affirmed. I was struck also by the way the channeled voice of her guide gave Brennan a gentle, roundabout way of
criticizing herself. When she returned from the heights of her trance, taking some time to collect herself, I feared she regretted my having kept
her in an extremity of consciousness. But she did not. What she regretted was having to come back.

I mentioned the change I'd felt in my body.

"You were sitting in my aura," she said.

It was not something that would show up on the tape, and yet it
seemed as important as anything she had said. She walked me to the door.
It was a frigid night. A new moon had risen.

6. THE GODDESS

On the morning of the Goddess Healing, Alix Harnden and I found seats a few minutes before nine. We removed our shoes and stowed our notebooks and papers under the chairs. There was a feeling of expectancy in the ballroom, where the combined freshman and sophomore classes—some 250 people—were already immersed in meditation. The temperature was growing warmer by the minute, and there was something churchly and hushed in the air. Onstage, two candles burned; Marjorie Valeri was seated at the burnished harp. Marjorie was a healer and teacher at the school, and at the time she also had a regular gig playing teatime at the St. Regis hotel in Manhattan. Usually her hands got tired after thirty minutes of show tunes and she'd take a break, but during Goddess Healings, she told me, she channeled the music and could play two hours nonstop.

The more "open" students could become on their own, prior to Brennan's arrival, the less work she would have to do to hold the energies on site. What Brennan did during these events was not the one-on-one stuff of healing-table diagnosis and treatment, Alix told me, but the effects could be extremely powerful all the same. One of the teachers had brought her scoliotic daughter to a Goddess Healing. She was X-rayed afterwards, and her spine was found to have undergone a fifteen-degree correction.

Ten minutes later, Brennan entered unceremoniously, took a seat onstage, and kicked off her white flats. She was all in white, like an angel in a church play. The candle flames shivered as Marjorie excited the harp. Meditation, candles, harps: Were these the instruments of energy medicine? Tonal arpeggios were soaring through the room. Brennan's eyelids fluttered; her breath rasped loudly. She raised her hands in benediction, then rose and came forward on the stage, arms outstretched like a conductor cuing an orchestra. The music rose a key in tandem, and with each key change, each vaulting chord, it seemed to step up the energy in the room. Brennan gingerly made her way down from the stage and began to move along the row of people in the front, stopping briefly to frame the crown of each person's head with her hands. Her fingers tickled the space above their scalps. It looked as if she were giving each person a shampoo, but rather than wearing the bored-stiff expression of a professional hairdresser, her face was aglow with the same beatific look I'd once seen on a statue of Kwan Chi, the Chinese female Buddha.

So she went, row by row through the ballroom. People began to sniffle and blow their noses. Somewhere in the back, a woman sobbed unabashedly. A kind of antiphonal chorus of grief rose and fell. Just as I was about to succumb to the mood, I remembered that at least half of my life had been one long clown show, and I started to laugh, and then strove to repress the feeling, because laughing seemed far more subversive than weeping. Alix in the next seat picked up the vibration. If we hadn't stifled ourselves, we could have tripped off the row, and maybe that whole section of the room. Half an hour later, I felt Brennan approach from behind, and opened my eyes, dumbfounded to see her standing *in front* of me. She was working on the student at my left. As she moved to me, her presence felt like the brush of a tulle curtain. She placed her hands around the crown of my head. Her fingers moved as if she were touch-typing on a hard-to-reach laptop. Her face was lost in rapture, her skin vividly flushed. Most of the time, she briefly held her hands above the heads of the students and then moved on, but in my case, she stepped back and plucked the air in front of my chest, as if she were unbuttoning a peacoat.

And then she traipsed away to the far side of the room to work on some of the teachers. Was that it? That was zapped? That was what I hoped would be the climax of my profile? There didn't seem to be anything especially profound about it. As woo-woo states of consciousness went, it didn't seem any deeper than what I could have achieved with an afternoon of pick-up basketball and two Advil. I had a clairvoyant vision of a long *New Yorker* piece being winnowed down to a short column in "Talk of the Town," and my days suddenly being devoted to finding kids who did drugs with their parents . . .

But when Brennan was on the far side of the room, posed against the nondescript backdrop of the wall, I was startled by something I saw. Startled, and then thrilled, and then shocked, and then I would say even dismayed. What I saw was an acetylene-blue glow around Brennan's head and arms. I saw it before I caught myself seeing it, and when I caught myself seeing it I thought, *I can't be seeing this*, and obediently it went away. I tried to see it again, and saw nothing. Then I stopped trying to see it, and lo! it reappeared—a magnificent molten blue light of the sort that blazes up in a garage where welders are working, only softer, with none of that industrial fierceness. What did it mean that when I tried to see it, it disappeared, but when I *allowed* myself to see, it was as conspicuous as Marjorie's harp? Did it mean I had to report myself to the National Council Against Health Fraud? Brennan put her hands over the head of a teacher in the corner of the room, and the light flowed around his head and shoulders. When she returned to the stage, she worked on Marjorie, who continued to play. Marjorie's field was greatly expanded, and to "touch" her, Brennan placed her hands six feet away.

Finally, Marjorie withdrew her hands from the harp, and Brennan returned to her seat onstage and sat there for a number of minutes at the center of an enormous silence. Then she picked up a little bell and dinged it three times, the sweet notes drawing the whole strange business to a close.

7. OLD PAIN

We reason of these things with later reason," the poet Wallace Stevens once wrote, "And we make of what we see, what we see clearly and have seen, a place dependent on ourselves." For my part, I still had historical ambitions, and no yearning for one of E. M. Cioran's metaphysical careers. I was still on assignment, holding fast to the mast. Following up that first Goddess Healing, I attended two more. At the second one, I was an observer again, auditing more classes at the Radisson

Hotel in Hauppauge. The third time, at a hotel in San Diego, I pinned an oversized name tag on my lapel and fixed a cup of herbal tea and milled about the department of subtle energy as a participant in a four-day introductory healing seminar. In San Diego, I was also chelated twice. It was basic, standardized preparatory treatment, but for a hands-on technique that was the psychic equivalent of being scrubbed for surgery, it seemed amazingly powerful, even when done by a fellow tyro who went through the steps following the now-hear-this commands given over a public address system by one of the teachers.

"Now move your hands up to the right knee!"

"Now place your hands on the heart chakra!"

And so forth. The convention room at the San Diego hotel was filled with people and more than one hundred healing tables. It looked, I imagine, like a Moonie wedding. But when, after an hour, I opened my eyes, I found myself transfixed by the acoustic tile on the ceiling of the convention room. I had never seen acoustic ceiling tile so beautiful, so exquisitely pitted and flecked, so luminous. This was ceiling tile by Cézanne, ceiling tile that would fetch millions at auction and inspire murder plots in the lower chakras of covetous connoisseurs. And of course this became—as how could it not?—yet another turn in the ongoing clown show. A man falls in love with a piece of acoustic ceiling tile. Sees the universe in a shard of fire-resistant, code-approved building product. Oh, the bathos!

Later that afternoon, all of us watched rather solemnly and with a little awe as Brennan worked on one of the participants, a sixty-two-year-old father of three from Mexico named Raul. Raul, I learned later, was a widower with a new girlfriend whom he'd wanted to marry. He'd had surgery for rectal cancer in June 1992 and February 1993, and when he filled out the application to Brennan's seminar, he complained of sexual impotence. Knowing his condition, Brennan made a point to work on him after the chelations. He was lying on a table. She stood over him, holding her hands above his body and rasping her breath. Her eyes were shut. After a while, she began to knit the air above his groin. This was her version of psychic surgery. It looked like a strange sort of pantomime complete with simulated sewing. Respect for convention prevented her from handling Raul's groin directly, so she worked above it. She brought in another teacher, Michael Spatuzzi, who set himself in the "horse stance" of a martial artist and held Raul's feet, thus boosting the energy. Brennan's breathing grew noisier, her hands twitched and flexed. She would tell me later that she had been extracting stagnant energy, and sewing tears in the aura, and straightening the lines of light that constitute the energy matrix of the human form.

"He was full of scar tissue," she said. "It was obvious he had had surgery. There was scar tissue in the pelvic area and no energy was flowing through. The vertical power current was cut off. The first chakra was destroyed; the second chakra was disconnected. The disconnections were causing the impotence. I cleaned the scar tissue out of the colon, rebuilt the lines in the second chakra. I had Michael hold his feet to help support the rebuilding of the second chakra."

Several months later, seeking an update, I spoke to Raul on the phone. Before the trip to San Diego, Raul said, his surgeons wanted him to have chemotherapy. He had refused, and sought out a Mexican spiritual healer, and then Barbara Brennan, whose books he had discovered. He had been very weak and would have to go back to bed sometimes in the morning. When he enrolled at the seminar in San Diego, the loss of his sexual potency had been his main concern; these were pre-Viagra days and the condition was jeopardizing his plans to marry his psychoanalyst girlfriend. He was very pleased with the results of Barbara's healing, and a half dozen follow-up healings performed at Brennan's suggestion by Michael Spatuzzi. "What Barbara did was outstanding," he said. "In the beginning, many times I would see a sexy movie with my girlfriend and nothing would happen. The doctors thought maybe there was some obstruction of the prostate, or that during surgery maybe they had taken some nerves. They didn't know. I feel very well now, and I have very good erections, and my energy is almost as good as it used to be before the surgery. My girlfriend thinks that many other things helped. She's a psychoanalyst—she doesn't believe in Barbara Brennan."

I might have said the same thing, but it seemed much too soon to be leaping to conclusions. In fact well into that spring of 1994 I was still trying to digest that first Goddess Healing back in December, not the immediate experience of the healing but what had followed soon after it. Of all the experiences I had among the Brennanites, the strange light included, it stood out the most. At first I had shrugged off the session; the allegedly "high energies" of the Goddess that had induced such heartrending moaning and wailing had gone right over my head. Afterwards, I lingered at the hotel to talk to students.

It was after eight at night when I finally got back on the Long Island Expressway, headed for home. I passed the miles in a pleasant daze, thinking about the healers I had met, how it was not in their nature to hold themselves back or hide; thinking of their intense, deep-striking eyes. In journalism, you're always watching, hanging back, throwing up a screen of questions, and trying to reserve judgment until the time is right to render it. Or you are pretending to have no judgment at all, to be an objective, value-free conduit like a phone line, not a sensibility that shapes and creates its world. *A place dependent on ourselves . . .* Journalism was beginning to seem a peculiar kind of life, a way of gaining intimacy and keeping distance at the same time, a way of being intimate without the real responsibilities of a relationship. It was striking to hear people use the word "soul" as if it denoted an actual essence and wasn't just some figure of speech to be sentimentally invoked at funerals. Healers were a frightfully earnest bunch, weren't they? Was it all their grappling with life and death, their endless reaching after the indefinable quotient of health? The brand of spirituality at the Radisson Hotel was hardly spilling over with brilliant speech, humor, or even the trickster spirit of the shamanism from which much of it stemmed. Were the Brennanites all trying to put a saintly foot forward? Did they all want to be the angel in the church play and get an "A" from God?

As I neared the city, an inexplicable euphoria took hold. It was deeper and clearer and stronger than the intoxication of wine, or even the bliss of those "hug drugs" that were legally prescribed until the government banned them a decade ago because, as I remember reading in *Time* magazine, some spiritual leader from the Drug Enforcement Administration had issued an encyclical saying that people shouldn't be allowed to find paradise in a drug. Oh, the killjoy bastard was probably right. God only knows what Puritan officialdom would say about the ecstasies of the heart chakra. The energies of the Goddess seemed to have taken my heart out of my chest and put it on my sleeve. The closer I got to New York, the more I felt joy mounting in my throat. I was overwhelmed with love for the silhouette of Manhattan rising on the horizon, for the traffic on the expressway, and even for the damn toll-booth, and when I got back to my apartment I could scarcely keep from sobbing for love of Clown Headquarters and my circumstances, which had seemed so meager, so full of failure, evasion, and estrangement. As they surely are, and yet somehow, that night and all the next week, they seemed immeasurably rich as well, rich beyond any reckoning I had ever dreamed of. Some flower had bloomed and put to rest all the quarrels of monks and clowns.

Later, trying to finish a draft of my article, I faxed a long list of questions to Barbara Brennan, and I asked her what she had done. "You had a block in your heart chakra," she wrote back. "It looked like you were very concerned about a particular relationship you were in. [The block] had been there for several years—perhaps three or four—but it is also connected to early childhood. The block had to do with commitment and the pain underneath your fear of commitment. It looked to me like you were considering what level of commitment was in a relationship, and if you were going to change that."

And I read this knowing that for all the unspecificity and triteness of the language, what she was saying was exactly right, right in a precisely vague sort of way, but right all the same. What she was saying was on the mark. For the last three years, I had been haunted by a decision to bolt an engagement. I had been trying to resurrect the relationship and by that December, the very month I had first visited the school, I knew but could not face the fact that it was not going to work. *I had had a dream that my fiancée had drowned in a lake, and I pulled her body out of the water, my whole family was there, we held her on our laps and put our hands on her and tried to warm her back to life, but there was nothing we could do, she was gone . . .*

Brennan went on: "I pulled the block and some of the associated old pain out of your heart so you could deal with the issue more clearly—to make your decision as well as feel your love more and be less afraid of loving another. So I would imagine after that healing that you probably would have entered into more process about the relationship. It seemed to be with a particular person. I did not look to see who, because I figured it wasn't any of my business." The point of the healing, she said, had been to show me that I "could experience love more or go through the process of learning to deepen love in relationship more."

Our whole family was there; there was nothing we could do, she was gone . . . so we started doing drugs together . . . And then one of us saw some paranormal light . . .

Alas, I did not see light again at the two other Goddess Healings. Nor did Barbara Brennan fiddle with the air above my heart. She left my fourth chakra alone, its seals or whatever intact. Maybe I was too busy making secret fun of people who use phrases like "in relationship" to experience love. Or too scared to do anything but make fun. (Did those phrases deserve to be mocked? Were my ready-made banalities any better?) Or maybe I already had enough to work on by myself. The last time I saw Brennan face to face, I asked why she had skipped the heart work in the subsequent Goddess ceremonies. She regarded me carefully and then said in a gentle voice, "I could see you were trying to maintain a healthy skepticism." Mine was an old struggle, she seemed to be saying. Everything in its time.

CHAPTER THREE

If a blind man came up to us and assured us that there was no such thing as ordinary physical sight, and that we were deluded in supposing that we possessed this faculty, we in our turn should probably not feel it worthwhile to argue at great length in defense of our supposed delusion. We should simply say: "I certainly do see, and it is useless to try to persuade me that I do not; I decline to be argued out of my definite knowledge of positive facts." Now this is precisely how the trained clairvoyant feels when ignorant people serenely pronounce that it is quite impossible that he should possess a power which he is at that very moment using to read the thoughts of those who deny it to him!

— C. W. LEADBEATER

1. OPRAH'S BASIC
SCIENCE HOUR

April 1994, Clown Headquarters. One of those afternoons of pro-crastination that dissolutely segue from *All My Children* to *One Life to Live*. My cableless TV with the rabbit-ear antennae groping for signals in the shadowy courtyard out back had developed high sense perception, clown-style: Blurry auric outlines were swimming around the light body of Erica Kane, and blurry snow-flicker ghosts were dogging the insuffer-able Viki Buchanan as she breathed fresh *pneuma* into Oscar Wilde's observation that all bad poetry is sincere.

A healer might have thought that Jupiter was misaligned with Mars or something, but the atmosphere of enervation in my home-office that afternoon had nothing to do with the stars. In fact, I had been going along productively, reading about the eighteenth-century career of Anton Mesmer, who had proposed theories and given treatments that were remarkably similar to what contemporary healers were doing. But then the mail came with news I'd been waiting for from *The New Yorker* about my piece. Kim Heron, a senior editor, had written a long letter. The gist of it was that the piece was a mess.

> I admit I represent the imprisoned psyche, [Kim wrote] but even we deserve clarity and comprehensiveness. . . . I think you have to find a way to tell this story without set-ting yourself the task of protecting Brennan from the pot-shotters or turning into an advocate, even just a wide-eyed

explorer advocate. What Brennan says about what she does is simply too farfetched, a lot of it at least, to be held up to very much judgment. As you point out, there's no real way to test what she says. I'm not in favor of gratuitous skepticism, but your own evident fascination with this kind of exploration is getting in the way of your telling the story. Rather than set a tone of indulgent bewilderment and awe, why not remove yourself almost entirely and just record what is going on around you. I *don't* think you're self-absorbed, but I do think that in a strange way this piece is too much about you; you're asking a whole lot of questions about the whole nature of inquiry and observation—basically the whole enterprise of journalism—so that you are putting a story together with one hand and taking it apart with the other. Does that make sense?

Unfortunately, it did. And it was so deftly written too—better written than the text it was addressed to. Kim was a genius, but I realized then there was no way even with her help that I could pin down all this nebulous material sufficiently to pass muster with Tina Brown. What had I been thinking! The very thought of having wasted what was now nearly six months was so depressing I lay down on my bed and flipped on the soaps.

And the next thing I knew, *Oprah* was on. Oprah herself was snowy and weirdly doubled, like Erica and Viki. Oprah's guest that afternoon (also snowy and weirdly doubled) was Larry Dossey, the physician and author who was preparing to launch *Alternative Therapies*, the first alternative medical journal to be indexed by MEDLINE. Dr. Dossey was promoting a new book, *Healing Words: The Power of Prayer and the Practice of Medicine*. Prayer was the first and last frontier of healing, the most farfetched brand of all. There was something about their conversation that made it seem like a surrealist play.

Oprah: OK. Now what is the bo—what is the thing—the experiment that excited you the most? There's so much to talk about, I'm trying to get it all in. What is the one that excited you the most? Praying for those seeds?

Dossey (*in a soft Texas accent*): Listen, that's close. Listen, you're going to think this is nuts.

Oprah: Yeah.

Dossey: But my favorite form of prayer-experiment involves not seeds, not even human beings, but I love those experiments with bacteria. It may be surprising to think that some people would feel warm and cuddly towards bacteria.

Oprah: You're going to lose me here. You're going to lose me.

Dossey: I know. I know. We're about to step over the line here.

Yes, they were, and if history was any clue, Dossey had better be careful, not just because he probably wanted to get one of those little red "As Seen on Oprah" stickers for the paperback of his book, but because doctors who stepped over the line were never treated kindly. Dossey would hardly be the first to risk the wrath of his professional fraternity. It was curious how powerful the status quo was in a field ostensibly devoted to discovery. Mesmer for example: his experiments had dismayed his peers, and he had eventually been run out of Vienna. Every fifty years or so, it seemed, somewhere in Europe or America, a well-known medical man or eminent scientist would emerge brandishing new claims about the vital force only to find he had offended the orthodoxies of the day.

Oprah: Yeah.

Dossey: But—but you pray for one batch of bacteria and not for the other batch. And the prayed-for bacteria germinate—or grow faster. They mutate faster and so on.

Oprah: Now when you say pray for it, what are—are you praying to the absolute?

Dossey: True. You pray . . .

Oprah: You're praying to God for the bacteria?

Dossey: Exactly.

Oprah: Isn't that a wasted prayer?

Dossey: Let—let me explain why we use bacteria.

Oprah: This woman said "No." But I've got other things to pray for than bacteria, though.

Dossey: Hang on.

Oprah: Yeah.

Dossey: Hang on. You see, in science, we try to deal with the skeptical cynical argument. Right?

Oprah: Right.

Dossey: And—and if you do these experiments on human beings, then people say, "Well, you know, the person was just thinking positive thoughts. It wasn't the prayer."

Oprah: Right.

Dossey: If you do the experiments with bacteria, you leapfrog a lot of these complaints and arguments because the bacteria . . .

Oprah (*eagerly, grasping the implications*): So you get two sets of bacteria.

Dossey: Right.

Oprah: Same conditions.

Dossey: Same conditions.

Oprah: Pray for some bacteria.

Dossey: Not for another.

Oprah: Not for another.

Dossey: And if the prayed-for bacteria grow faster, it wasn't due to the placebo response. You know they aren't praying for themselves. And their mommies—their fellow bacteria aren't praying for them. This couldn't enter into it. So if the bacteria respond, they you know you've really got something here and that you've shown that prayer really does something substantial.

Oprah: What is the prayer though? Doesn't it matter? Because we're going to talk about how we pray. And, see, I always think that your intention with the prayer is the thing that gets through. You know, I try to get through a direct line, not to go through Mary or nobody.

Dossey: (*unintelligible*)

Oprah: Yeah. Direct line. So I'm thinking that you have to be very clear about your intention.

Dossey: Mm-hmmm.

Was that one of Oprah's light bodies drifting off, or was it my astigmatic TV? Was part of Oprah wondering what the rest of her was talking about? I suddenly felt like Tina Brown. All this stuff about direct lines, intention, the Absolute, Mary, bacteria. Jesus, what the hell were they talking about? Did the studio audience have any idea? Maybe Oprah's producers should have set up their own experiment—Show A and Show B. Same studio, same guest, same audience, same questions, same graphics. Pray for one show, not for the other . . .

> Oprah: And for me, "Thy will be done" is always the best prayer. What is going to bring the most peace in this situation? How can I best be used in this situation? Not what my will is, not what I want. But you let me follow whatever is the divine course of action for my life. Now that seems to work for me.
> (*Applause*)
> Dossey: Yes. Yes.

It was a good question: What was going to bring the most peace? It suddenly occurred to me that my piece had been dead on arrival because I had not been scientific enough in my approach to the healing school. I had not been able to remove myself entirely and affect the magisterial objectivity of the white-coated scientist standing outside of nature. My motivation had been driven by the desire to understand how I might participate more deeply, not less. In essence, I had written the story *from the point of view of the wrong chakra*. To succeed in the fact-driven pages of a materialistically-oriented magazine, I should have approached the subject as any journalist who fancied the epaulets on his trench coat would, which is to say from the vantage of the third chakra, the chakra of mental conceptions, of opinions and ideas, of the self as intellect. I set out that way but got waylaid by weird personal experiences, and unexpectedly emotional responses, and by a philosophy of knowledge that challenged the distinctions between observer and subject that journalists typically made. In effect, to put it in the healing lexicon, I had gotten yanked down into the second chakra, the chakra of emotions—a messy, swampy, confusing place, especially dreadful if you come from a family of Connecticut WASPs. When I tried to go "up" to chakra number three to write my piece, I found I was bogged down in the clutches of chakra number two.

Then it occurred to me that I might as well go all the way down, back to the beginning, down to chakra number one, the root chakra, if you will, and look at the foundations of this ongoing quarrel between my monk and clown. And if I did that, I would be writing a book, not an article, and if I was going to write a book, I thought, why shouldn't it have a subtle energy system just like a body? It could be organized around the chakras; thematically guided by the chakras; energetically driven by the chakras. Why beat around the bush? In for a dime, in for a dollar. Having already destroyed his career as a dilettante magazine journalist, the author might as well make something of the wreckage. He could lay out the roots of his demise in the first chapter, and then unpack the emotional impetus behind it in the second chapter, and by the third he could finally get into the energy of the critical mind that tries to conceptualize these age-old monk-clown quandaries and quarrels.

And beyond the Manipura chakra was Anahata, the heart lotus, where the dialectics of the self were pitched headlong into the interpersonal mystery of love. And assuming anyone could get through that treacherous zone, the energies of the throat and brow and crown chakras all were beckoning with their varieties of insight and madness. *Baywatch* was coming on, but I flipped the set off and went back to work.

2. THIS MAD GLORY OF HANDS

For thousands of years, hands-on healing has thrived outside the compass of science, with no warrant of efficacy other than its apparent usefulness. What may be humanity's oldest therapy is depicted in fifteen-thousand-year-old Pyrenees cave images, and described in the Ebers papyrus of early Egypt, and the gray-beard literature of China and India, and the ancient texts of Judaism. Aristophanes noted a session in Athens twenty-four centuries ago when healers supposedly unblinded a man and cured a woman of infertility. Modern medicine, which honors Hippocrates as its father, prefers some of his insights to others: "It hath oft appeared that I could draw from the afflicted parts of my patients aches and impurities by laying my hands on them or moving them over the area concerned, as if my hands possessed some strange healing power." In Ireland, strange-power tradition extends from St. Patrick, said to have restored sight with his touch, to Valentine Greatraks, the seventeenth-century "Irish stroker" famous for a wide array of cures, to healers of the present day such as Finbarr Nolan, whose gift is attributed to his being born the seventh son of a seventh son. (So strong is the legend of the seventh son of a seventh son that when Nolan was two days old a woman came to his house to ask his mother if her son who was suffering from ringworm could touch the newborn baby.)

Even Christianity can be seen as the triumph of a healing cult organized around the handiwork of a talented carpenter's son—handiwork that so alarmed later church officials that starting with the Synod of Ancyra in 314 A.D., decrees were issued barring the practice of healing. The New Testament reports eight instances in which Jesus of Nazareth singled out someone for his healing touch, as well as many mass healings performed in impromptu clinics. Luke 4:40: "Now when the sun was setting, all they that had any sick with divers diseases brought them unto him; and he laid his hands on every one of them, and healed them."

Healers at hand, on hand, by hand. But how? By what means? Was there some science in this mad glory of hands? Churched or unchurched, hands-on healing has been hopelessly entangled in the myth and mishmash of religion, written off as irrational quackery or shamanism, the province of charlatans and revival-tent con artists playing on the hopes of desperate people. Its miracle cures have been discounted as suggestion, the placebo effect, the natural resolution of disease. Self-appointed quackbusters and vigilant Food and Drug commissioners were not around to debate the Son of God or fault his Apostles for the scientific sin of relying on "anecdotal" evidence. It would be seventeen hundred years after the birth of Christ before scientific inquiry would assume its modern guise, and almost two additional centuries before medicine really embraced the stringent contemporary standard of the randomized double-blind placebo-controlled clinical trial.

And so here was the question at the core of my quarrel: By our modern measures, by our vastly sophisticated science, our secular materialistic mode of inquiry, which exalts the Bunsen burner and the Erlenmeyer flask and would rather verify than trust—was there something in Hippocrates' hands other than his imagination? Did something flow from the palms of Joel Wallach and Barbara Brennan and the thousands of other practitioners of what is sometimes called "energy medicine" (fifty thousand in North America alone, according to an overview published by the NIH Office of Alternative Medicine)? Is there some kind of biological energy, subtle or not so subtle, that can be marshaled, and passed between people, and calibrated in the exchange as it melts tumors and allays headaches and alters the chemical characteristics of the blood, and that (to descend a moment from the Aesculapian temple to the kitchen) by some reports can even mummify bananas and mutton chops? Are there experimental results that can verify the currents of healing energy and the phenomena associated with it? Is there a remotely plausible theory that might account for the ability of clairvoyant healers to pluck details out of thin air or accurately diagnose illness over the telephone or tune in to videotapes of Chinese martial artists or stand in hotel rooms off the Long Island Expressway and interface with mothers in Wisconsin? If these are not the least extravagant examples, neither are they the most. Many physicians would settle for a scientific explanation of how hypnosis can cure viral warts or speed the healing of burns. Or how relaxation techniques can lower a diabetic's need for insulin.

Ach, we're back in the borderland between physics and metaphysics, grappling yet again with the quandary of vital force. Strictly speaking, energy, whether in the form of lightning or a lightning bug, is the ability to do work. It is not a thing but a potential, not stuff but performance; it's movement, change, action, a flow of electrons, a force unleashed. We know it by its results: the eyelids lift, the arm draws a match across the stove, the air warms in the one-room schoolhouse.

One of the paramount achievements of twentieth-century physics was to define energy as an aspect of matter, and matter, in turn, as an aspect of energy. We know the human body generates ten to twelve watts of bioelectricity. We know that like most appliances we are ringed by an electromagnetic field; each cell in the body has a north and south magnetic pole. We know that as we are bombarded by energy from without—cosmic rays, microwaves, cell-phone transmissions—we also radiate energy from within, an envelope of heat from the breakdown of food, sound and electromagnetic energy from the pulsing heart, bursts of electrical activity from the moody brain, whose current oscillates at between two and twenty cycles per second. Perhaps there are other frequencies of energy coming off us as well, which appear to "sensitives" as concentric auras of color wreathing the body—perhaps there actually are the halos, aureoles, and glories reported in religious literature. Perhaps there are emanations like the "bright strong light" that some witnesses observed around the left hand of Therese Neumann, the farmer's daughter and legendary stigmatic from Bavaria whose wounds were studied for thirty-five years until her death in 1962.

Like Prometheus, who tamed fire without knowing the principles of combustion, we have been using energy as medicine despite our paltry understanding of its stimulating role in our peculiarly stimulated condition. Energy medicine in its early forms exploited (to uncertain effect) the natural magnetism of the lodestone. The early Romans treated gout with the electricity of decapitated torpedo fish. As new forms of energy were discovered, new cure-alls emerged. The last two centuries have seen therapies based on chemical energy, X rays, radioactivity—all external to the body. The question again is: Is there some energy that comes from inside? Some bioenergy that healers can generate and harness?

Many religions would demur that the distinction between external and internal—or between healer and patient—is artificial, the product of narrow scientific assumptions and illusory conceits. Science arrived late to the quandary of hands-on healing, but in truth it makes more sense to say that science created the quandary when it divided mind and body. Science separated what hands-on healers would insist are indivisible. In making the body an object, science draws lines that do not exist in nature. Suddenly there are distinctions between "organic" and "psychogenic" illness that are foreign to healers; there is the idea that some illnesses are not as "real" as others. There is the bias that says that "real" disease has a physical pathogenic existence in the dense stuff of the genes or in the tissues of the body, and that anything born of belief or imagination or the less dense, nonstuff stuff of the mind doesn't count as much.

These perennial mind-body questions, which may forever roil the sleep of philosophers and physicians, were not approached scientifically until 1784. That was the remarkable year when in Paris a commission chartered by the last French king undertook what might be called the first systematic study of hands-on healing in history. Anticipating by more than 150 years the sort of biomedical evaluations taken for granted today, nine savants convened in the capital of the Enlightenment to weigh and measure whatever mysterious force it was that was inspiring legions of Parisians to put themselves in the hands of Franz Anton Mesmer.

3. CHAIN OF THUMBS

The august members of the commission appointed by Louis XVI in March of 1784 were nearly as renowned as the great mesmerizer himself. Chairman Benjamin Franklin, then the seventy-eight-year-old U.S. representative in Paris, had called electricity out of the sky with the invention of the lightning rod; Antoine Lavoisier had given oxygen its name and established the principles of modern chemistry; Jean-Sylvain Bailly was the leading French astronomer and future Mayor of Paris. Among the others were four physicians including Joseph Guillotin, who would share with Mesmer the distinction of having his name become a pungent English verb. (And a decade hence, when the French monarchy had been swept away by the Revolution, Lavoisier and Bailly would die in the contraption that Guillotin had persuaded the state to adopt as a humane alternative to the headsman's axe.)

Mesmer did not participate in the commission's work—that job fell to his chief student, the French court physician, Charles D'Elson, who had written to the king requesting an official review. However, Mesmer's genius was everywhere at issue. Was he, as he would "dare to flatter" himself years later in an autobiographical account, a man whose discoveries would "push back the boundaries of our knowledge of physics as did the invention of microscopes and telescopes"? Or was he a spell-casting charlatan in a lilac robe, enriching himself at the expense of suffering dupes and bored aristocrats? Herewith sounds the theme of all medical heresy, now as then.

Mesmer was born in Germany in a small village on Lake Constance, the third of nine children. He rejected the priesthood to study medicine at the University of Vienna, where he wrote a thesis on the influence of the moon and stars on the course of disease. Mesmer launched his practice in Vienna and at age thirty-four married Maria Anna von Bosch, a wealthy aristocratic widow ten years his senior. They set up house in a luxe, music-filled mansion near the Danube. The young Mozart often stayed with the doctor and his wife, and his opera *Bastien und Bastienne* was premiered at an outdoor theater on the grounds of Mesmer's estate. Mesmer himself was a talented musician; Mozart's father said Mesmer was the only person in Vienna who could really play the glass harmonica, a strange concentric array of spinning glass bowls that resonated ethereally like wineglasses rubbed with a wet finger. Benjamin Franklin, who would sit in judgment of Mesmer's ideas, is credited with redesigning in 1761 the instrument that Mesmer preferred above all others.

Influenced by the writings of Paracelsus and ancient beliefs surrounding magnetism, Mesmer began to experiment with magnets. In July 1774, he successfully treated a patient with magnets obtained from a Jesuit priest with the forbidding name of Maximilian Hell. Before long, he noticed that he could achieve results simply by laying his hands on patients. After one session of hands-on healing, the director of the Munich Academy, lame in both legs and losing his sight, was able to walk and see better. Mesmer treated dozens of illnesses, many of which doctors today would consider psychosomatic. Though his cures often seemed miraculous, especially given the impotence of competing treatments, Mesmer took a strictly naturalistic view of illness and cure. "Mesmer's first claim to our remembrance lies in this—that he wrested the privilege of healing away from the Churches," wrote Frank Podmore, one of the founders of the London-based Society for Psychical Research, in his 1909 book *From Mesmer to Christian Science*.

Mesmer supposed that his healing success was based on his ability to marshal a flow of an invisible magnetic fluid that pervaded the universe.

He called it "animal magnetism." It could be stored in people, animals, silk, stone, glass; it could be enhanced by music and intensified by mirrors. Disease arose from blocks in the flow of the fluid, and a healing "crisis" often was provoked when the flow was restored. "Mesmer looked upon himself as a scientist whose observations had led him to important theoretical and practical discoveries," noted Alan Gauld in his 1992 book *A History of Hypnotism*, but he "had an inner tendency towards mysticism. . . . He felt the pulsations of the cosmic fluid, suffusing and uniting all things, especially all living things, and he felt it flow with peculiar strength through him. He knew the theory to be true, and facts, observations, cases were simply fitted to it."

In essence, Mesmer reframed the Hippocratic idea of nature's healing power in rationalized, naturalistic terms, terms in tune with the tenor of the times. Substitute the Chinese concept of *chi* or Western energy lingo for "animal magnetism," and there's little in Mesmer's vitalist ideas of health that modern-day healers would quarrel with. Wrong theory, right practice, they might say. Or, judging by the plethora of magnetic healing gizmos advertised in holistic tabloids, maybe they'd say right theory, right practice.

Why Parisians took to Mesmer more ardently than the Viennese remains a question. Were the French more susceptible to the occult element in Mesmer's ideas, the intimation of divine agency in animal magnetism? Conversely, did they resonate with the theory's scientific overtones? Gauld wonders if Mesmer's success wasn't due to a plentiful supply "of wealthy, bored, and indolent persons, over-fed, under-exercised, and prone to constipation, indigestion, hypochondria and the vapours."

It may be that Mesmer illustrated as few before him the truth of Voltaire's remark that "the art of medicine consists of amusing the patient while nature cures the disease." Mesmer had arrived in Paris in February of 1778, the year Voltaire died. Within months, he had entranced the aristocracy and alienated the city's powerful physicians. He allowed his pride to be outraged when the French medical academies declined to recognize his "discoveries," and at one point he threatened to quit Paris. Marie Antoinette offered him a handsome annuity to stay. He was the darling of grateful farceurs who satirized him as "the true model of science and zeal." Ladies-in-waiting referred to him as "the divine Mesmer." Pamphlets were published comparing him to Socrates.

Mesmer's modest offices in the place Vendôme had been quickly overwhelmed by patients, and he had been obliged to rent the Hotel Bouillon on the rue Montmartre. When the crowds grew so large that he was unable to magnetize patients individually, he fashioned the *baquet*, "a kind of travesty of the galvanic cell," as the historian Podmore put it. He filled a large oak-planked tub with bottles of magnetized water, pulverized glass, and iron filings. Patients were arrayed in a circle outside the *baquet*, lashed together with "the rope of communication" and fitted between projecting iron rods. They linked their hands, thumb to forefinger, making what was soon known as "the chain of thumbs."

The atmosphere was nothing if not dramatic. The *baquet* salons were curtained and dimly lit. Astrological glyphs adorned the walls; thick carpets covered the floor. Music drifted in from a pianoforte or a choir, or sometimes from Mesmer himself, serenading his patients on the glass harmonica. Dressed in long theatrical robes of lilac-colored silk, he glided about, making magnetizing passes with his hands or an ivory wand. He had only to point a finger and some patients would immediately go into convulsions—a contagious Mesmeric crisis of sighs and weeping and laughter. Wealthier patients were privileged with individual attention, taking seats in chairs, their backs to the north, with Mesmer sitting opposite them, pressing his knees to their knees, holding their eyes with his most mesmerizing gaze. He would pass his hands over their abdomens, or hold both hands in the shape of a pyramid and traverse the length of their bodies. In other rooms, *baquets* were reserved for the lower classes and the poor. Mesmer even magnetized a tree in the Bois de Boulogne at the end of rue Bondi, passing his hands along the branch tips and working down the trunk to the roots. Thousands of people attached themselves to it by ropes in the wild hope of siphoning off some animal magnetism. Mesmer's tree was quickly mythologized as the last to lose its leaves in the fall and the first to blossom in the spring.

It was in September of that inaugural year in Paris that Mesmer found his first pupil, his foremost champion, and his eventual rival: Charles D'Elson, physician to the king's brother and respected member of the French medical academy. D'Elson had been impressed with Mesmer's success treating some of the cases D'Elson had pronounced hopeless, especially that of a ten-year-old boy who had been wasting away with fever for forty-five days. Mesmer took up the boy's hands, and D'Elson was amazed to see the child break into a sweat; for the first time in weeks, the boy showed signs of appetite, consenting to eat some crabmeat and drink a little watered champagne. D'Elson tried to interest his colleagues in the medical establishment in Mesmer's work, difficult as he knew that would be. "I thought [Mesmer] might more easily make the four great rivers of France run in the same bed than to get the savants together in good faith to judge a matter that was outside their fundamental concepts," he wrote in 1780, two years after Mesmer's arrival in Paris. He even anticipated by four years one of the objections made by the royal commission: "If M. Mesmer had no other secret than how to put the imagination into motion effectively, for health purposes, would not that still be a marvelous thing? For if the medicine of imagination were the best, why would not we be doing the medicine of the imagination?"

As it turned out, D'Elson got little thanks for his efforts. The moody, egotistical Mesmer accused him of coveting his business and his ideas. He and D'Elson had a falling out. D'Elson was censured by his colleagues, and his advocacy of animal magnetism eventually cost him his position in the medical academy.

Why doctors were not practicing the medicine of the imagination was not the question the king's commission set out to answer. The members were less interested in whether Mesmer's or D'Elson's cures worked than whether they worked for the reason Mesmer and D'Elson said they did—which is to say, the commissioners were concerned with the existence of animal magnetism, not with its utility. As the astronomer Bailly, who wrote the commission's now classic report, put it: "Animal magnetism may well exist without being useful, but it cannot be useful if it does not exist."

Over a period of five months, the commissioners conducted sixteen experiments devised largely by Lavoisier. They worked with the agreeable D'Elson, who had campaigned for such a review. The Austrian doctor was displeased at first, but later, when the commission's critical findings were published, he could argue that *his* discovery had not been refuted, and that responsibility for the poor showing lay with D'Elson's faulty skills and not with any fundamental error in the theory of animal magnetism itself. The commissioners visited D'Elson's *baquets*; they observed the standard eighteenth-century methods of magnetizing, which bear an uncanny resemblance to contemporary healers' laboring over the second and third chakras: "Above all, the patients are magnetized by the laying of hands & the pressure of fingers on the hypochondria [the area immediately below the sternum] & lower abdominal areas; the contact [is] often maintained for a considerable time, sometimes a few hours." It was clear the commissioners were amazed by the variety and extremity of emotions D'Elson seemed able to elicit with animal magnetism, especially during the "crises":

> Nothing is more astonishing than the spectacle of these convulsions; without seeing it, it cannot be imagined: & in watching it, one is equally surprised by the profound repose of some of these patients & the agitation that animates others; the various reactions that are repeated, the fellow feeling that sets in. One sees patients specifically searching for others & while rushing toward each other, smile, speak with affection & mutually soothe their crises. All submit to the magnetizer; even though they may appear to be asleep, his voice, a look, a signal pulls them out of it. Because of these constant effects, one cannot help but acknowledge the presence of a great power which moves & controls patients, & which resides in the magnetizer.

The commissioners tested the vats for electricity and found none. They took pains to have themselves magnetized, assuming positions around a special *baquet* set aside for them by Dr. D'Elson. They sat for two and a half hours, bound together by "the rope of communication" and "from time to time making the chain of thumbs." And they felt . . . nothing, nothing they could attribute to the action of magnetism. They repaired to Franklin's estate in Passy and arranged with D'Elson to test "commoners"—an asthmatic widow; a woman with a lump in her thigh; a scrofulous little six-year-old named Claude Renard, who was emaciated and had a swollen knee; a man with a tumor in his right eye; a woman

who had been knocked against a beam by a cow. Some of the commoners felt something; some were unmoved. The commissioners turned to
patients "of a more distinguished class." To forestall offense, the better-
born were denoted only by initials in the commissioner's report. A Mr.
M felt some heat on his kneecap—a rare positive result. The commissioners explained it with reasoning that seems steeped more in hidebound
value judgments about the worth of kinesthetic awareness than in science: "We may suspect," wrote Bailly, "that it comes from the cause
described above, that is, from too much attention paid to observing one-
self." Which is to say what, exactly? That the overexamined life is not
worth living?

Soon the commission shifted its focus from exploring the hypothesis that animal magnetism was causing the remarkable scenes in the salons
of mesmerists to the possibility that the effects were produced by what
the commissioners called "imagination." D'Elson brought to Franklin's
estate in Passy a twelve-year-old boy known to be especially sensitive to
animal magnetism. D'Elson magnetized one of the apricot trees in
Franklin's orchard. The boy was led blindfolded into the orchard and
asked to stand in front of four trees that had not been magnetized, and
then to hug them for a couple of minutes. At the first tree, he began to
sweat and cough, and confessed to feeling a pain in his head. At the second tree, he felt giddy. At the third, he grew dizzy, and his head ached.
He confided that he was closing in on the magnetized tree, when in fact
the distance had been increasing.

> Finally, at the fourth nonmagnetized tree, & about
> twenty-four feet from the magnetized one, the young man
> had a crisis; he lost consciousness, his limbs stiffened & he was
> carried to a nearby lawn, where M. D'Elson gave him first aid
> & revived him. The result of this experiment is totally con-
> trary to magnetism. M. D'Elson tried to explain what hap-
> pened by saying that all trees are naturally magnetized & that
> their own magnetism was strengthened by his presence. But
> in that case, anyone sensitive to magnetism could not chance
> going into a garden without incurring the risk of convulsions,
> an assertion contradicted by everyday experience.

So it went all summer, until the commissioners were satisfied that "touching," "imagination," and "imitation," were "the real causes of the effects attributed to this new agent, known under the name animal magnetism." Bailly wrote: "This agent, this fluid, does not exist, but as chimerical as it is, the idea of it is not new. Magnetism . . . is only an old error. This theory is being presented today with a more impressive apparatus, necessary in a more enlightened century; but it is not for that reason less false. Man seizes, abandons, takes up again the error that gratifies him."

Imagination, the commissioners concluded, was the strongest of the three causes. So strong they saw fit to warn the king of the dangers inherent in the Mesmeric methods and to attach a secret report, which today illustrates the blinders of that era, an era whose luminaries could on one hand take pride in their rational method and their scientific discoveries, and on the other could complacently mistake class pretensions and cultural prejudices for facts of nature. "Women," the commissioners reported, "have as a rule more mobile nerves; their imagination is more lively and more easily excited. . . . It has been observed that women are like musical strings stretched in perfect unison; when one is moved all others are instantly affected." Given the uselessness of conventional medicine, which relied mostly on bleeding, drugging, and cauterizing patients, the commissioners were on thin ice asserting that "there are no real cures and the treatment is tedious and unprofitable. There are patients who have been under treatment for eighteen months or two years without deriving any benefit from it."

The Bailly report in August 1784 was followed by another report, prepared for the Royal Society of Medicine in November. It took an equally dim view of magnetism, and in 1909 Podmore observed that it was of value only "because these interested witnesses have so few definite facts to urge against the treatment." Both reports provoked angry comments and replies, especially from patients, and there were many— Mesmer and D'Elson alone treated eight thousand people in 1784—who felt themselves to have been helped by the magnetizers. (D'Elson had more than 160 pupils; Mesmer taught his techniques to more than 300 physicians and practitioners organized into Societies of Harmony, which, as Henri Ellenberger describes them, were "a strange mixture of business school, private enterprise, and Masonic Lodge.")

D'Elson prepared a supplement to the report that offered 115 cases of cures using the mesmeric method, including colic in an infant and fever in a toddler, that seemed to preclude the role of imagination. The patient's point of view was summed up in one brilliantly sarcastic testimonial: "If I owe the health I enjoy to an illusion, I humbly ask the savants, who see so clearly, not to destroy the illusion. While they enlighten the universe, let them leave me to my error and permit me, in my simplicity, frailty, and ignorance, to make use of an invisible agent that does not exist and yet heals me."

If animal magnetism was an error, a lawyer from Grenoble wrote, it was the most useful of errors. And that was the point. The commissioners were more interested in debunking an unfounded physical theory than exploring what was obviously a method for enhancing health that was considerably more humane and, apparently, in many cases, more effective than contemporary medical practice. "Probably what will most strike the modern student in reading the reports of 1784," Podmore wrote, "is that the commissioners, in the course of the five months over which their inquiry extended, found so little to excite their curiosity."

The vogue of mesmerism passed. While the physical existence of animal magnetism had been discredited, its psychological implications were only beginning to dawn. Out in the French countryside, Armand Chastenet, the Marquis de Puysegur, who had been a pupil of Mesmer's, discovered artificial somnambulism, the trance state of "magnetic sleep" that several generations later was renamed "hypnosis" by the English doctor James Braid. The water had suddenly become transparent and the marvelously strange submarine grottoes of the unconscious mind were now visible to many Enlightenment scientists rowing along in their glass-bottomed boats. By the end of the century, hypnotists had discovered the fish trails that led Freud to psychoanalysis, and Mary Baker Eddy to the uncompromising extremes of Christian Science, and had showed countless doctors the possibilities of suggestion (or the placebo effect, "to please the doctor," as it came to be called)—the power of the mind's ability to heal illness, control pain, and sometimes even reconfigure reality. Who doesn't marvel even today at the power of hypnotic suggestion to make the eye on one occasion respond to a stinging whiff of ammonia as if it were no more irritating than the perfume of lavender water, and on another turn lavender water into ammonia?

The commission's report is heralded today as a masterpiece of well-founded skepticism in the face of mass folly. It's "an enduring testimony to the power and beauty of reason," wrote the evolutionary biologist and author Stephen Jay Gould. It should be "translated into all languages and reprinted by organizations dedicated to the unmasking of quackery and the defense of rational thought." But for all its common sense, sound reasoning, and elegant, even beautiful writing, the commission's report conveyed no sense that what was happening around the *baquets* and all over France was important. It conveyed no sense that the phenomena Mesmer and company were eliciting held any scientific interest. This, when in fact, the phenomena gave birth to psychology. For all of their openmindedness, their willingness to be magnetized, the commissioners indeed seemed strangely incurious. From the airy brushing-off of mesmeric effects as "imagination," you would not have guessed that within a generation mesmerism would be routinely used to produce the first effective method of surgical anesthesia. At a time when surgery was an agony that often ended in death and the only effective form of anesthesia was sousing the patient with whiskey, you would not have guessed that in eight months in India surgeon James Esdaile would be able, with a minimum of pain and bleeding, to amputate one arm, one breast, and two penises; to excise three cataracts, extract three teeth, remove five toenails by the roots, make a six-inch incision in a sinus, and cut out one large leg tumor and fourteen scrotal tumors (including one that weighed a rather incredible eighty pounds). You would not have guessed the phenomenon of mesmerism contained anything of scientific or medical interest. Here in its first guise was an extraordinary therapy used today for pain control, relief of skin diseases, control of blood during surgery, control of stomach acid, asthma, herpes, burns, musculoskeletal disorders. Organizations devoted to the unmasking of quackery might well look to the report not just for the quackery that skeptics are so confident was exposed but for dogmatic tendencies and a kind of complacent omniscience that habitually plague science. Its contemporary lesson may lie less in the folly of quack beliefs than in the folly of treating a method of knowledge as an ideology. History loves humbling yesterday's know-it-alls.

As for Mesmer, if from our vantage he sometimes seems like a proto–New Age prophet, a California guru before there was a California, he hit notes on his glass harmonica that inescapably mark him as a man of his time. A year after he arrived in Paris, Mesmer published a memoir on the discovery of animal magnetism, in which he asserted the primacy of subjective experience. "Animal magnetism," he wrote, "must be considered, in my hands, as a sixth, 'artificial' sense. The senses can neither be defined nor described: they are experienced. It would be useless to try to explain the theory of colors to a person blind from birth. It is necessary that he see them; that is to say, they must be experienced. It is the same with animal magnetism. It must, in the first place, be transmitted by experience. Experience alone can render my theory intelligible."

Well, maybe not. It's one thing to assert the primacy of the subjective, which is still the beautiful and endlessly problematic principle of all hands-on healing. It's another to insist that subjective experience can give any guidance or support to a theory about experience. The raw sensory input of experience, as we know, says the sun rises out of the ocean and circles the earth. For all his pseudoscience, Mesmer still believed in the eighteenth-century idea of the scientist who stands outside nature and makes his measurements and prepares his all-encompassing theory. That Mesmer emphasized the subjective data of "experience" and not data gleaned by objective methods only meant that his theory unraveled faster. Had he turned up two hundred years later in California, he might have converted his *baquets* to hot tubs and endorsed a brand of hydrotherapy based on water-activated *chi*. But how would the poor doctor have coped with our postmodern spirit, which attacks the idea of scientific authority and teaches that, despite our ability to pinpoint the distance between molecules, our experience is fundamentally unintelligible and that the only thing to do, short of going gaga for God or developing into a *Bay Watch* sociopath, is to hold on like Beckett's clowns with some pitiful bit of existential style?

In his fashion, Mesmer held on. No amount of rational analysis or experimentation could disabuse him of his belief in—his experience of—the physical reality of animal magnetism. A gypsy in Paris had predicted the doctor would die in his eighty-first year. He left the city in 1802 and eventually returned to the town of Meersburg on Lake

Constance, not far from his birthplace. Summing up his impact, Henri Ellenberger wrote that "Mesmer's theories were rejected, the organization he had founded was short-lived, and his therapeutic techniques were modified by his disciples. Nevertheless, he had provided the decisive impulse toward the elaboration of dynamic psychiatry, even though it would be a century before the findings of his disciples were to be integrated into the official corpus of neuropsychiatry."

Near the end, Mesmer sent for a friend, a Catholic priest who was a skilled musician and could play the glass harmonica. Mesmer wanted to hear one last song on his beloved instrument. Sad to say, the priest arrived too late to unwind anything but a threnody. Here's to the gypsy: Mesmer was eighty-one.

4. ABSOLUTE MAYBES

Maybe the star-struck mayor of Paris was right: People seize, abandon, and take up again the error that gratifies them. Or maybe it's not the error they take up, but some tantalizing crumb of evidence. Where the science of hands and the search for healing energies were concerned, the chain of thumbs would not be broken. In 1932, a century and a half after the commission's report to Louis XVI, the biographer Stefan Zweig, seeking to rehabilitate Mesmer's reputation, raised anew the possibility that some vital physical force might one day be confirmed.

> Why [he wondered] should not the proximity of the human body, which can restore the brilliancy of a faded pearl, exert upon a neighboring human body, by means of an aura or radiation, an influence which stimulates or tranquilizes the other's nerves? . . . Who shall venture, in this sphere, to utter an absolute yes or an absolute no? It may well be that some day, with more delicate apparatus than we now possess, a physi-

cist will be able to demonstrate that there is something substantial in the forces which we at present incline to regard as purely spiritual and immaterial; that laboratory evidence will demonstrate as real that which . . . has come to be regarded as superstitious folly.

Such were the mid–nineteenth century hopes of Karl von Reichenbach, next after Mesmer in the chain of thumbs. History has forgotten his name, but at one time he was among the most famous scientists in Europe, a metallurgist, a chemist, inventor of kerosene and paraffin, and one of the foremost experts on meteorites. (He left the Austrian government his large collection of those falling stones that Lavoisier scoffed could not exist, because logic forbade stones to fall from a place where there were no stones.)

In April 1844 in Vienna, Reichenbach was introduced to a high-strung twenty-five-year-old named Mary Nowotny, who had an unusual sensitivity to the energy of magnets. Reichenbach combed Vienna for other "sensitives," and a month later, he made a dramatic test, which he describes in the English translation of his book *The Odic Force*:

> I took an immensely large mountain-crystal with me on a visit to a highly sensitive girl, Miss Angelica Sturmann; her doctor, Professor Lippich, a man celebrated as a pathologist, was present on the occasion. We put two rooms into complete darkness, and in one of them I placed the crystal, in a spot unknown to the others. After pausing a little, to allow our eyes to get accustomed to the dark, we brought the girl into the room where the crystal was. Only a short time elapsed before she told me the place where I had set it down. The whole body of the crystal, she said, was glowing through and through with a fine light, while a body of blue light, the size of one's hand, was streaming out of its peak, in constant motion, to and fro, and occasionally emitting sparks; it was tulip-shaped, and disappearing in fine vapour at the summit.

So began what some consider the first scientific investigations of the phenomena of the aura. Sensitives reported seeing colors not only around magnets but around people's hands and shoulders and heads. They reported feelings of heat and cold and tingling sensations. After some experiments, Reichenbach was convinced the phenomena were not caused by magnetic energies but by a new force, which he named the "odic force" or "od" after the Norse god Odin, the father of all gods, maker of Valhalla and husband of Frigga, the rare unimpeachable clairvoyant who could foresee the destinies of all men but refused to disclose her insights, not even for money. Od had many of the properties of Mesmer's animal magnetism. It radiated from all substances—crystals, plants, the human body. It could be conducted. It displayed polarity—negatively charged in a person's right hand, positively charged in the left.

Might od constitute an absolute yes? Reichenbach thought so. He published his experiments in 1845 in a book which was translated into English in 1850 as *Researches on Magnetism, Electricity, Heat, and Light in Their Relations to Vital Forces*. It caused a sensation in Germany, where the metaphysical implications of od jibed with the spirit of German Romanticism. But Reichenbach completely misread the extent to which his treatise would upset the scientific anthill. Former colleagues shunned his invitations. Many condemned the theory without bothering to study the evidence. A Dr. Dubois-Raymond dismissed the book as "an absurd romance," and "the most deplorable aberration that has, for a long time, affected a human brain." Reichenbach was so piqued by the critique that he wrote a long rebuttal in the introduction to a later edition. Insisting that he had repeated every experiment "ten, twenty, a hundred times," Reichenbach pressed on, and by 1856 he had done experiments with more than two hundred self-proclaimed sensitives, many of whom were physicians, chemists, mathematicians, and philosophers. Scientists, in other words, and therefore indubitably reliable.

But for all his excellence elsewhere in science, Reichenbach seems to have foundered on psychical research and has to be counted as an absolute maybe-not. One obvious error in his experiments was pinpointed as early as 1846 by the English physician James Braid, who helped move mesmeric phenomena from the marketplace to the scientific domain. As Alan Gauld notes in *A History of Hypnotism*, Braid had a "much firmer grasp than anyone who had preceded him, or than anyone who was to succeed him in the rest of the century, of the readiness with which psychological experiments, especially ones involving mesmerism or hypnosis, may be contaminated by 'experimenter effect' or 'doctrinal compliance.' " Simply by shaping subjects' expectations, the English physician showed that they could be prompted to see flames guttering atop magnets or crystals, even when no magnets or crystals were present. They could be induced to feel flows of heat tingling in their hands. Braid's experiments echoed the research of the king's commission. Which is not to say that Reichenbach's sensitives did not in fact sense the phenomena they reported; rather that Reichenbach was under an obligation (which he seems not to have met) to rule out his role in contributing to, if not creating altogether, the effects he was studying, however unwitting that role might be.

Years later, the London-based Society of Psychical Research tried to replicate his work. Of forty-five sensitives tested, only three demonstrated the ability to sense the phenomena Reichenbach claimed for evidence of od. The brief entry under the great chemist's name in the *Encyclopedia of Occultism and Parapsychology* can pass as a caution to anyone odd enough to brave the scientific outlands of energy research. "While [Reichenbach] could and did produce a wide range of positive results he was never able to demonstrate his major causative agent, the od. He was never able to eliminate a variety of possible causes, both paranormal and mundane, for the effects."

So we move ahead another half-century to the next hand in the chain of thumbs: Walter J. Kilner, a British physician who worked for much of his career at St. Thomas's Hospital in London, where he supervised the introduction of newly discovered X rays into clinical practice. This was the racy era of "scientific medicine" celebrated by Abraham Flexner in America. X-ray technology had made Kilner curious about the ultraviolet end of the visible light spectrum, and he'd wondered if the just-out-of-sight frequencies might account for the aura phenomena reported by Reichenbach and the occult literature of the spiritualist Theosophical Society (notably Charles W. Leadbeater's pamphlet on the aura, published in 1895).

In 1908, Kilner began to experiment with light-screens made with a dye derived from coal tar, called dicynanin, which he obtained from a German chemical supply company. When he looked through the glass-

and-dicynanin screens, Kilner discovered effects similar to what Reichenbach's sensitives had reported. Here, it seemed, was a way of viewing and describing the aura directly without a neurasthenic go-between. The screens showed three concentric outlines of light. In experiments that followed, Kilner found the nebulous silhouettes could be affected by electricity; magnets altered their depth; they seemed to disappear when a negative charge was applied to the body of a subject. When subjects were hypnotized, the auras viewed through the screens lost some of their brilliance. Kilner was persuaded that the approach of death was signaled by a reduction in the size of the auras.

Convinced of the diagnostic usefulness of his aura screens, Kilner published his work in 1911 in a book initially entitled *The Human Atmosphere* (it was reissued in 1965 as *The Human Aura*). The word "atmosphere" had fewer occult connotations than "aura," and Kilner was at pains to distinguish his findings from the esoteric reports on the subject. All the same, the reviewers were dubious. "Dr. Kilner has failed to convince us that his aura is more real than Macbeth's visionary dagger," wrote one in the January 1912 issue of the *British Medical Journal*. But the skeptical opinion hardly damped enthusiasm among the aura-prone. Kilner's awkward screens were trimmed into goggles by a British spiritualist named Harry Boddington and patented under the name Aurospecs; a later version that did away with the expensive dicynanin dye was called Kilnascrenes.

So can we say that in 1911 a clever physician came up with an absolute yes? Even today, a number of psychically minded people take Kilner's findings as evidence of the physical existence of the aura. Barbara Brennan's textbook uncritically cites Kilner's work, as does the *Encyclopedia of Occultism and Parapsychology*.

But as recently as September 1962, in a paper published in the *British Journal of the Society for Psychical Research*, Arthur J. Ellison, a lecturer in electrical engineering at the University of London, reported a number of experiments he and colleagues had conducted hoping to resolve the aura of doubt around the various quasi- or pseudoscientific proofs of the aura. One experiment tested a sensitive or "medium" who claimed to see streams of blue-gray light flowing from the fingertips when someone held his hands close together—a common indicator of what healers call the "etheric body" and a claim that I was no longer in a position to ridicule, having seen something very much like that myself. Ellison introduced the simple control of concealing the position of his hands under cardboard boxes. He slit the boxes to allow any energy to flow between his hands and restricted the medium's vision to the space between the boxes. Ellison put his own hands under the boxes, and the medium described the emanations he could see via his high sense perception.

"His remarks bore no relationship whatever to the position of my fingers," Ellison said. "At the end I surreptitiously removed them from the box and folded them on my lap. He continued to describe the colors which appeared and disappeared at the slit according to his psychic vision. The result of this experiment was quite unequivocal. There was no correlation between the psychic vision and the position of the fingers."

Even more pertinent was Ellison's explanation of the auras seen by Walter Kilner. Studying a pair of Kilner goggles, one of Ellison's colleagues found that the lenses admitted a large amount of infrared light and blocked out most of the middle spectrum of visible light, blocked all but a narrow band of red and blue—two skinny bookends framing an empty shelf:

> If the image is correctly focussed on the retina for one of these bands, it will be slightly out of focus for the other, the eye having a certain amount of chromatic aberration. The image which is out of focus will appear as a blurred outline superimposed on the other image. . . . The aura seen with the goggles appears to be a pseudo-aura. It is most surprising that it did not occur to Kilner to check by means of a simple experiment that the auras he was observing had objective reality; he merely makes this gratuitous assumption of objective reality throughout his work. . . . It appears to be only too easy to go astray in this way if one's initial work is insufficiently fundamental.

So much for Kilner, dismissed for cause.

Again another fifty years; again another link in the chain of thumbs. This one the formidable Wilhelm Reich, the brilliant heretical Austrian psychiatrist, one-time disciple of Freud, and discoverer in 1939 of "orgone" energy. An encompassing od-like life force, orgone had all the customary properties and some special ones, such as the one that allowed it to be collected in custom-designed metal-and-wood boxes called "orgone accumulators" and another that allowed it to be projected through Flintstone-style antiaircraft guns called cloud-busters, which Reich believed could affect the weather by draining or adding orgone to clouds. The techno-shaman had more than a few people convinced too. Blueberry growers in Maine paid him to make rain.

Reich rivals Mesmer for the mantle of most creative figure in the last two hundred years' worth of vitalism theorists and energy healers. His reputation still swings between the poles of screwball and genius, but he advanced profound and influential ideas about the manifestation of mental energy in the body. He broke from the Freudian camp to emphasize a patient's underlying "character structure" rather than his neurotic symptoms. Many energy healers, aura balancers, people who practice the deep-muscle massage of Rolfing, subscribe to Reich's view that emotional trauma is locked in tissue and that disease results when the "body armor" of physical patterns and habits obstructs the flow of bioenergy, or "orgone," as Reich insisted on calling it. Distinct from a number of neovitalists, Reich argued that the illimitable force of orgone was not part of the electromagnetic spectrum but was the ground out of which the electromagnetic spectrum itself emerged—an idea which, by definition, is the property of metaphysics. Could orgone have had conventional electromagnetic aspects? Reich claimed positive results treating cancer and arthritis with orgone. Some other experiments concluded that protozoa grew more slowly inside the orgone accumulators and that mice with malignant tumors lived longer after a daily half-hour exposure to the energy.

To the extent it's known at all, orgone is remembered more for the political response it provoked in the U.S. Food and Drug Administration than for any unique or carefully documented healing benefits. In March 1954, the FDA got a federal district court injunction ordering Reich to stop trading in the accumulators and to make no further claims about orgone's efficacy or existence. The charges, notes the sympathetic *Encyclopedia of Occultism and Parapsychology*, stemmed from the federal agency's "tragi-comic misunderstanding of Reich's theories of cosmic orgone energy in relation to a cure for cancer." In any event, Reich refused to comply, noting in a letter to Judge John D. Clifford that "no one, no matter who he is, has the power or legal right to enjoin the study and observation of natural phenomena including Life within and without man; [or to stop] the communication to others of knowledge of these natural phenomena so rich in the manifestations of an existent, concrete, cosmic Life Energy." After a trial in May 1956, Reich was sentenced to two years in jail for contempt of court. He died in the federal penitentiary at Lewisburg, Pennsylvania, of heart disease, on November 3, 1957, a day before he was supposed to be released. His books had been burned by the Nazis in a previous decade. Once again they were seized by government authorities and thrown into the fire, this time under the supervision of Food and Drug Administration agents at the Gansevoort Incinerator in Brooklyn. Copies of works that made any mention of orgone were destroyed up until 1960, when the vital energies of FDA vigilance were shunted off—perhaps by the impending nationwide seawater swindle—and the task of protecting the public from the deviant orgone of Wilhelm Reich was abandoned.

5. MUMMIFIED BANANAS

That nature doesn't always behave as we expect disorients the mind; that it doesn't always behave as we would like disillusions the heart. The former knows, the latter hopes, and the rivalry between knowing and hoping runs through the history of healing. It is expressed in what we have heard homeopathy historian Harris Coulter call the schism between rational and empirical medicine—between therapies that "make sense" and methods that seem to work, sense be damned.

But Coulter's notion of a "divided legacy" between the rational and empirical spirit of medicine can be extended to describe a much larger division between the medicine of the West, with its emphasis on the mechanics of matter, and the medicine of the East, with its emphasis on the dance of energy. Mesmer and his scientific offspring explored the different nature of the body implicit in these two philosophies. They tried to reconcile the differences, which were great then and remain great today. The controversies they aroused and the blunders they committed have shed much light on the politics of science and the fallibility of scientists, but perhaps more than anything else they have illuminated the inhuman effort required to engage antithetical ideas. D'Elson knew whereof he spoke: We might as soon put the four rivers of France in one bed as step outside our training and apprehend creation in a new way.

Short of proof based on the ABCs of rationalist science, the medical mainstream is bound to look askance at the mavericks of energy medicine; until recently it viewed healers working in the alien paradigm with undisguised contempt. "Healers can't cure organic diseases. Physicians can," wrote William Nolen, exemplifying the hard line of many doctors. (Dim view and all, Nolen's 1974 book *A Doctor in Search of a Miracle* was until recently one of the few books about psychic healing written by a physician.) Doctors tended to dismiss healing as a fantasy because it "couldn't" be real. Anecdotal claims and practical merits aside, it didn't make sense, and scientific medicine abhors therapies that don't make sense. The skeptic would rather rationalize healing results as products of superstition, imagination, suggestion, the placebo effect, than entertain unproven theories of energies that defy the laws of physics. And perhaps that caution is the better part of valor. But attributing a result to suggestion doesn't explain it; it simply substitutes one enigma for another.

As for evidence of a healing energy? Mainstream medicine has regarded it as presumptively suspect. It's not "hard" enough. If outright fraud is not involved, experiments purporting to show healing energy are taken as the result of some error, or flaw, or artifact of poor experimental design. When something "can't" be real, anyone bothering to study it can't have much of a grip on reality either. Ergo, experimenters in this sphere are suspect too. The onus is on them to prove they haven't succumbed to "unconscious dramatization" or let their covert mystical tendencies contaminate the data. Healing researchers are obliged by their deviation to be even more hardheaded than scientists working within the conventional point of view, and to strive for unassailably hard data. (Given the prevalence of the hard/soft metaphor, God knows what fearsome male sublimations are at work stiffening up the search for nature's secrets.)

But even as Wilhelm Reich's books were roasting in the Gansevoort fires—one measure of the heat that heretical views of health and the human body can generate—the chain of thumbs tendered a new link: a Canadian biologist named Bernard Grad, whose careful, ingenious studies still stand as some of the best and most persuasive healing research ever done. His ground-breaking work forty years ago may one day bring fame to his university. For the time being, Grad's achievements are proclaimed in mossy places like the *Encyclopedia of Occultism and Parapsychology*, where his name falls between "Graal, Lost book of . . ." and "Grail, Holy." Acknowledged or not, he is, in a phrase, the father of hands-on healing science.

And unlike his forebears in the chain of thumbs, he was still being propelled around his hometown of Montreal by the vital force. In 1995, eager to escape the library, I arranged to visit Grad at his home. Inspired by Abraham Flexner, who rode the rails all over the continent, I boarded the Montrealer in Penn Station on a November morning. The trip quickly turned into an ordeal of delays and breakdowns that made Flexner's turn-of-the-century faith in technological progress seem infuriatingly naive, at least insofar as it could have been stretched to include Amtrak.

It was dark and snow was falling when the train skulked into Montreal, hours overdue. I hadn't reserved a room anywhere, and hadn't been to Montreal, and didn't know east from west, but I was possessed to set out on foot, thinking that if homing pigeons could orient themselves to the earth's magnetic field, I with high sense perception ought to be able to find a cheap motel. The travail of the experimental method and the dismal limits of my ability were soon apparent. I flapped around for an hour and finally staggered into the first place I spotted, a painfully over-priced Holiday Inn.

The following morning, I went by subway to an unassuming neighborhood not far from McGill University. Bernard Grad, born and raised in Montreal, had worked for thirty-six years as a professor at McGill, investigating hormones, cancer, and the aging process as a researcher in the gerontology unit of the Allan Memorial Institute of Psychiatry. He retired in 1985. He published more than ninety papers in his field and won a number of awards, including the 1954–55 CIBA Foundation Award for work in age-related changes in thyroid function. Against the advice of colleagues, and in all likelihood at the cost of a full professorship, he also published thirty-six papers in the field of hands-on healing.

He met me on the porch of the house where he lived with his wife, Renée, a painter, and one of his sons, Willis, who worked as a doctor in the emergency room of a local hospital. (His other son, Roland, also was a doctor, in family practice.) Grad is an intensely compassionate man, and it shows in his face. That winter he was seventy-five, agile and full of humor, with a thick shock of white hair and long sideburns and dark wise eyes enlarged by wire-framed glasses. He was wearing slippers, a bow tie, and an argyle sweater. We sat down in a book-cluttered living room filled with Renée's paintings. I noticed a photograph taken when Grad was in high school.

"What do you see when you look at that picture?" I asked.

"I see somebody who had a lot to learn," he said with a laugh.

Grad was an only child of Jewish parents, but he never knew his father, who died in the 1918 flu epidemic, before Grad was born. He was raised by his mother, who struggled to make ends meet on the meager salary she earned in a clothing store. Unable to afford the twenty-five cents a week for carfare, Grad blazed a footpath to school over one of Montreal's substantial hills. All through his boyhood, he was unselfconsciously attuned to nature, to what he felt as a kind of force around him. One of his most vivid memories was of being four years old in a Montreal park and feeling the emanations of the grass and the paving stones; he could see some vitality in the air, hear it murmuring like the wave-wash sound of a sea shell; sometimes he had the sense of it rushing up his back. "Schooling tended to take those feelings out of me," he recalled. In high school he took to science; he also made a name as a sports star, running track and playing left outside forward on a team that won the city soccer championship four years in a row. In 1937, he graduated at the top of his class with a scholarship to McGill. College coursework in science further buried the vitalistic experiences of his boyhood. Grad recalled the time a medical student told him of William Osler's belief in the importance of bedside manner; Grad derided the idea as "witchcraft."

But in time he found himself growing disenchanted with the study of physical chemistry at the university. He turned to biochemistry, thinking it would be livelier. "To my horror, biochemistry wasn't alive," he recalled. And as if in the midst of some incipient spiritual crisis that could be resolved in no other way, Grad began to spit up blood a month before his twenty-first birthday. He was diagnosed with TB in one lung, an often-lethal illness in those pre-war days before antibiotics were clinically available. Doctors collapsed the lung and packed Grad off to a sanitorium, sixty miles north of Montreal in the Laurentian mountains. There he spent the next two and a half years, the first sixteen months of which he was confined to bed.

"I came very close to death," he said. "I saw all my athletic hopes dashed. I had thirty-two months of enforced silence. I read the *American Journal of Tuberculosis*, and Emily Brontë and Jane Austen, and books on pollution and nutrition and growing things naturally. I read a book called *Doctors, Disease and Health* that suggested you should be eating fruits and vegetables and grains. Remember, this was in 1942 and people weren't thinking about diet that way. As I got better, I started to feel the energy again in my body, a flow of it at certain times of the day, an afflux that corresponded to the way I felt. The disease awakened me to paranormal things. I rediscovered the child in myself. When I went back to the university and to my education, I had some hesitation, but I had no advisers. What I had was this contact with nature, which I couldn't verbalize."

He got his B.S. in 1944, and began a Ph.D. in the department of anatomy. The next summer, the energy that had flowed through his youth and nearly dried up during his education and his illness burst forth in a startling flood. "When I left the sanitorium, if I got a cold, I was supposed to stay home in bed for four days. I was lying in bed when suddenly I felt a current go from my head down through my heart, down my left leg, cross over to the right leg, come up the right side, and go through the heart again. It was like putting your finger in an electric socket. It made a clockwise circuit, like something moving through me, and when it passed through my heart, I felt as if I might die. It upset and frightened me. I called a doctor, who was puzzled, and he called his doctor who scolded me. My own claim is that it was a ball of energy. It convinced me that there was an energy in the body. It was very strange, because I experienced it the very day and almost the very hour that the bomb was dropped on Hiroshima."

Grad sought books about energy and people who had any expertise on the subject. There weren't many of either. "I was looking for answers to questions I didn't yet know how to formulate," he recalled. And then he happened upon two books by Wilhelm Reich, *The Cancer Biopathy* and *Ether, God and Devil*. A week after he got his doctorate in 1949, graduating magna cum laude with a thesis on the interaction of thyroid and testes hormones, Grad took a bus more than two hundred miles to Reich's Institute of Orgone Energy in Rangeley, Maine. Reich made as deep an impression on the young scientist as he had on the American psychiatrists he had trained when he was working with Freud. Grad returned periodically over the next five years to visit and study with Reich. He watched Reich work with the body energy of patients and saw some of Reich's more farfetched ideas in action, like orgone cloudbusting.

"That contact with Reich was really an informal training in how to study life-energy," Grad said. "In all my academic training, all consideration of energy went out the window. Reich had showed a number of properties of orgone energy in his work. I was convinced by my own work that orgone existed. I did an experiment with AKR mice, which are bred to develop leukemia at about six months of age. By thirteen months, ninety percent of the mice will be dead of leukemia. I built an orgone accumulator according to Reich's design, and was able to reduce the incidence of leukemia by twenty percent. But there was no change overall in lifespan—the mice had liver and kidney problems."

As he was discovering Reich's work, he was also beginning a two-year self-analysis. He reserved an hour a day for free associating; he would write and talk to himself as if he were a character on a stage. "I had three laboratories," he recalled. "One where I did conventional research. One where I did bioenergetic research. And one inside of me."

The work in the last was of necessity. In 1957, Grad's oldest daughter, Julie Ann, three and a half years old, died of acute laryngitis. He and Renée found some consolation in Subud, a spiritual practice that seeks to renew "contact with the essential force of life." It had been developed by an Indonesian man with the enervating mouthful of a name

Muhammad Subuh Sumohadiwidjojo. Followers of Subud would meet two or three times a week, stand together in groups for about thirty minutes, and allow themselves to be drawn into the silent presence of others.

First his daughter in May; then, in November of that year, another death, this one fixed in Grad's memory after the coincidence of a portentous dream. "I was lying on an operating table, and Reich was operating on me, opening up my body, pulling out my intestines and pointing to something inside me. I could hear myself saying to Reich, 'You opened me up, now close me.' Reich smiled, and closed the incision, and then went out the door. I received a phone call that night telling me that Reich had died."

He went to the funeral, half wondering if someone of Reich's charisma and vital force really could die. Reich's work and influence had affected Grad so much that he felt increasingly at odds with himself, obliged to acknowledge phenomena that his scientific training had no room for. Years later, in 1971, when his mother was dying of breast cancer, Grad saw an expression of joy and surprise ignite her eyes during her last moments. "It was as if she'd seen somebody," he recalled. "And then I saw a kind of shadow, moving up her feet and her body and out through the top of her head, and when her eyes closed, she was finished."

However, Grad was too much a product of the scientific temperament to take subjective experiences as proof of anything. It was one thing to talk about energy, live with it, even see it gathered up as a shadowy evacuation at the point of death. It was another thing entirely to nail the stuff down in a lab.

In October 1957, a few weeks before Reich died, Grad had gotten into a conversation with a Hungarian lab technician who mentioned that the wife of a friend had been healed of arthritis by a man from his home country. The man arranged an introduction, and Grad met the healer who would be known in the literature of hands-on healing as Mr. E.

Oskar Estebany had emigrated to Montreal to join his son after the Soviet invasion of Hungary, in 1956. He was a Catholic. He'd fought in the Hungarian military as a lieutenant in World War I, and had made a career in uniform to the disappointment of his parents, who had hoped he'd be a priest or doctor. During the 1930s, when he was a cavalry officer teaching in a military academy, Estebany noticed that the horses he rode never seemed to tucker out or get sick, while the horses his students rode often pulled up lame or became exhausted. When he rubbed the animals down, he noticed that his hands got very hot and the horses returned to form much faster than when other officers massaged them. When Estebany's son was twelve, he came down with diphtheria; Estebany held the boy in his lap for two days, and his son recovered from what at the time was often a deadly illness. He began to lay his hands on people in the 1940s—accepting no money for the work—and found he was able to diagnose problems by sensing changes in the body's heat. After 1947, when he treated the son of Dr. Babits Antal, a physician at a urology clinic, he developed a reputation among half a dozen physicians in Budapest. He found he was particularly useful helping people with thyroid and kidney disease.

In Canada, Estebany worked as a cabinet maker. He told Grad at their first meeting that when he healed he felt heat and vibrations, and he believed that his hands radiated some kind of energy that could boost a person's recuperative powers. It seemed to him that he drew this energy from the environment. "Estebany was the first healer I met," Grad said. "He talked about the energy in his hands the way Reich had talked about cosmic orgone energy." Looking to extend the experiments he'd been doing since his exposure to Reich's ideas, Grad took what he later called "a fateful step" and invited Estebany to take part in some studies.

The first week in November 1957, a day before Reich died, Grad began his collaboration with Mr. E. Professionally, these new studies would not help his career. Experimentally, he was somewhat in the position of Columbus sailing toward the edge of the earth: one foot on the bedrock of conventional science, the other on the moonbeams of the occult.

"I wanted to create some unfavorable conditions that healers could overcome—conditions that required healing," Grad recalled. His first concern was to eliminate the possibility that any experimental effects could be ascribed to the power of suggestion. Consequently, he began with mice. (It's generally agreed that animals can't be suggested back to health, but it should be said that this is a problematic assumption built on the same mind-body quicksand as Descartes' assertion, by way of Aquinas, that animals don't have souls. Bacteria, fruit flies, mice, dogs, chimpanzees, humans: Is drawing the line on suggestibility any more scientific and therefore less arbitrary than drawing it on soulfulness? Soul and suggestibility both seem doubtful circular ideas that depend on Cartesian dualism, which is to say a special kind of dissociative self-consciousness that splits the mind from the body and enables a mental part to observe "objectively," or with various portions of terror and pity, as the poor mortal corpus troops off to economics class or a baby shower or the guillotine. Who can prove that soul and suggestibility aren't one and the same? That they are not simply artifacts of a disastrously unnatural fragmentation? It's not as if Descartes offered a lot of evidence for the soul as an entity apart from the entity that takes suggestions and the entity that can read and write in French. . . . But *je pense* this parenthesis has gone on too long. All I want to suggest about suggestion is that only one species has reliably displayed the degree of intransigence over the centuries that proves it is utterly impervious to suggestion, and anyone who has ever lived with a house cat will agree.)

In any event, Grad used six- to nine-week-old Cadworth Farm No. 1 female mice from the Canadian Breeding Laboratories. To get a rough idea of what Mr. E could do, he set up two preliminary experiments. The results were astonishing. The mice that had been deliberately inflicted with skin wounds and treated from the outside of their cages twice a day for twenty minutes by Mr. E healed much faster than mice that didn't get the treatment or another group of mice that had been artificially warmed up.

With two other experimenters from the University of Manitoba, Grad began a third study that would introduce more stringent controls. The wounds would be measured by people who didn't know which mice were getting treatment and which weren't, thus preventing any subtle biases from creeping into their analysis of the wound sizes. Estebany's contact with the mice would be further restricted by concealing the cages inside paper bags; Mr. E would not be able to see the mice he was treating; for some of the groups the bags would be stapled shut so that his healing energy would have to penetrate the paper. Papering over the cages would also guard against the chance that the assistants would let the conditions of the mice affect the way they handled the cages when the mice were brought into the treatment room. And, finally, Grad and his colleagues would introduce simulated healings by people who didn't claim to have gifted hands. This also would insure that all the mice were handled uniformly, neutralizing the so-called handling effects. (The effects themselves may have healing-related potentials: Some studies have reported that gentling a mouse in your hands increases stress resistance, raises growth rates, lowers "emotionality," enhances immune function, and helps some mice with implanted tumors live longer. Lest this seem too unequivocal, other studies have found that mice with leukemia die faster when handled, so go figure.)

There were three hundred mice in ten cages; each mouse in each cage had her own little berth, isolating her from her sisters. The cages were divided into three groups. One group got twice-a-day fifteen-minute sessions with Mr. E, each session five hours apart; one got a similar regimen of treatment from the nonhealers; one got no treatment at all; but the mice in the control group were watered, fed, and moved around just as the mice in the other groups were. Each mouse was anesthetized with ether, the hair on her back was shaved, and then an oval patch of skin was snipped off with scissors. The outline of the wound was traced onto transparent plastic with a grease pencil and then its area was calculated. To make sure any variation in the size of the wounds did not compromise the results, the three mice with the largest wounds were randomly distributed to the three treatment groups; the next three were similarly assigned, and so forth until the entire brigade had been parceled out.

The healings were performed for the next twenty days. Mr. E was unusual, Grad told me, because his interest in science was such that he was willing to put in long hours doing the tedious work necessary to get a large, statistically robust sample. After the fifth day, the wounds were traced and measured daily for the next fifteen days. Over the first two weeks, the mice in all three groups healed at about the same rate. The cuts that all started out as about three-tenths of a square inch shrank to a little less than one third that size. But by day fourteen, the wounds on the mice getting treatment from Mr. E were smaller. Mr. E's mice were about one to two days ahead of their sisters.

"I remember seeing the data, and it really surprised me," Grad said. "The odds of this happening by chance were less than one in a hundred.

It was one of the mind-boggling experiments of the 1950s. The fact that one could do a thing like that still agitates me."

In scientific lingo, the wounds on the mice that Mr. E was treating with his hands inside the bags (but outside the cages) were "very significantly" smaller. (Significance is a term of art that describes the chances that data are due to chance; the generally accepted threshold at which experimental effects become "significant" is five percent or less, which is to say that if you did the experiment twenty times you'd get the same outcome nineteen times, and there would only be a one in twenty chance that it was all a fluke. If you ran it two hundred times and got the same outcome one hundred and ninety-nine times, the results would be even less likely to have happened by chance and thus even more significant.) In the series where Mr. E treated groups of mice with his hands outside the stapled bag, the results were not statistically significant, but the average size of the wounds was smaller.

Under some conditions, then, it seemed Mr. E had markedly speeded up the healing time of wounded mice. Grad and his University of Manitoba colleagues, Remi J. Cadoret, a physician, and G. I. Paul, a statistician, published their findings four years later in a 1961 volume of the *International Journal of Parapsychology*:

> The results of this experiment, in addition to the two smaller experiments with a similar outcome, give considerable backing to Mr. E's claim to possess some influence over at least one type of healing. It seems unlikely that suggestion operating through language or symbols would be effective in animal experiments of this type in causing these treatment effects. . . . The failure to find a suitable explanation at present might tempt one to call this healing effect "supernatural." However, use of this term merely indicates a lack of factual information which would enable us to explain the effect in terms of presently understood mechanisms.

What was the mechanism? Grad was convinced that however spiritual traditions might define healing, it had to have a physical basis. Attempting to tease out the properties of the healing hand, he went on to conduct and publish even more striking experiments with Mr. E and

other healers, studies that appeared not only to defeat the idea that healing was synonymous with suggestion but to open up wholly paradoxical
new vistas. Healing energy, in Grad's understanding, seemed to have a
mind of its own, to know what to do. Sometimes it stimulated healthy
processes, like skin repair, and sometimes it inhibited unhealthy processes.
Grad found that Mr. E could slow the development of goiter in mice that
were being fed an iodine-deficient diet—in essence, he could help the
mice compensate for the lack of a vital chemical nutrient. He discovered
that Mr. E could mitigate the growth-inhibiting influence of saltwater on
sprouting barley seeds, essentially by making saline solution less toxic.
Grad tested the effect of healer-treated water on the body weight of rats
and its influence on the rate at which yeast can produce carbon dioxide
from glucose.

In the barley-seed experiment, Estebany held a beaker of one-
percent saline solution for thirty minutes. The water was poured over
barley seeds implanted in pots of peat moss. Untreated saline was poured
over a control group, and then both groups of plants were cultivated
under identical conditions for two weeks. (It was the same basic experimental protocol that would later get Oprah Winfrey excited about
bacteria-prayer studies.) The result was more than just the mitigation
of the growth-inhibiting effect of saline: "Significant acceleration of
growth" had occurred in the plants that began life in the peat with a
sip of Mr. E's water. Grad imposed more stringent controls, giving Mr.
E sealed bottles of saline to hold. Again the results were significant. If
Estebany were emitting some energy, Grad concluded, it was capable of
penetrating glass.

Even stranger were the results from pilot studies using a couple of
psychiatric patients suffering from depression, and a first-year medical
student openly skeptical of the concept of hands-on healing. These preliminary findings suggested that the energy of people in negative states
could have a negative influence on wound healing and plant growth,
and concomitantly that the enthusiasm, confidence, and intention of a
positively-minded "healer" might be a crucial factor in the outcome of
a healing. In other words, the very mind-stuff that had been pushed to
the margins of materialist science was turning out to matter, or so it
seemed. The point was anecdotally driven home to Grad once when he

observed a healer with hypertension trying to heal a rat. The rat died shortly after the treatment. "I hate rats," the healer confessed.

Some months after meeting Grad, I came across a speech he had delivered in 1988 at the thirty-first convention of the Parapsychological Association that summed up his conclusions about his out-of-bounds explorations:

> After studying this effect on animals, plants, and nonliving material for more than thirty-one years, I have come to the conviction that there is indeed a healer phenomenon, which is not just suggestion or the placebo effect and which could be usefully investigated scientifically. [It was based on an energy, he told the convention.] Although much remains to be discovered about the properties of the energy, the groundwork has been laid. . . . It is pulsatory in nature and is associated not just with the brain but with the entire organism. The solar plexus in humans plays a critical role in its action and it would appear to be strongly associated with the emotions, but [it] is not at all irrational. On the contrary, it acts as if "it knows what to do." That is, it . . . carries within itself both intelligence and information. This is very apparent in the healing process, during which time the healer simply transmits the energy or stimulates it within the body of the patient. From then on, the energy appears to know what to do on its own, without the healer's being involved.

The day was almost gone. Renée Grad had fixed us lunch, and the afternoon had whisked past as quickly as the morning. The Grads were headed out that night, but before they left there was one last set of experiments I wanted to ask about, the ones with George Ille.

"George Ille came to the lab in 1982, out of the blue," Grad recalled. "He's a Hungarian. His father was in the Hungarian military. Until he was seventeen or eighteen, he lived in Russia. He fought in the Korean War on the side of North Korea when he was nineteen years old. He left Hungary when Estebany did. In Montreal he met a psychiatrist who worked at the Allan Institute, and he told him about some experiences he was having. Images of Egyptian gods and goddesses were coming to

him—he was an atheist—and then he found that he could mummify bits
of chicken and meat. I think he was afraid he was going nuts. The psychiatrist said, what the hell, let him go and see Grad. Ille brought in bits
of chicken and small fish that he had preserved. I was a total skeptic, but
I set up some experiments. We first tried to see if he could mummify
beef, but the untreated beef hardened too quickly and we needed it to
rot for a control. We tried pork, we tried horse meat. I knew bananas rot-
ted. I studied the rate of spoilage. They lose weight in a straight line. So
we started off with green cooking bananas—green, not yellow. We usually did an experiment with two groups of four bananas each. Ille held
each banana seven times for two and a half minutes, with a minute inter-
val between each treatment. The average total treatment time was seventeen minutes. There was little difference in their size or color at the start,
but the bananas Ille held started turning black faster. They went from
green to black without going through yellow. They lost water at double
and triple the rate of the unheld bananas and then, after three or four
weeks, they got hard like wood. I actually have bananas that are at least
six or seven years old now."

Grad pulled out his keys. They hung from a ring that was chained to
a small banana, dark brown and hard as a walnut. He seemed amused by
my bug-eyed reaction. I asked if the same result could be gotten from an
oven.

"Yes, but the temperature has to be sixty degrees centigrade."

"What's the temperature of the hand?" I asked, forgetting all those
long-gone days of adding lame harmony as Question Mark and the
Mysterians sang "98.6." Chalk it up to Centigrade-Fahrenheit confusion,
and all those metric distances on the highway signs, not that I had
encountered many of them in the Montreal subway. Or chalk it up to the
disorientation of holding a petrified banana.

"The temperature of the hand is thirty-one to thirty-three," Grad
said, kindly.

"Could a chemical do this?"

"I don't know of one. I had Ille wash his hands every three minutes.
He said he would sometimes wake up in the middle of the night so hot
he had to wrap himself in a wet towel. But it's not heat or rubbing or
pressure. I believe it was an energy process, but as to the nature of the

energy . . ." He shrugged. "I've tried other healers with bananas, and it doesn't work out."

In 1990, Oskar Estebany died in Montreal of prostate cancer. He was ninety-three. "He used to say that healers couldn't heal themselves," Grad said. (Estebany felt the flow in his hands up until the end. An hour before he died, he put his hands on a friend and exclaimed, "It is still there!") Ille still lives in Canada, and makes skillfully sculpted American Indian figures. Grad's work inspired Sister Justa Smith, a Franciscan nun and Ph.D. biochemist who obtained Estebany's services in 1967. Smith was able to show not only that Mr. E could increase the activity of the enzyme trypsin by ten percent after seventy-five minutes of hands-on healing, but that he could restore ninety percent of the enzyme's catalytic ability in trypsin samples denatured by ultraviolet light, an experiment Grad had suggested.

Grad's work also inspired the pioneering studies of Dr. Dolores Krieger, now an emeritus professor at New York University and one of the major figures in hands-on healing. In an experiment in 1971, Krieger found that patients who received hands-on treatments in addition to their regular nursing care had markedly higher levels of hemoglobin in their blood. She knew that hands-on healing and chakras had been described for thousands of years, but she called the procedure that seemed to evoke these biochemical changes "therapeutic touch" (TT) in the hope of making it more palatable to adherents of Western medicine. Nurses performing TT on premature babies found that the infants gained weight faster and developed more quickly. It has proved useful in calming people in the emergency room, and has been shown to be especially effective in treating dysfunctions of the autonomic-nervous, lymphatic, and circulatory systems. While skeptics continue to fault the methodology of the research on which TT is based, and to criticize advocates for ignoring or downplaying studies that show no significant effects, Krieger and others have trained more than 47,000 health-care professionals in TT, and the procedure has been the subject of some twenty-two doctoral theses. Krieger developed TT with clairvoyant healer Dora van Gelder Kunz, but she refused to copyright it. To her way of thinking—she's a Buddhist—it was nothing new.

On the train south the next morning, I found myself wishing I had asked Grad less about his scientific work and more about his own healing ability. He had discovered in the course of his research that he had a gift too, and when we did go into the topic, he seemed a little embarrassed, as if it were unseemly for a scientist to be a healer. Or maybe the sudden shyness he showed had to do with the fact that the energy he was able to muster did not come from his hands but from his feet, like Pyrrhus, King of Epirus, who according to Plutarch could cure ailing spleens and ease colic by passing his big toe over the trouble. Grad's curiosity had cost him professionally. In the early 1960s, his boss had urged Renée Grad to persuade her husband to give up healing research. And in 1970, the man confronted Grad directly: "Do you still believe in this stuff?" Grad had replied, "I know what you're asking me, and I know what kind of answer you want me to give. But nothing will change my mind about what I've seen in the last fifteen years." He held on to his job, but he was never made more than associate professor.

What stayed with me, though, all the length of that long ride south through the winter woods, was a moment late in the morning when Grad's son Willis came home after a night shift in the emergency room. A young woman had been rushed in with anaphylactic shock after unwittingly eating something with peanut sauce in it. Her body was in a death struggle with one of its designated enemies. Willis had seen a case of this kind of shock before in a young doctor who had arrived from Calgary to start work at the hospital; he had spent three months in a coma and had eventually gone back home much the worse for wear. From that case Willis had learned how little time there was to intervene. A number of drugs had to be precisely deployed. He gave the woman a shot of adrenaline and a muscle relaxant; he worked by hand a breathing bag that contained one hundred percent oxygen. He administered some other drugs. It was touch and go. She hovered on the edge of a coma, but she stayed conscious. She lived. In almost any other system of medicine she probably would have died. He was too modest to say so, but Willis had saved her life. For an hour or so after he went upstairs to sleep, all the discussion of healing that his father and I were having seemed pale and beside the point. At times, there was nothing subtle about the vital energy of life. And I suppose that moment would have been what I remembered most on the train ride home, the note that would have overshadowed everything else, had it not been for the feel in my hands of that unutterably strange banana.

CHAPTER FOUR

In this body, in this town of Spirit, there is a little house shaped like a lotus, and in that house there is a little space. One should know what is there.

What is there? Why is it so important?

There is as much there in that little space within the heart as there is in the whole world outside. Heaven, earth, fire, wind, sun, moon, lightning, stars; whatever is and whatever is not, everything is there.

—CHHĀNDÔGYA UPANISHAD

1. VALENTINE/PUMP

Even before Mrs. Denadio was wheeled into Operating Room 21 and the dire circumstances of her heart were made manifest in the blooms of blood and the odor of sawed bone and cauterized flesh, I found myself wondering about the status of my own heart—not its life as a valentine, or a doormat, or a demilitarized zone, but its life as a pump. Which is to say, not the mind's heart, the psychic locus of love, courage, grief and yearning; not the heart that waxes glad at roses and wedding vows and in its more preposterous moments palpitates over Hallmark poetry and the theme song from *Hair*; not the heart known to the healer's hand as a plexus of frequencies whirling over the chest, or the clairvoyant's heart heralded as the gateway of the astral plane, or the heart envisioned by yogi masters as the twelve-petaled chakra Anahata with a goddess bathing in nectar that drips down from the pineal gland on a spindle of light. Not the mind's heart, which has a thousand guises, but the body's heart, which has but one: the dogged pump, the cause for wonder.

Given the setting, an operating room at New York's Columbia Presbyterian Medical Center, April, 1995, how could it be otherwise? Everything in OR 21, from the refrigerated air to the flensing light, was set up to help the body's heart survive its strictest crisis. Everything underscored the materiality of the surgical view and made all the subtler dimensions of the heart, such as they might be, seem illusive and trivial—fey conceits that would collapse at the first sign of chest pain.

Chest pain or perhaps even nothing more dramatic than close inspection: I remembered a story I'd read about the young ascetic Dayānand Sarasvatī, who lived in India in the nineteenth century, an era when the heart chakra was supposed to have a material existence—to be as physical as the bone of the ribs or the protective shroud of the pericardium. Dayānand discovered a corpse in a river one day, and thinking he might have a closer look at the physical structure of the chakras, he began to dissect it. Only there wasn't a chakra to be found, at the heart or anywhere else the wheels of light were supposed to be spinning and distributing *prana*. While Dayānand may have based his subtle-energy anatomy on the wrong assumptions, his disenchantment ran deep, and out of it was born the reform Hindu sect called Arya Samaj.

So it goes, time and again: facts indifferent to theories, the mind's ideas dashed on the body's truths. In the name of science you try to sweep away the valentines—the myths, the fanciful ideas, Aristotle's heart as the seat of the soul, Galen's "Prince of All Bowels" heart with its egregiously confused blueprint for the circulating blood. You try to see the pump for what it is. To see the tissue without the prejudice of dreams, like Thoreau on Mt. Katahdin, driven half out of his mind by the actual earth, the stone-force and glory of the real.

And yet they cannot be dismissed entirely, these fey conceits, for they seem to lie at the heart of what we think we are. And even the effort to see without conceptions itself depends on a conception. Some habit, some countervailing perversity or froward spirit rises up, and you find yourself reaching for the pulse of a valentine in a room dedicated to the exigencies of a pump. Valentine/pump, valentine/pump: The refrain thumped in my head like the mocking chant of "either/or, either/or" that the little ruffians shouted at Kierkegaard as the brokenhearted philosopher wandered the streets of Copenhagen, distraught because he had disengaged his fiancée and sacrificed marital happiness to pursue the queer and lonely work of founding existentialism.

Equate your identity with the memorabilia of the valentine heart and you may have to reckon with the possibility that there is no *there* there, that it's all a fiction. I know I felt some presentiment of the void growing as I watched the nurses rack the scalpels and the clamps and the sterile towels, and saw the perfusionists at the heart-lung machine whispering over a thicket of tubes, and followed the doctors in the blue gowns and white masks and blood-spattered rubber clogs as they scrubbed under their nails and soaped their arms and then entered the OR holding their wet hands aloft, looking, for the moment, like cormorants drying their wings. Would Descartes have dared define reality as thought in the razor-light of OR 21? Nothing untangles the knots of the mind-body problem faster than a scalpel.

I suppose I was afraid—for Mrs. Denadio on the brink of her ordeal; for the cormorant surgeons for whom her coronary bypass was just another death-defying stroll on the high-wire of modern medicine; for myself, some kind of queasy illusion-mantled greenhorn awaiting whatever revelations were to be found in the heart's exposure . . .

The head anesthesiologist arrived, a bluff woman named Samantha Mullis, in her late thirties. Her eyes cut around the room.

"You I know, you I know, you I know," she said. She turned to me. "You I don't."

I explained I had been invited to watch the operation by the head surgeon that morning, Dr. Mehmet Oz. The prerogatives of a successful surgeon like Oz are akin to those of a ship captain in the nineteenth century. Dr. Mullis smiled—or seemed to behind her mask—and asked if I would be all right with the sight of blood.

In a grim sort of way, I was keen on it, as if nothing short of blood and the literal tissue of the pump itself could break open the sorrows of the valentine, the heart pain I had buried but was loath to feel. *We held her on our laps and put our hands on her and tried to warm her back to life, but there was nothing we could do, she was gone* . . . At the risk of taking apart with one hand the story I have been putting together with the other, I was beginning to understand that much of my intellectual quandary was based on emotional numbness and ignorance of the heart—my heart, other hearts, hearts in all their guises. In the paradigm of energy healing, I would have been diagnosed as having a kind of subtle heart disease. Or not so subtle, as the case may be. The ecstatic expansion that had occurred on Joel Wallach's healing table had not lasted, nor had the rush of heartfelt love that swept over Clown Headquarters after Barbara Brennan monkeyed with my fourth chakra. Those experiences cast long shadows even in recession. They were the two free issues you got with a trial magazine subscription—a couple of psychic joyrides, courtesy of the universe. For more, you had to pay, and not with an AmEx card. Pay by working. You had to do the work. But what was the work? It wasn't trotting to the library to dig through the history of the vital force, or mulling over the careers of the genius crackpots who got caught up in the illimitable whirlwind. I had begun a meditation practice. I sat in silence for half an hour every morning. It seemed an important discovery to learn that the Chinese phrase for "meditation" was "remembering truths of the heart." And I was struck by the tenet in Buddhism that holds that the process of waking up often starts with suffering. In our private suffering we develop compassion for the pain that binds all sentient creatures. But in meditation I had not been able to recapture the intensity of those altered states induced by healers. On my own, it seemed, I could not engage the heart, my heart, as it had been engaged in the two healings. In a way, I was trained to disengage; in a way, I was my own anesthesiologist. Numbness was very useful, or had been until the consequences of living with a chronic leeriness of emotions began to pile up. At the time, I hardly grasped my own unwillingness to face the heart directly—my heart, the valentine heart—or why I was loath to risk presenting it without the ironic mediation of clown metaphors—"doormat," "demilitarized zone"—figures of speech that made light of heavy emotions. What I could grasp was that OR 21 was a theater dedicated to the ultimate heart trouble and to a level of suffering that was grave enough to make a dozen other brands of pain, my own included, seem almost like blessings in disguise. Blood? I nodded to the anesthesiologist. Let it flow.

Promptly at 7:30, two attendants wheeled in the forty-nine-year-old computer operator from Nutley, New Jersey. Joyce Denadio had diabetes; she was a lifelong smoker. A week earlier, she had gotten an urgent bulletin from her heart in the form of severe chest pain. Chest pain is one of the most common symptoms that sends people to the doctor, but in more than half the cases, no cause related to the body's heart can be found. The body's heart is simply expressing some agitation of the mind's. Mrs. Denadio would have been overjoyed to discover her pain was only, say, a panic disorder registering on the exquisitely sensitive seismograph of her heart, but the angiogram revealed that hardly any blood was getting through the three main arteries that fed her left ventricle: She had a myocardial infarction. Her heart, the undeniably material heart that pumps, was dying for want of oxygen.

As one of 300,000 coronary bypasses performed annually in the U.S., the operation that morning was run-of-the-mill stuff: bread-and-butter work for Dr. Oz; another day's lesson in the art of patching hearts for his team of medical students, residents, and fellows, who would handle much of the preliminary cutting and snipping. But in one respect, the script was unlike any other. Oz had added a wild card to the cast, a brown-haired, fifty-three-year-old hands-on healer named Julie Motz. With Oz's blessing and the patient's permission, Julie was planning to lay hands on Mrs. Denadio for the duration of her eight hours under the knife.

This was the angle that had caught my interest, at least on the surface: the cultural incongruity of a hands-on practitioner in the inner sanctum of a modern medical temple. I don't want to further belabor the tension between mainstream medicine and the fringe. It's clear many hospitals have reformed their ideas of care in the two decades since a bunch of Therapeutic Touch nurses returned from a weekend training seminar to find a sternly dizzy memo from their administrator saying "There will be no healing in this hospital!" Orthodoxies change. In an article in the March 1997 issue of *Clinical Cardiology*, editor-in-chief C. Richard Conti wrote: "About twenty years ago I took care of a patient who was admitted into our Coronary Care Unit with an uncomplicated myocardial infarction. On day two of his infarction, I noted that he had a peculiar yellow cast to his skin. I subsequently learned that his wife had rubbed Vitamin E all over his body. At the time I thought the patient's wife was slightly crazy. Maybe she knew something I didn't." Today Vitamin E is a staple of heart-conscious diets; and Therapeutic Touch is practiced in many hospitals, including Columbia Presbyterian. But installing a hands-on healer in an operating room of a university medical center remains a radical departure. That spring day in 1995 when I witnessed Joyce Denadio's operation at Columbia, it was almost, well, sacrilegious—akin to letting a clown help out at a Catholic mass.

The heart Julie Motz proposed to monitor had never been approached before in OR 21. Under the prevailing medical model, its very existence was in doubt. Anyone was well within his rights to ask how relevant the mind's heart was to a bypass operation, to the health of a heart that was incontrovertibly physical. Wasn't the mind's heart, whatever its actual nature, part of that dream country on the far side of the Cartesian divide and thus incapable of influencing the function of the pump? Julie Motz was claiming that the mind's heart could affect the material welfare of the body's heart, but what evidence suggested the dream-drenched valentine and the pump were linked? Or supported her contention that the apparent differences of the mind's heart and the body's heart had nothing to do with the actual nature of the organ but with the various ways one might touch it?

"For every physical event there is a corresponding emotional and mental event," Motz had told me a few days earlier. "That's what I'm working on. It's not weird. If we were educated in an intuitive culture for twelve years the way we are in an analytical culture, it wouldn't seem all that strange. Thought and feeling are energy, and what I'm trying to do is pick up the energy of those thoughts and feelings, and feed them back to the patient. It's very logical." She believed that by feeding a patient's thoughts and feelings back to the heart—and sending along a supplemental flow of love, some inmost sympathy communicated via the hands and the mind's intention—she could fortify the body's heart. Or at least understand its predicaments a little better.

As ever, it sounded nice in theory, but with precious little to say that energy work would make a difference, Motz had to rely on Mehmet Oz's willingness to sail uncharted waters. In most hospitals, the only way a healer can participate in cardiac surgery is to have a heart attack. Oz was not interested in alternative medicine just because it was different. Mainstream studies in cardiac surgery had shown depression to be a key indicator of how long patients would survive after open-heart surgery; surgeons ignored the emotional and mental states of patients at their patient's peril. In Oz's view, anything that could be done before or after the operation to mitigate the sense of psychic trauma ought to be investigated. Maybe Motz could give him some insights into his patient in the course of the operation. Maybe she could even increase the patient's chances of getting off the table. The surgical personnel would tolerate her if it was his pleasure to have her attending.

Motz had donned the green scrubs for the first time some months before, during one of Oz's transplant operations. It was sort of like bringing a play-by-play announcer versed in cricket down onto the field to comment on the action during a baseball game. Motz relayed changes she was able to sense in the patient's energy field. (Though not awake, the patient probably retained some subconscious awareness, most likely smell, and perhaps hearing. Open-heart patients are often fitted with headphones and provided with tapes to "listen" to.) As a bit of a maverick, bright but impolitic, used to pressing ahead without a lot of support or concern for the consensus opinion, Motz urged Oz to talk directly to the hearts he was transplanting. Oz replied that he would be laughed out of the operating room. His surgical teams were already fighting the temptation to joke about the healer as they listened to her report what she believed were patients' moods and emotions registering in her own body. During that first transplant operation, she said she could sense the patient's anger as roughness in her chest and his anxiety as turbulence in her stomach. At one point during her debut, Oz saw that Motz was beginning to look a little green around the gills. He asked a burly perfusionist named Jimmy Beck to take her outside for some air. When Beck returned, his clown got the better of him. "I sense a change in my stomach," he said. "It's a tenseness . . . No, it's a growling . . . No, wait a minute . . . I'm just hungry!"

The attendants lifted Mrs. Denadio from the gurney onto the narrow operating table and bundled her in a blanket. With her arms lashed onto perpendicular rests, she looked vaguely like a martyr on a cross. She was wired up to a sophisticated computerized system of sensors that brought her vital signs online. A mask went over her face, a catheter into her arm; a saline drip was started. A large-bore catheter that would provide electronic reports of blood pressure and other crucial information had to be inserted into her right jugular vein and then threaded down into her heart—probably the most painful part of the operation she would undergo prior to anesthesia. Julie Motz was holding her hand.

"Now Mrs. Denadio . . ." said an anesthesiology resident in a saccharine voice. "You'll feel a little prick."

Blood gushed over Mrs. Denadio's neck; she winced and rolled her head away and squeezed Motz's hand.

The resident tried again, but he couldn't get the catheter into the vein. Mrs. Denadio's neck was beginning to look like something out of an Arnold Schwarzenegger movie. Motz crouched beside her and whispered encouragement. It was clear that of the dozen or so people in the room—each with a precisely defined part to play in an intricate min-

uet—none had the time or inclination to offer any but the most per-
functory reassurance to Mrs. Denadio. Motz at that point had nothing to
offer but reassurance. She took time, she poured herself into the connection, giving her complete attention to Mrs. Denadio. Does it sound
trite? I am worried such phrases cannot do justice to what seemed an act
of witnessing. It was not that Motz alone understood what Mrs. Denadio
might be going through in a general way, but that she had visited Mrs.
Denadio in the hospital before the surgery, and had gotten to know her,
and in a specific way understood the impact of this procedure at this time
on this woman—not "the patient," not "Denadio J," social security number such and such, but the soul of the woman in all its subtleties, Joyce,
with her thinning brown hair, and her worried husband, Joe, and her bad
habits, and her friends at work who sent in cards; Joyce, who missed her
Yorkshire terrier, Bo, and who found herself crying when she got to the
hospital but didn't know why . . .

And Mrs. Denadio seemed deeply grateful to have the healer there,
holding her hand and whispering into her ear that it would all right, *it
would be all right*. It struck me that you did not have to buy any of the
way-out stuff about subtle energy or energy medicine or know anything
about the heart chakra to see the effect of one woman's presence on
another and to understand the beauty and the power inherent in that act
of empathy. You did not have to know anything about medicine East or
West to glimpse what it meant for one frightened human being to hold
the hand of another at T minus zero.

This is not to say that hand-holding obviated the need for the enor-
mously complex operation or that the loving presence of a healer could
in any way substitute for the procedure. A chauvinist of Western medicine would argue that the technology itself was humane. Unlike at
London Hospital in 1791, there was no bell to ring in OR 21 that would
summon the attendants needed to hold the patient down when the surgeon was ready to begin. What Julie Motz was doing—was it anything
more than being there?—was not the last word in the therapy that morning. But if it was not the whole of medicine, perhaps it had something to
do with the heart of it.

Rather than cause her any more pain, the doctors decided to forgo
the chance to get pre-anesthesia data on Mrs. Denadio's heart and to

insert the catheter once she had been put under. "Okay, Mrs. Denadio, we'll see you tomorrow morning," said one of the residents. Mrs. Denadio's eyes fell shut.

Dr. Mullis looked at the bank of computer monitors. "She's out," she said.

Mrs. Denadio's passage from subject to object was breathtakingly swift. The blanket was unceremoniously shucked off, leaving her body naked on the table, like a corpse stretched out for autopsy. The armrests were folded up, and her arms were packed in towels tight against her side. A catheter to take away her urine was established. A mustard-colored wash of iodine was sluiced across her chest, and then a giant piece of adhesive plastic was laid over the skin to keep it from falling away from the incision. The route of the cut was outlined with a Derma-marker pen to make sure the scar would not show afterwards when she unbuttoned the top of her blouse. Her face was screened from her chest by a green cloth that established one boundary of the sterile field.

And then Oz pushed through the swinging doors, arms uplifted, his wet life-giving hands ready for a towel and latex gloves. You could be forgiven for thinking that Oz was showing off his hands. He carries $180,000 of annual post-tax disability insurance on them. He owed not just his livelihood but his very being to the art of sewing: Mehmet's mother, partial to handmade dresses, had met his father in Turkey through the elder Oz's sister, who was a seamstress. And while the theater of his entrance in OR 21 had much to do with the gravity of the morning's work and the godlike authority accorded the head surgeon, it reflected more than a little of Oz's own charisma too. I had trailed him on rounds for a few days and found that he was one of those freaks of nature who seem to have no capacity for sloth. Say you are thinking well of yourself because you have washed the dishes and sharpened all the pencils; his secretary phones with an update on *his* morning: "He's doing a heart transplant right now, and he's got a double lung transplant waiting, and those are in addition to his two regularly scheduled open-hearts, and then at three he's supposed to fly to Boston to deliver a lecture." In two months he would be thirty-five years old. His colleagues were using his energy as a benchmark, correlating their own vitality as a fraction of a "full Mehmet unit." At the scrub sink they would ask, "What are you today?"

and maybe one would reply, "Uh, I'm about a point three." Or maybe a "point seven" if they'd had a double latte and a diet Coke. "He runs down lobs," his tennis partner Eric Rose sighed, as if there were no greater testimony to Oz's vitality. (Along with being Oz's mentor and department chairman, Rose also happens to be one of the top heart-transplant surgeons in the world.)

To see what could be done on a full Mehmet unit, a week before Mrs. Denadio's surgery I had waited in Oz's heavily trafficked office for the printer to disgorge his curriculum vitae. It seemed to take the better part of the morning: Harvard graduate magna cum laude; medical school at the University of Pennsylvania, where he was class chairman and school president, and also managed to squeeze in an MBA from Wharton. During his residency at Columbia he won the prestigious Blakemore research award four times. He was an Irving Assistant Professor of Surgery at the College of Physicians and Surgeons. He held three patents, two for dye techniques that facilitate the use of medical lasers and one for a solution that preserves transplant organs. At the time—spring of 1995—he'd made twenty-three noteworthy presentations to professional societies, contributed chapters to eight books, written fifty-six abstracts and one hundred and thirty-one papers; he was doing about 250 operations a year. Amid all this he had found the time to marry and father three kids, and to preserve his claim to some family property in Turkey, and had even ducked off to serve two and a half months in the Turkish army. Oz became the leader of seven thousand troops, thanks to his height. At six feet, he was a giant among Turks. Technically, his training had been in vascular surgery, but during his time in the army, he did dozens of circumcisions on soldiers in their late teens—a free circumcision is one of the sought-after perks of military service.

"That's not vascular surgery, is it?" I asked.

"It can be," Oz said.

What a résumé can't convey is Oz's enthusiasm and—no other phrase seems so apt—his openheartedness. A career spent with his hands on the body's heart had not diminished his feeling for the mind's heart, scarce as the indications of it were in the medical literature. Julie Motz told me one day that when she first saw Oz do surgery she was deeply moved by the tenderness of his touch. I was struck by his lack of pretention. One day in his office he said, "I used to bicycle to work across the George Washington Bridge, but my wife told me it wasn't professional. And my chairman backed her up." All of lost youth and the weight of adulthood hung in a note of rue, and then he shrugged cheerfully and laughed, and reached into a drawer for a bag of Turkish apricots and almonds sent by a grateful bypass patient. Streams of colleagues and students wandered in to discuss cases, cadge almonds, and rib him about a recent appearance on the evening news in which his work with mechanical hearts was accompanied by footage of the Tin Man from *The Wizard of Oz*.

Now in OR 21, Oz wanted to see how the early stages of the operation were progressing. The lower-ranking surgeons would open and close Mrs. Denadio's chest; surgical residents would harvest the vein grafts from her left leg. Oz would handle or supervise the most delicate sections: He would shift Mrs. Denadio's heartbeat over to the heart-lung machine, and then chill and stop her heart; he would sew the bypasses around her coronary arteries. Once those alterations were done, he would try to get her off-bypass and start her heart back on the job it had never abandoned before.

Julie Motz had taken up a position at Mrs. Denadio's head, outside the sterile field where the anesthesiologist and her assistant were working; Motz had enlisted a partner, Sally Smith, a second-year medical student who had overcome her concern that her interest in healing might harm her young reputation as a doctor-in-training. Smith had scrubbed as thoroughly as the surgeons and stood inside the sterile field with her hands settled on Mrs. Denadio's feet. There the two healers stood for most of the next seven hours.

I watched the younger surgeons make the first cuts in Mrs. Denadio's leg. As the glistening tissue fell open, the focus of my personal understanding of the mind-body problem began to slide from my brain toward my stomach. The flesh of the leg looked too much like hamburger. Once at a summer camp in Vermont where I worked as a counselor, a kid had impaled his leg on a piece of metal; I had to drive him to the hospital. The gash didn't seem too bad, a frown of weird red subterranean stuff erupting from the netherworld of the body, but when the nurse began sewing the lips of the wound together, I was suddenly down near the floor, my head snapping back with some ammoniacal genie in my nose, and the nurse who held the smelling salts sighing sweetly and saying in a condescending voice, "It's always the men . . ." As the surgeons got ready to harrow the chest with a small power saw, I realized the hardest sight was not the prospect of the open chest itself but the transition to it, the assault on flesh. Maybe there was no need to see that. Even first-year medical students in anatomy class usually start dissecting the back of their cadavers, and approach the face, where the vestiges of personhood inhere, with some uneasiness and reservations. I was going back and forth in my mind. Oz was shuttling among three operating rooms, and when he asked if I wanted to pop over to OR 23 to look in on a lung biopsy, I said sure.

It was the family of Oz's wife, Lisa Lamole, who piqued his interest in alternative medicine. Lisa's father, Gerald, was one of the top heart surgeons in the country—a member of the first heart-transplant team in Texas—but he had also been called "Rock a Doc" by *Rolling Stone* magazine for playing music in the OR to relax patients. He and his wife, Emily Jane, were vegetarians and followers of the spiritual philosophy of Emanuel Swedenborg. Mrs. Lamole developed a special low-fat diet for her husband's cardiac patients and held her ground when some of her husband's colleagues said they would not refer patients if Dr. Lamole prescribed low-fat diets, which today are gospel. When she herself was a candidate for gall-bladder surgery, she refused the knife, preferring to handle gallstones by modifying her diet. Her kids got penicillin for strep throats, but their bellyaches she treated with herbal tea, their earaches with garlic and olive oil, and their sore muscles with arnica gel.

Oz had set up the Cardiac Complementary Medicine Study Group in 1994. He called it complementary because he wanted to build on Western medicine, not abandon it. "Meditation didn't cure polio," he said. He mailed letters to one hundred cardiologists, outlining a program to study therapies in four areas: diet, meditation and hypnosis, manual therapies like massage, and energy medicine of the sort practiced by hands-on healers.

"I didn't feel there was a huge downside," he recalled. "I felt secure with my colleagues. If I kept doing what I was paid to do, the most they could do is caution me in a brotherly way. I would say to them, 'I know you think this is a little crazy, but I feel we are neglecting our patients in a crucial way.' "

He heard from excited doctors who had been interested in alternative techniques and from doctors who wanted to make sure he wasn't opening the door to the fringes of healing without a lot of reflection. Dr. Myron Weisfeldt, the chairman of medicine at Columbia Presbyterian, asked: "Is this something we want to do?" Dr. Oz said he would give grand rounds in the fields he was looking at and stressed what he believed was the "institution's responsibility to evaluate this stuff."

For the first study, he wanted a project that would be a solid bet. Julie Motz, who was studying for a master's degree in public health, had suggested a list of possible experiments, from aromatherapy to hypnosis. One of the perfusionists in the heart unit, Jery Whitworth, was also interested in hypnosis and wanted to explore new approaches to cardiac care in memory of his father, who had died of inoperable heart disease. Most doctors were familiar with hypnosis from medical school; it didn't entail any major revisions in the materialist paradigm, no science-straining leaps of faith. The Complementary Study Group enrolled twenty-two patients scheduled for surgery at the hospital. Nine were designated as a control group; the remaining thirteen were taught to hypnotize themselves. The instructors focused on getting the people to relax their jaw and throat muscles in hopes of lessening the stress of having a breathing tube inserted down the throat. They suggested that the patients try to extend their hypnotic state to the surgery itself, in essence to program themselves to minimize their bleeding, maintain normal blood pressure, and in some unknown subliminal way, reduce their experience of pain and discomfort. After the ordeal was over, the patients were to concentrate on healing quickly, minimizing pain and discomfort, and normalizing blood pressure. The goal was to see how hypnosis changed the patients' "quality of life"—an outcome Oz and his colleagues assessed by having patients check off their levels of stress and depression on a standard psychological mood inventory. The results suggested that patients who were taught hypnosis relaxation techniques were significantly less tense after the operation than patients who didn't have the training. Their scores for depression and fatigue were also lower.

When we returned to OR 21, there was a terrible odor of burned flesh in the air, and Mrs. Denadio's breastbone had been riven in two and her ribs spread apart by the cage of a stainless-steel retractor; the surgeons were about to cut into the pericardium, the tough membrane around the heart. A whole new set of blue towels had been carefully laid over the drab green ones, building up a sort of stage for the delicate work to come. I went around the edge of the room to where Julie Motz and the anesthesiologist were standing, and peered over the edge of my mask down into the open chest, and suddenly I understood the depths of the word *apocalypse*, from the Greek *apokalyptein,* meaning "unveiled." The surgeon's scalpel pierced the pericardium. Gloved hands flashed, needles were expertly worked through the membrane and then drawn back with tails of silk thread that were pulled tight and clamped off so they held the pericardium out of the way like guy lines on a tent.

And there was Mrs. Denadio's heart.

If you want to know what the soul looks like, look at the body, said Wittgenstein. But we don't, we look everywhere else, or don't look at all, as if we can't bear the idea that the two are even implicated in each other, much less one and the same. No improviser's truck-cum-trumpet word game was necessary to make the world seem new. Here was a terrible breach opening with the strangeness of tissue and dream compounded, an intimacy of mind and body that was too intense, too claustrophobic, too morbid for everyday life. Suddenly I was confronted by my own complicity in the fiction of dualism, how much all of us require the configuration of mind *and* body, how eagerly we embrace the refuge of that Cartesian partition which holistic medicine is so quick to deplore. Can the comfort of the division really be that much of a surprise? The separation we establish between mind and body is like a piece of Sheetrock that divides a one-room house and affords us the means for keeping what we do not want to face at some remove, safely quartered in the other room. The mind defines the otherness of the body, and mind remains mantled in the dream of its separate life until some crisis collapses the wall, and the ghost in the machine suddenly staggers under the weight of its chains and stumbles in the chalky rubble of its conceits, pierced by its inescapable relation and the implication that it is the lesser of two realities, that perhaps it was never anything but an artifact of the flesh, an illusion. For such hard lessons in the nature of duality, Buddhist monks are sometimes dispatched to meditate among the corpses in the charnel house. They might find the same insights contemplating the excavated heart.

It looked like a small animal suddenly unearthed, a mole blinking in the bright ruin of a roofless lair. It beat on bravely in the third-degree light, flexing and kicking, undaunted by the flood of unfamiliar air. It seemed almost foolhardy pressing on in the face of such great peril. It was the size and color of a mango, and the way it looked, streaked and smeared with blood, it could have been a mango floating in a compote of mashed strawberries.

Hours passed. Mesmerized by the body's heart, I had the unsettling sense it was not just the mind's heart that was vaporous, but that the mind itself—mind, self, soul, psyche, all the pronoun agencies and whatchamacallits of self-consciousness that had been nattering for centuries about the phenomenology of forms and essences and reason and free will and choice and anxiety—all of them suddenly seemed as delusional as characters in a movie speculating on the nature of their existence apart from the projector. Where was the valentine now? What life was there apart from the pump?

Meditative hours passing in the pure concentration of work: The surgeons rerouted Mrs. Denadio's blood, rigging the tubes that would carry it to the bypass machine and back. When a cannula was slipped into the great arch of the aorta, a geyser of blood sprayed up and flecked the goggles of the people leaning in to assist Dr. Oz. Long red strands of Mrs. Denadio's saphenous vein were snipped out of her leg and dropped into a saline solution in a cup. Her circulation was shifted onto the machine, and Oz began the procedures that would cool and slow the heart, the heart that had first begun to beat when the cells that formed Mrs. Denadio's body were twenty-five days old, the heart that had been pushing out five quarts of blood a minute, seventy-five gallons an hour, seventy barrels a day, never stopping, year after year after year. And now with a dose of potassium chloride, the same compound used in intravenous executions, Mrs. Denadio's heart came to a stop. It was ready to be repaired. Oz clamped a section of the vein from Mrs. Denadio's leg and began to sew the graft into the slippery vessels. He liked to have his hands in a "flow" state, and toward that end he would often start surgeries with Bruce Springsteen playing on the tape deck and close them with Vivaldi. He peered intently through head loupes that magnified three and a half times the slippery red tissue of Mrs. Denadio's heart. He requested sutures and clamps and, later, units of lidocaine. At one tense point he brought Mrs. Denadio's heart off the bypass machine, and it began to beat chaotically. He snapped at a surgical nurse for failing to test the defibrillator: "If it doesn't defibrillate, it's not a defibrillator!"

All the while, Julie Motz periodically called out soft directions to Sally Smith to move her hands. Julie floated her hands above Mrs. Denadio's temples, and squatted down and held the woman's shoulders, and touched the crown of her head. Sally held Mrs. Denadio's ankles, then switched from the small toe of Mrs. Denadio's right foot to a point on the sole known as the "bubbling spring." The bubbling spring was the terminus of the kidney meridian, and in Julie's experience, it usually felt flat and undercharged in heart patients. She looked up at Sally, and said quietly, "Did you feel that?"

Sally nodded.

"It felt like the energy picked up—there was a smoothness to it," Julie said.

You had to mark their dedication if nothing else. They both stood there through the long hours of the operation, witnessing something that seemed too intangible to matter in the OR. Anyone untrained in the art of hands-on healing might wonder what they were doing. Even knowing a little bit about what they believed they were doing wouldn't clarify it much, as the metaphors of running energy, holding energy, and checking energy could only breed more metaphors. Maybe the healers were up on the promenade deck of the S.S. *Denadio*, arranging recliners, while Oz and company were down at the waterline trying to repair the rips and keep the good ship afloat. Perhaps they would have been just as effective had they been priestesses chanting the pain-allaying words of the Heart Sutra, which ends: "Gone gone gone beyond gone altogether beyond, O what an awakening, all hail!" Or the beautiful heart prayer from the Egyptian Book of the Dead: "My heart, my mother; twice. My heart, my coming into existence. Not be there resistance to me in the judgment. Not be there repulse to me by the divine chiefs. Not make thy separation from me in the presence of the Keeper of the Scales. Thou art the double within my body forming and making strong my limbs."

If the body's heart does in fact have a double life, if there is such a thing as the mind's heart (can anyone who has ever loved doubt this?), if there is such a thing as the fourth chakra, the "high heart," the seat of the soul, perhaps it can be found in the feeling of heartache and the concomitant idea of shared fate, of compassion born out of the understanding that when you stare into the mortality of someone else's heart, the mortality of your own stares back. *Thou art the double within my body . . .*

A week later, Mrs. Denadio was sitting in her hospital room with her husband, Joe, who worked as a parking enforcement officer. She'd climbed a set of stairs and traveled the length of the hospital solarium. She'd washed her hair. Her appetite was back. The zipper-like wounds on her chest and left leg were mending nicely. She was eager to sleep in her own bed, and sit on her deck, and squeeze her dog, Bo.

Dr. Oz and Julie Motz and Sally Smith stopped by to see her. Oz said she'd be going home soon. He was wearing blood-stained clogs and his white coat with the heart ornament pinned to the lapel. He lingered for a bit, then ducked out to check on other patients.

"She's euphoric now," he said to me. "I want her to get greedy. Her purpose is not just to survive, it's to go out and do great things."

Julie Motz and Sally Smith stayed with Mrs. Denadio a while longer.

"When I moved my hands to your kidney meridian I felt that something was making you angry," Motz said. "And I whispered to you: 'Joyce, I want you to roar, I want you to push the anger out through your chest.' It seemed like there was some old anger. I got an image of a car. Does that make any sense?"

Mrs. Denadio looked puzzled, but then she said, "When I was six my parents drove off without me once—left me up at Lake Hopatcong. I was abandoned out by all the cars."

"Were you angry?"

"Maybe I was," she said. But it was recent history that seemed to be preoccupying her now.

"It was like a blessing to have you there," she said to Motz. "I was so afraid, and you made me feel relaxed. I was so at peace because I knew you were there."

"She was definitely scared, and it relaxed her," said her husband.

"Thank God they did not wheel me in there by myself," she said.

I asked how it had relaxed her.

"Julie was saying that my veins were going to take over the work of arteries, and I just started to float. At last somebody wasn't telling me what was going to hurt, but what was positive. She has such a wonderful touch. I told my girlfriend about it on the phone and she said, 'What is she?' And I said, 'I don't know.' "

Julie Motz and Sally Smith smiled. Mrs. Denadio searched their eyes with much gratitude and feeling; Mr. Denadio squeezed her hand. *Gone gone beyond gone altogether . . .*

"They were sort of doing inspirational work," Joe Denadio explained. It seemed that what he said was as much for himself and what he didn't understand about the fate of hearts as for anyone else in the room.

2. INTERLUDE WITH A GHOST

Some time after Mrs. Denadio's surgery, Julie Motz invited me to attend what was a sort of counseling-and-healing session she was holding every Wednesday afternoon in the Milstein Pavilion at Columbia Presbyterian Hospital. She had been working for a number of months without pay with patients who had undergone or were waiting for open-heart surgery—men and women who needed new valves, coronary bypasses, in some cases entire new hearts. Many of the transplant patients were being kept alive by mechanical pumps—left-ventricle-assist devices that did what their own left ventricles no longer could. The so-called LVADs, saucer-sized pucks of stainless steel, had been stitched into their abdomens and connected to their diseased hearts by a tube; the pumps were powered by portable batteries, which the patients pushed around like shopping carts. Some had been in the hospital for months waiting for their name to come up on the transplant list. They were in limbo, sustained by machines, waiting for hearts; some were depressed, some numb with dread. Tethered to their carts, they shuffled around the ward, like doomed invalids pacing the attic of a gothic house.

The session was in a conference room in the Milstein Pavilion. Motz had everyone pair up and one member of each pair lay hands on the other. I stood behind a middle-aged former New York City cop and put my hands on his shoulders. He seemed to have retreated so far inside himself that there was hardly any light coming out of his eyes. I guess I pitied him: He was my age, a cop, a black man; he seemed hopelessly estranged—from others, from himself. It was as if he no longer had the key to his own body but was standing outside in the street, looking up at the windows of the house he used to live in. Vitalizing and life-saving as it might be, the pulse in his body wasn't his own. It belonged to a machine. It sustained him, but it did not affirm him or define him or uplift him in any way. I could feel it jerking in his flesh, remorselessly mechanical, indifferent to his being. It slapped back and forth like a windshield wiper. No wonder he was depressed. You may not understand until such an encounter how sensitive and changeable the organic pulse of the heart is, how it quickens or slows with moods, how its responsiveness is crucial to the sense of self we organize; in some way, perhaps the variability of the heartbeat even defines who we are. We are registered in the pattern of our flux.

After ten minutes, Motz had the people with their hands on change places, and I met the eyes of the ghostly man. They were heartbreaking, for their glimmer of recognition, the faint light of fellowship, and the memory of the pain those bonds entailed.

"Thank you," he said.

That was all I knew about him—the pattern of his pulse, the faint light of fellowship in his eyes. I didn't even know his name. I found out much later that he waited six months on the ward before a suitable heart was found. The transplant came off okay, but after a year he developed an aneurysm, and he died. His name was Vincent.

3. THOU ART
THE DOUBLE

With that call to settle my hands on a stranger, I had crossed the continental divide and was now treading on new and perilous ground. I could no longer get off with the dodge of being an observer; I had to weigh the responsibilities of being a participant, even a practitioner. It was a small step but a profound distinction, as sharp and frightening as the line between the anonymity of the audience and the exposure of the stage. You're in the stands, you're watching a World Series game, and suddenly with the gliding logic of a dream, you're standing at the plate pinch-hitting, and it's the bottom of the ninth, and then suddenly the coach tells you it's not the World Series, it's a cricket championship . . .

I didn't think there was any harm in casually laying hands on fellow tyros at introductory healing seminars where the rudiments of energy medicine were, generally speaking, being taught to people whose main interest and concern seemed to be spiritual enhancement, not medical treatment. But to feign expertise with a ghost who was one failed battery from death? This wasn't a game.

In the United States, unlike England and Europe, no board certifies healers. If you are looking for a healer in the U.S., it's impossible to know who is good and who isn't. You might think, given their beliefs, that all healers would have uncommonly high levels of integrity and not be as encumbered by the fetters of egotism as the rest of us, but their rivalries can sometimes be as bitchy as those among any bunch of professors or magazine writers. Some months later, several new healers had volunteered at the Complementary Care Center at Columbia Presbyterian. When I asked one what she thought of Julie Motz's healing abilities, she gave me a sharp look and said that Julie seemed very sincere but when they had done some healings together patients had asked afterwards why the new healer's hands were so hot and Julie's weren't. "Warm heart, cold hands." It was something Bette Davis could have said in *All About Eve*.

Would it have been better to confess my inexperience? To disabuse Vincent of any misconceptions he might have had about my ungifted hands? I hope not; I don't think so. I can't see that he expected much from a session of hands-on healing, other than that it might assuage his loneliness. He could have easily looked at me as if to say "Who is this clown?" but he didn't, and it occurs to me now, reflecting on that afternoon, that his heart was in no shape for sarcasm. Unlike the stand-back, smart-mouthed journalist, he was no connoisseur of irony with a heart too refined for Hallmark cards; there must have been plenty of songs and lyrics that would moisten his eyes.

But in truth, I can't see that my amateur effort could have caused him any harm—how much worse could things get? He was already in the hospital, already in the midst of a health catastrophe, already waiting for a last-chance, life-sustaining operation that was unthinkable forty years ago. And some of the presumably best medical care in the world was available just outside the conference-room door. Still, I felt a responsibility toward him, no less significant for its being short-lived. I think it was the desire of the novice practitioner not just to aid and comfort, or do what can be done, but to do everything possible under the sun, do it perfectly, righter than right, and to know everything about what is being done, and to radiate a certain faith in the benefit of the procedure. In truth, I knew virtually nothing, and probably radiated only uncertainty. It was clear that there were limits to what you could learn about hands-on healing simply as a client lying on a table. You had to get up and change places with the healer. But when you did that, when you took even one step in that direction, from the dark anonymity of the audience toward the light of the stage, you ran into the strangest heart of all.

In a way, this crossover was not a surprise. It had been spelled out years ago, before Barbara Brennan had fiddled with my heart chakra, even before my personal cosmology was cracked by a lily and the Queen of Enemas decamped for California. It had been spelled out in what I had always thought of as a heart dream. After all, the heart is both the issue and the forum in many energy-medicine philosophies that envision an alchemical transition from the physical to the spiritual.

The dream went like this: I was being guided down a long hall by an old actor. We were related, though not so you'd notice. He was handsome, trimly built, could quote Shakespeare, and moved like a cougar; I was gangly, plain, tripped over my words, and time and again clocked my head on the ceiling ducts in the hall. Whack! Ow! Bang! Ow! There seemed no end to those ceiling ducts. At last we reached a darkened theater, where an outsized bowl of whipped cream was sitting onstage in a pool of light. My blood relative dipped his hand in and began to eat, sighing as if nothing in the universe tasted better. I asked if I could have some whipped cream too—weren't we family, after all? He shook his head. He said I had to go through a door at the back of the stage. He pointed to what seemed to be a blank wall. On closer inspection, I noticed the faint outline of the word "Heart" stenciled like a star's name on the door of a dressing room. I pushed and suddenly the theater was gone, and I was wading knee-deep in a warm green sea. In the distance there was a young woman; she was naked and disarmingly beautiful (or beautiful and disarmingly naked). She had long tawny hair and serene green eyes, which she fixed on me. Mary Tyler Moore was standing next to her, wearing knee socks and a kilt and spanking her with a long-stemmed rose . . .

I raise this here as a roundabout way back to the valentine heart, which seems to hold many of the secrets of healing when it is not busy being the thing that aches with love, and breaks when things go to hell, and roams about at night conscripting icons of primness to play whip-happy sidekicks in aquatic sex fantasies. I woke from that dream and within a few months had quit my job, moved to a new city, and enrolled in an acting class. Following my heart, as it were. Never was there an organ with more stupid ideas. Prince of the Bowels indeed. You'd have to look a long time to find a worse actor. I had a teacher who remarked one day, "You're not using your imagination to personify the character, you're using it to avoid pain."

Ten years later, her psychological insight began to make sense physically. I was sitting with a healer named Michael Mamas in a mostly deserted oceanside restaurant north of San Diego. A wintry day, white surf raking the empty beach. Mamas had just left his teaching job at the

Brennan School to launch a school of his own, the School for Enlightenment and Healing he was calling it, and thus making overt the intriguing but uncertain connection between health and higher states of consciousness. Mamas was a talented healer, and unlike many, articulate. He had studied physics and spent many years in an ashram; his second sight was impressively advanced. We had been talking for several hours, and I imposed on him—I asked him what was going on energetically in my body. He said he didn't like to read people in restaurants. What healers do shouldn't be turned into some party trick for entertainment. I must have appeared disappointed, or maybe I had piqued his ego.

"Well, all right," he said.

And out the diagnosis came, chop chop chop, all matter-of-fact, cut-and-dried as anything a car mechanic might offer after a look-see under the hood.

"You have a kink in your vertical power current," he said. "It's sort of like a kink in a garden hose. The main flow of energy goes up your body and then veers off to the right when it gets to the heart chakra, which is why there's less energy in your left shoulder and arm than in the right."

Wow! How about that! I was struck not just by what he said but by how obvious it all seemed to him. Plain as day, he could see the current of my life detouring around my heart, denying my left arm its full complement of juice. And it made some sense too; my left shoulder and arm didn't have the vigor of the right one. I had a dip in my spine; caddying once when I was fourteen, I had permanently wrenched ligaments on the left side of my middle back. Fluid had once accumulated mysteriously in my left elbow. The rheumatologist who drained it with a needle prepared a culture on the assumption that it was caused by some common bacterial infection, but he had been puzzled to find that nothing appeared in the petri dish; he shrugged and chalked it up to causes unknown and said maybe I would need a shot of cortisone if it happened again. That was that as far as Western medicine was concerned. Was there a pattern the more Eastern mind might uncover in these ailments that was not something it was imposing to gin up meanings and amuse itself? Energetic evidence, perhaps, of a swordfight three hundred years ago, a wound carried through incarnations? I swear, for years I have had the hard-to-describe sense of having less flow and vigor in my left arm than in the right, a deficit I feel goes beyond what might be expected from the dissimilarities of handedness. (Or does it? Disabled once by a broken right finger, I was forced to shave with my left hand for a month, and to sign checks, and to use my left arm in ways I never had before, and I don't remember once feeling this same weakness on the sinister side . . .)

The heart chakra that was diverting energy probably wasn't always closed, Michael Mamas said. Its condition reflected the way I had developed. But since from his point of view "all was chosen," the detour must be significant and intentional. It must have been created as a way of coping with the exigencies of feeling, a strategy for surviving, an energetic defense, and thus ultimately what we were talking about was a karmic problem, a life task to be worked out. In other words: I had performed a kind of subtle heart bypass on myself, which shunted the flow of "energy" around my heart. In other words: I did not *live* much in my heart, or let its presence suffuse my life, and any changes I was bound for, or could hope to make, would come out of engaging that fundamental fact.

4. HALF MOON BAY

I have been unpacking this story as if it were a steady progression toward a known end, one event following another in a shapely line, so that Monday's acorn became Tuesday's seedling and Sunday was implicit with the sweet deep shade of a grandfather oak. But of course this is the prescription for the illusioning poetics of Aristotle, who said narratives must unfold in linear rhythmic sequences comprising starts and middles and ends. Which is to say that how a story gets staged hasn't much to do with how it's lived. I would like to convey the impression that as I scampered up the chakras, I raised new insights and correspondingly new questions, and that each step I took and each choice I made emerged coherently from the one before and pointed ineluctably to the one ahead. It would be nice to say that at the heart chakra the past made way for the future in seemly fashion, and neat valentine lessons arrived just in time to produce the felicities of love. How little justice that would do to the way it actually was—to the tangled skeins of incident, to revelations delivered in revision, to the long dull stretches of unconsciousness that possess the gleam of latency in retrospect. The very idea of achieving wholeness by orderly piecemeal steps seems paradoxical. Wholeness is always present, or not at all; only the perception of it shifts.

In November 1995, I arranged to attend a week-long energy anatomy and physiology class for hands-on healers taught by Shelby Hammitt, a healer in her early fifties. My goals are easier to see now than they were at the time. Most obviously, I wanted to get a better handle on energy; I wanted to know what I was doing when I was trying to do whatever healers were doing when they said they were doing something. In this sense, the attraction of the class was akin to the attraction of piano lessons. More deeply, I wanted to undo the heart bypass that had sent me spiraling into middle age with the emotional maturity of a college freshman. It wasn't falling in love that was the problem, it was sustaining it. I was old enough to be a husband but still unwed; I was old enough to be a parent but still childless; I was old enough to love wisely and well and yet from some of the evidence it seemed there was more feeling in a left-ventricle-assist device than in my heart. And, of course, as in the example of the dry-eyed dictator who dispatches people to their death but weeps over a lost cat, the other side of such hard-heartedness is bathos, a crippling attachment to a sentimentalized past. I had framed my own confusions about pumps and valentines as part of the ancient schism of mind and body, but deep down I suppose it was no more than not wanting to live a dream-haunted life of regret and guilt. On many levels, there were bridges to build and marriages to make.

As for why I put myself in the hands of Shelby Hammitt, I could say that she had been described as one of the best healers in the country who still had a regular practice—she wasn't preoccupied with running schools or traveling all over the world. She was approachable. On those occasions when she did hold classes, such as her Anatomy and Physiology for Healers, she was well known for letting greenhorns put their hands on her back and arms as she worked so they could feel what she was doing, feel the kind of energy she was running. (It was sort of like Miles Davis letting a young trumpeter sit in with his band.) But these are all, well, *reasons*, and I don't think the decision was based on the faculty of reason, at least as it is conventionally construed. Heaven forfend it look as if I were following an intuition. And then there was the astonishing synchronicity of our socks . . .

When I flew to San Francisco and headed south in a rented car, I found I couldn't focus on the week ahead. The radio was full of distracting news about the CIA, which had spent $20 million on psychic research and had concluded that clairvoyants were accurate fifteen percent of the time. Even more distracting were the ups and downs of Micron Technology, an Idaho-based company that made random-access memory chips. I had been obsessively tracking the stock price of this one-time highflier, hoping to jump in at the bottom of its steep decline and ride a bungee rebound back to financial security, which was looming as a concern now that my judgment as a magazine writer had proved questionable. Micron, or MU on the New York Stock Exchange, had closed two days before at forty-eight dollars a share. My intuition, silent on so many other subjects, had shouted itself hoarse hollering "Buy! Buy! Buy!" But no, I didn't buy. And, of course, in that morning's paper I read that the accursed stock had rocketed up five bucks. I was swimming in rue. Why why why hadn't I listened to my intuition? Why did the wretched doubt factory of my head always get in the way? Even with a measly hundred shares, I could have covered the cost of Shelby Hammitt's healing class, alchemizing tuition from intuition in the crucible of Wall Street. The failure to heed the prompt of some inner knowing seemed grave and vast beyond the missed upsurge in MU, or the numerous examples of its converse—those times when no inner conviction warned me off financial turkeys. It seemed to point to a larger dereliction, a chronic inability to trust my gut sense of things, the folly of letting my head get in the way— bang! ow!—and proceeding blindly without those heartsome guides so esteemed in the healing community.

I swung west on Highway 92, a hairpinned, light-dappled road that climbed under canopies of eucalyptus and crested high in the coastal mountains. You come over that divide where the land tumbles toward the blue immensity of the Pacific, and catch the whiff of early morning mists dissolving in cypress and eucalyptus trees, and something breaks inside you; base preoccupations melt away.

Half Moon Bay Motor Lodge was set back on a bluff not far from the ocean. As I was early, I parked out front and found a table at the lodge's restaurant. I ordered what turned out to be a plate of prefab hash browns and eggs that tasted like a neoprene wet suit, and to kill time I began to wonder which of the people in the restaurant were healing students and which were just locals having a miserable breakfast. The long-haired guy in the purple fleece jacket? Maybe. The overweight man in the yellow aviator glasses? Doubtful. The bony, bright-looking woman in the red cotton blouse? Possibly. The heavy-set woman smoking in a black nylon jumpsuit? Very doubtful.

Generally speaking, in California you can get a sense of the hands-on healing culture from its practitioners' habits and preferred fabrics and favorite foods; certain beliefs about body and mind often are related to the degree of luminousness in the eyes. Black Nylon and Yellow Specs, I daresay, didn't have enough light in their eyes to be healers. But maybe Purple Fleece and Red Cotton had too much; maybe they were cult members or fitness nuts who owed their incandescence to overdoses of ginseng or stratospheric DHEA levels boosted by wild yam supplements. Is having not enough eye-light worse than having too much? Does having more make you a better person? Give you the authority to write your own story or set yourself up as a healer? Does it make you less likely to be one of fate's pawns? Surely Purple Fleece and Red Cotton thought they were steering, not drifting. And maybe Black Nylon and Yellow Specs would confess that things just happened to them, that they were just sort of drifting along. I felt somewhere in the middle: hoped not to be counted in the drifter's camp, whose pale-faced members seemed to think that they had no choice but to fork up ersatz eggs placidly, but not really qualified to be counted in the steering camp either. The steering camp was filled with fleecy create-your-own-reality people who believed the magic of "synchronicity" delivered whatever they needed in their lives, and that some tribunal of angels and guides and spiritual entities existed not only to match them up with their soul mates and help them summon subtle energies to treat disease, but to find them parking spaces right in front of the cineplex.

Surrender the hyper-vigilant observer mode? Not without a fight. But as Blake once said, to generalize is to be an idiot, and the results of my speculations were humbling. In the conference room at the lodge, people were trickling in and taking seats in a circle of chairs; none of my breakfast suspects was among them. A small table was set with the usual hodgepodge of totems that spoke to the eclectic spirituality and idiosyncratic rituals of healers: flowers, a snakeskin rattle, framed pictures of the Indian holy woman Gurumai and the healer Rosalyn Bruyere. Shelby Hammitt came in and took a seat at the top of the circle and hooked up a small microphone. The room quieted down. At the back of the room, fellow healer Susan Brown, who was assisting Hammitt, switched on a tape machine. Hammitt closed her eyes for a moment, and when she opened them she seemed to reach around the room.

"Hello," she said.

She was dressed in a loose purple blouse and matching pants that allowed her to sit with her legs open in a meditation pose meant to keep the energy flowing freely through the first chakra. Her eyes were a penetrating blue-violet color. Her gray hair was pulled back in a ponytail. There was a faintly hawkish cast about her face that seemed to bespeak focus and attention to detail: As I got to know her, I associated the expression with an economy of being, a hard-won simplicity all the more impressive for being born of struggle. She sipped from a big cup of diet Coke—she was gripped by a most unenlightened addiction to the stuff. Her hands were incongruously small—soft and pink and fleshy like the hands of an adolescent girl—but their size belied their strength and mysterious ability.

There were thirty-five of us in the class. We went around the circle introducing ourselves and offering up brief bits of background. Some of the student healers had come from as far as Germany and Switzerland. Only five were men, all of them with serious eye luminosity; I recalled something I'd read in an acupuncture textbook once, a Sinhala aphorism from 500 B.C.: "If you cannot be the king, be a healer."

Most of the women were in their thirties or forties; some looked as if they had been steering for years, and some looked as if they had been drifting and were very tired of it, tired of things not going right, tired of

their no-account husbands, of experiences they couldn't share with anyone, of sensations that made them wonder if they were crazy. To the
extent that delving into the anatomy and physiology of the body's energy
was a kind of inner empiricism—a set of skills, a spiritual training, a philosophy of knowledge that fortified the self by aligning it with luck and
fate and metaphysical proceedings—maybe the class did promise to help
them get their hands on the rudder. All the quavering and doubt at the
outset was oddly reassuring to me. Even healers sometimes wondered if
what they did was nuts:

"I'm afraid when I'm healing that it's all a dream, that's it's not real."

"I know when I have my hands on someone that I'm in the body,
but I don't know exactly where I am."

"I have a lot of fears about the physical and emotional incursion."

Hammitt nodded, drew conversations out, and where possible connected them to what she declared would be the theme for the week. "The
big question for this class is why do we have to be here on this plane, in
this life," she said. "As healers we try to experience realms that aren't
physical, but the various layers of the energy field, the various realms, the
various energy bodies, are all right here—wherever here is."

In the parlance, Hammitt carried a big field: She could hold a lot of
energy. So much, in fact, that she claimed she often inadvertently demag-
netized her bank and credit cards. Though she lived in Los Angeles, most
of her healing practice was based in New York, and when she rode the
subway, she liked to play with her energy, and sometimes tried to see if
she could energetically induce people sitting across from her to scratch
their noses. Her field was not always so mischievously inclined or that
strong. Her own background described the archetypal story of the
"wounded healer" who makes her way through a wilderness of breakdowns and bad scenes in search of a new and deeper awareness, forging
a new self from the ruins of the old. Hammitt had grown up in Rye, New
York, in a privileged family, and had attended private schools, and college
in Boston in the 1960s. She wanted to be a doctor, but she suffered from
attention deficit disorder and bouts of severe depression. In her early
twenties, she fell into an abusive relationship with a drug-addicted jazz
musician and found herself living a marginal life amid the squalor and
violence of Harlem. She spent a year in "the loony bin," as she put it.

Two marriages ended in divorce. She bore two sons and raised them without much help. Both were now teenagers.

The foundation of Hammitt's healing work had been laid under the guidance of Rosalyn Bruyere, who had also been one of Barbara Brennan's teachers. Hammitt began studying with Bruyere in 1983. Unlike students at the Brennan School who graduated after their training, students completing the program at Bruyere's Healing Light Center Church are ordained. Light Center healers had taken part in research projects, notably a wound-healing experiment by California-based researcher Daniel Wirth, which was one of the few replications of Bernard Grad's work, and the only one in which the wounds were inflicted on human volunteers rather than mice. (The results confirmed Grad's findings.) For a number of years, Bruyere herself had participated as one of nine so-called world-class healers in experiments at the Menninger Institute in Topeka, Kansas, run by Elmer Green, the father of biofeedback. After reading about Buddhist monks who enhanced their energy sensitivity by meditating in front of copper walls while seated on stools insulated from ground currents by glass bowls, Green built a copper-walled laboratory known as a *mu* room (*mu* and MU: synchronicity alert!). He had wired Bruyere and other healers up to highly sensitive instruments that measured changes in brain states and electromagnetic fields. One of his findings was that healers show different brainwave tendencies. Most people exhibit delta waves, which are associated with creativity, only in deep sleep. Green discovered that Bruyere can run delta fully awake for several hours a day.

Hammitt had been ordained a minister in Bruyere's church in 1988. But she still had some of that "healthy skepticism" Barbara Brennan had alluded to, and acknowledged the possibility that her beliefs were as liable to be a part of maya—the realm of illusion—as anyone else's. Where younger and more impressionable healers sometimes got snared in the glamour of psychic adventures and seemed loath to question the validity of subjective experience, Hammitt went out of her way to maintain a casual and undramatizing attitude toward convention-shattering phenomena. She seemed to me from the very start to be approachable and down-to-earth, uninterested in wowing people. It wouldn't serve her purposes as a healer to boggle clients with stuff they couldn't handle or freak them out with concepts they had no means of integrating.

"I'll be giving you assignments to help you all lose your minds this week," she was saying now. "We'll be traveling the Way of Disorientation. Your nervous systems get accustomed to habitual responses, and with the habits comes unconsciousness. There are parts of your mind you don't have access to because you've become unconscious. One of the things you can do right away is change hands—brush your teeth, comb your hair, hold your fork with the hand you don't normally use. What we're looking for are ways to open up the energy field, deeper ways of letting new experience in."

The way of disorientation was like the truck-is-a-trumpet improvisation exercise. As with the word games, the purpose was to defamiliarize the commonplace, strip away old routines and ingrained patterns, and reinfuse the world with its forgotten freshness. Changing hands was only one of the discombobulating tricks. Sometimes Hammitt wore socks whose colors didn't match. As did I, but out of sloth, not calculation. The first time I met her, she was wearing a red sock on one foot and a purple sock on the other, and by some light-of-the-lily coincidence, I was too. Synchronicity in excelsis!

But adding disorientation seemed almost unfair, given how disoriented any greenhorn was likely to be already. Next to the veterans in the class, I was handicapped by primitive energy-sensing abilities, not to mention lingering chronic misgivings about the premises of the whole business. The course was designed for sophisticated healing students who needed to satisfy anatomy and physiology requirements to graduate from various healing schools. The work was unsettlingly far from the rigorous but conventional anatomy and physiology instruction you'd find at a university. No formaldehyde science, no textbooks of irrefutable truth. We were supposed to be coloring in diagrams from the Anatomy Coloring Book, a kind of interactive textbook widely used in medical schools. But the heart of the work was in real time, hands-on; we would learn the energy signatures of body tissues and organs— the anatomy of tuning in, not the anatomy of cutting open. The dynamic anatomy of living tissue, not the static anatomy of dead. Our tools were hands, not scalpels.

On the second day of class, Hammitt taught the group to do what she called a spinal expansion. She went over the steps. We were to generate "matrix energy" of any color or frequency, then juice up the disks in the spine, energetically connect to the cerebrospinal fluid and the sacrum, attune to the pulse, and gently feed energy into the skull joints. She had already had the class trying to feel and—perhaps the more difficult task—describe the various layers of bone tissue. The periosteum, in Hammitt's experience, often had a cool slippery texture; the cancellus was dry and shardlike; the marrow juicy, sort of like lava, rumbling with a rough red guttural quality, like a motorcycle, a big chugging Harley Davidson hog. Hammitt demonstrated the technique on Cynthia Reynolds, a student from San Francisco, who had recently been in a car accident. Once she started, Hammitt quickly identified an area where compression in the spine had backed the cerebrospinal fluid up into the fourth ventricle of the brain. Her aim now was to open that compressed area and restore the unimpeded flow of the fluid. It took about an hour, and when Cynthia got off the table, she looked transformed. How to put it? There was more of her in her eyes.

The class divided into groups of three: Guinea pigs lay down on one of the dozen tables; one student stood in support at the feet of the person being healed, and the designated healer proceeded with the spinal expansion. When it was my turn to put my hands on a fellow student's back, Hammitt sidled over. She watched with an assessing eye for a moment, then eased her hand onto my shoulder. She had said that she was most effective not talking about her work but teaching via "direct transmission"—which is to say she could accomplish the most by letting students experience the "frequencies" she was generating, the vibrations, the energies, the sound, the light, the God-knows-what that she had developed and found useful in her practice. I would say she was like a vocal coach teaching pupils how to sing. Within seconds of her settling her hand on my shoulder, I could feel her influence. It was startlingly distinct. Where before I'd been like a little boat dawdling along with its spinnaker luffing, suddenly there was a sharp snap, and a strong gust of fresh wind bellied the sail taut, and the vessel surged forward . . .

But how were you supposed to generate these energies in the first place? How were you supposed to pinpoint and maintain specific frequencies? The question seemed not to have an answer other than that generating energies is just one of the abilities of a human being, as second nature to life as generating the notes of a song is to the throat. Making energy—channeling it, focusing it, sailing it, using it—was no more or no less mysterious than the agency that allows us to sing. It was having to translate these vibrations into the do-re-mi of language that introduced the headaches. How did you describe what perhaps could be conveyed only by experience? You had to trust in what Hammitt kept calling "conjoint reality"—you had to believe that you were picking up the same stuff as the next person, sharing the same understanding, an understanding of a phenomenon that was deeper than any intellectual conception of it, the same unsaid unsayable understanding at the heart of existentialism.

Oh, how maddening it is to try to do justice to this stuff in words! It seemed to me that energy in the body—to the degree that it could be sensed and distinguished immediately without years of training—could no more be corralled in language than the essence of a smell. No wonder the Chinese had such trouble capturing the variations of the pulse, grasping at metaphors like shipwrecked sailors at any passing log or floating chest. When I thought I had tuned in to the marrow and was somehow sensing the core of the bone in one of my fellow student's femurs, I got the impression of a drunk stumbling through wind chimes, an image that could be useful only to me, an image that, unlike the number on a radio dial, could not help anyone else find the station broadcasting from the femur. The continual struggle to translate the ineffable into language knotted Hammitt's forehead and balled up her sentences. I look back at my notes from that week and find my own hermetic descriptions and am hard-pressed to know now what they mean: The trauma in Cynthia's back felt like when you go from a paved road to gravel. Cancer felt like dancing in a mosh pit. The voice of the liver was like a cassette playing too slowly in a Walkman with rundown batteries. The pancreas had an agile, hyper feeling. Lymph nodes felt like a humid wind blowing over small grapes.

"Every cell in the body has a sound, even the molecules," Shelby had said. "You can work with the DNA by tapping in to the resonance of the molecule. As you expand the number of frequencies your nervous system can hang out in, you increase the possibility of using all your high senses—kinesthetic, visual, auditory."

But what did healers actually do? someone asked.

"They create a flow of energy," Hammitt said, "and an environment in which the actual healing takes place. We're just facilitators."

"So why bother to actively restructure chakras if healing can be accomplished by just sitting with the cerebrospinal fluid?"

"Good question," Hammitt replied, and said nothing else.

Because it didn't seem like an answer and I suspected there might be some method to her silence, I asked if she were letting the question hang out there like a pair of unmatched socks in order to thwart the rational process and thus facilitate the Way of Disorientation.

"No, I mean it; it is a good question," she said. "And I don't want to put my foot in my mouth. I've given up textbook answers. Healing is a living thing. Asking the right questions can set things in motion, but imposing the wrong framework can shut things down."

That first day, in which she had demonstrated the Spinal Expansion, Hammitt said that all of us together would be building the energy of the class and that it was very important to pay attention to this cultivation. Each of our fields would be getting bigger and more sensitive in the course of the week; we had to be aware of where we walked and how we went in and out of the conference room, had to be careful not to pull our hands too quickly out of someone's field when we were working on them. Much later, someone asked me why, and the only explanation I could think of was that pulling your hand away too fast was as palpably raw and unsettling as hanging up the phone after a long talk without saying good-bye. Some ceremony of departure is wanted. Hammitt gave us dream assignments. We were to request a dream from our bones the first night, and a dream from whatever community was formed by the pancreas and the liver the next.

After two days, I was beginning to mark changes in my own "energy field." I could hardly feel it at all in the morning after swimming in the hotel's chlorinated pool, but by evening, after the long concentrated hours of standing in silence, holding feet, holding legs, holding flanks and heads and arms and settling my hands on the chakras of the torso, I could point my right hand at my own left thumb, which was still restricted after being jammed in a basketball game, and I could feel the force of my fingers wedging into the joint like a needle. It was too obvious to dispute, and too much of a commonplace even to get worked up about, but exhilarating nonetheless, like being on a bicycle and rolling for the first time.

Maybe training a professional healer ought to be considered on par with training a highly skilled athlete. Think of the years it took Michael Jordan to educate his body, to go from a toddler who could hardly walk to the slashing, darting, leaping whippet- and leopard-like champion— thousands and thousands of hours of practice and play, of drill and study, native ability realized through brutal work. Mastering energy might be no different than mastering any performance, singing, painting, writing, doctoring. It is not a matter of drenching yourself in information but of patiently over the years imbuing the hand with some incommunicable wisdom.

And when Hammitt showed us a frequency which in her view was a vibe that could help oxygenate tissue, I had for the first time a sense that I knew what I was doing—not in any rational way, but rather in the way of speaking a language when you are nine or ten years old, with no conscious knowledge of how to use the word "mores" but it pops out of your mouth in a sentence anyway. How could anyone make oxygen with their hands? I don't know. I don't even know if I was making oxygen or nitrogen or methane, but when I put my hand on Shelby's back while she demonstrated what she had found to be a useful frequency that appeared to have the effect of perfusing the tissues with oxygen, a strong, sharp, crystalline image of a drizzly wet-cypress-tree morning welled up out of nowhere, and the idea occurred to me that I could summon up that image and then just let my hands go with it, in effect let my hands rain, and that if I let my hands rain, I would be doing whatever it was that Shelby was doing when she was making oxygen. I extended my arms and tried to let my hands rain, thinking perhaps that it was only folly that was reigning. "Shelby," I said. "Can you tell me if this is right?" I put my hands on her hands and let them rain, and she looked a little shocked and said, "That's it."

So we all went, deeper into the disorienting garden. Friday morning we stood in a circle, and Shelby said a prayer for the father of one of the students who had not waked up after surgery—he had a coronary bypass like Mrs. Denadio, and a heart valve replacement to boot. "Grandfather, Grandmother, Powers of the Four Directions . . ." Shelby said. A fly buzzed loudly around the center of the circle. Micron Technology had slid back five-eighths, but never did the fervor seem so trivial, so far away. I did not quite understand the technique of requesting dreams on the liver/pancreas themes, but that night I found myself on some island in the arctic, ringed by ice floes. I was making a movie with a hand-held camera but hadn't mastered the zoom lens and so was zooming erratically. Past the thin margin of grass and soil lay great floes and sheets of sea ice, ice heaped and jumbled, and shining brilliantly under the sun; gaps were opening in the ice; meltwater was running everywhere. A woman was sitting by the ocean like an umpire in a chair at a tennis match, but the chair she was sitting on seemed to be made of frozen menstrual blood, and was not long for the world. "Look!" she commanded, pointing to the south. Mount Everest towered on the horizon. She referred to it by its Tibetan name, Chomolungma, "Mother Goddess of the World." It was terribly foreshortened, austere, wreathed in mist and blindingly white where the sky was clear, and it seemed to me a kind of revelation of some terrible truce between the physical and the spiritual. Nowhere else on earth could you be so grounded and so ethereal at once.

We had probed the bones, the spine, the lymph, the liver, the pancreas, and the lungs. On the last day, the most extraordinary of the week, we turned to the heart. All week I had felt myself making a turtle's progress, marking some new abilities and a willingness to entertain heretical beliefs, but never completely free of doubt. Sometimes trying to discriminate among the layers of a tissue, trying to detect the tip of the pancreas and the kidney, trying to flush out the liver with some enigmatic purgative made of magnetism or heat or whatever vital forces of matter and spirit enlivened the hand seemed to require a level of imagination or sensitivity or credulity I was not capable of. Reach blindly into a bowl of cooked DeCecco pasta and tell me you can ascertain whether it's Linguine No. 7 or Linguine No. 8. People solemnly crowded around Shelby like piglets, trying to get into their hands the feel of what she was doing. During one of the discussions, I was hissed for suggesting that maybe sometimes healers used the concept of karma to excuse their failures—saying there was nothing they could do because the illness was in the person's karma. What surgeon who had botched a bypass could get away with telling the relatives that the patient's death was "God's will"?

But then we came to the heart, and the method in the madness was not hard to see. The week of field-building, the emphasis on the etiquette of connecting and disconnecting made sense. Our purpose was nothing more than to explore the heart. Shelby began by demonstrating on one of the women, Sue O'Neill. One table in the middle of the room: the lot of us gathered round, taking care to move gingerly, conscious of the gathered presences. I can say that the mood shifted profoundly; an air of sacredness came on like evening, a stealthy yet immense possession. Shelby first cupped her hands over Sue's chest, fashioning in miniature the *temenos* (the Greek word for "sacred space") she had worked hard to construct over the past week in our conference room at Half Moon Bay. And then, as she told us in a quiet voice that seemed to float out of her, she allowed her energy, her current, the life in her hands, to sink through Sue's chest and down into the heart muscle, taking note of the tissue and the chambers. The quality of her energy was like velvet, but the fine points of her technique were lost on me as I found myself swept up in a rush of emotions, joy surging so intensely I scarcely knew what to do with it. I began to smile as if I'd won some great prize. I started to giggle and then gulped back some guffaws and desperately tried to restrain the urge to collapse in a cackling roar. I didn't have room for this flood of happiness. The laughter was all the more amazing for being completely inexplicable—no one was saying anything funny, no one was saying anything at all, and here I was about to die from trying to stifle myself. It was contagious too, it started to spill over, clowns kept coming out of the kiddie car. I looked over at Colette Martin, a student from New Mexico who had sold her house to pay for her tuition to the Brennan School, and when she caught my eye she began to sputter and shake too, and that tripped off Danielle, a French-Canadian student and healer who was dressed in a violet suede jacket. What was this ecstasy rippling through the room, pulsing from what seemed to be nothing more than a good strong bond between Shelby's hands and the center of Sue's chest? Joy welled up, wave after wave. Shelby invited us to lay our hands on hers, but scolded people who moved too quickly, oblivious of the energy, of the expanded state of Sue and Shelby together. I edged my hand in. The muddy currents of the liver, the manic feeling of the pancreas, the rainforestlike quality of the lungs—all seemed straightforward compared to the textures of Sue's heart.

When it was our turn to have a go, I teamed up with Colette and

Danielle, the clown gang, giddy with the pleasure of trying not to laugh in church. Colette lay on the table first, Danielle held her feet, and I approached her heart. Oddly, it was easier to sense activity with my hand above her chest than with my hand directly on the skin. Maybe it was some vestigial connotation of sex getting in the way; I had to shift my hand awkwardly between her breasts. Per instructions, I tried to let my energy sink in, seeing if I could distinguish the sternum from the heart muscle beneath it, and as Shelby had, find the ventricles and valves. The value of the exercise as an anatomy lesson was suddenly eclipsed when Colette began to weep. The skin around her eyes bunched up and tears flowed. Having my hands on—or evidently in—her heart elicited strong emotions in her, she said.

"Can you feel me in your heart?"

"Yes," she said.

Still with her eyes closed and evidently awash in sorrow and heartache, she said that she had only known a total openness of the heart once in her life. More than anything, she wanted to achieve that state again, but she was too frightened to risk it.

"I want what's inside my heart to be on the outside," she said, her face glistening with tears.

I was not about to start weeping—*too many years of hardboiled voices telling me "Turn off the waterworks!"*—but I felt a compassion for her, and an intimacy that was as intense as sex, sex without jungle frenzy, only the exquisite tenderness. As I was to learn when I was on the table, it was more moving for me to be the one making the connection than to be the recipient of it. I was able to raise my hands above Colette's chest and still maintain from both our points of view the intercourse between us. Now my hands were a foot above her body, but I still felt them to be deeply connected to her—her what? Her heart? Her essence? Her emotional dopp kit? Or maybe it was what everybody in the room from Shelby and her assistant Susan Brown on down would say it was: the heart chakra. In different schools and traditions you found different chakra locations. But what about all the chakra discrepancies and contradictions? What kind of anatomy and physiology class couldn't agree whether the first chakra hung between the legs like a downward-facing funnel or was set perpendicular to the midline of the body? Shelby chalked such discrepancies up to the paradoxes at the heart of healing, but you could be forgiven if you were dyspeptically reminded of the caption E. B. White once wrote under a cartoon of a kid frowning over a plate of vegetables: "I say it's spinach, and I say the hell with it." If thousands of years of clairvoyant sages and saints and all-seeing know-it-alls and super-omniscient prophets can't settle on the whereabouts of the first chakra, why shouldn't the rest of us dismiss the whole business? Why shouldn't the rest of us take after Dayānand Sarasvatī and reform ourselves?

I would have liked Dayānand to have felt what I could feel with my hands now two and a half feet over Colette's body, and to have experienced the same weird urge I had to move my fingers as if they were entangled in a cat's cradle of fine thread. For the record, I was still exploring, mapping the territory; I was not functioning in the capacity of a healer. I could feel a funnel-shaped area above her heart where the air had definite density and texture. Could I be more vague? Certainly. It seemed that I was no longer inside the heart that could be hooked up to a bypass machine, but it was an organ nonetheless. Emotional, not physical. It did not pump or beat or bleed. It broke and ached and loved. It was easily denied, but its essence was undeniable. Now my hands, my presence, were touching some part of it, sharing some of Colette's life. And something wanted to be done. My fingers were doing it. I didn't have to do it. My job, if you could call it that, was to keep up a stream of chatter about how embarrassed I felt to be mimicking the goofy-looking finger-twiddling abracadabra stuff that it sometimes seemed healers did because they needed to look busy. But does a child who can't talk quarrel with the process of mimicry? Don't we learn language by mimicking incomprehensible sounds? Science is a social consensus forged of observations and falsifiable hypotheses. Here was a social consensus forged of empirical observations made by people who were confirming their findings with each other. Their hypothesis could not be falsified, but did that make the whole enterprise any less rational, especially given that it seemed to be a skill or sensitivity that could be learned? I'll venture to say my hands had fastened on to some micron technology known only to them, off-limits to my rational understanding. Either that or they had had a nervous breakdown and were semaphoring pure gibberish. But it felt right to move my fingers in the air above Colette's heart. It felt right.

5. WHITE WORLD WITH A COW

On the plane east, I could still feel Colette's heart in my hands. A couple of brokers in the row ahead of me were talking about a stock they were dying to buy but were damned if they were going to pay more than nine dollars a share for. They kept punching it up on their screens, and dangling buy offers. They couldn't get over the fact that nobody had bitten. Nobody would part with the stuff; it was the damnedest thing. Getting that stock for nine dollars a share was their whole reason for being. I studied them carefully because they seemed the product of some ghastly modern cloning experiment in which the heads of donkeys had been affixed to the bodies of men.

Over the course of the next year, Micron Technology resumed its descent, sinking downward to darkness on extended wings. Maybe my intuition had been operating after all, taking the long view in eschewing that pigeon. That year, Shelby Hammitt traveled to India and in the presence of the Indian holy man Sai Baba had what amounted to an epiphany. To some, Sri Satya Sai Baba, who claims to be the reincarnation of Sai Baba of Shirdi, who died in 1916, is a magician and a fraud; to others, an avatar. After her encounter with him, Hammitt felt her abilities deepen in ways that almost mocked the hard work and incremental progress she'd made in eighteen years of energy healing. "Sai Baba had the biggest energy field I have ever seen," she said. "His body was like a drop of water in an iceberg. It seemed to me he encompassed all frequencies that have ever been or ever will be. I could feel that he constituted this place that was at the center of the universe. All things were connected to him, and with each of his movements, everything moved. After Sai Baba, my own frequencies changed so much I didn't have the access to my normal guides, but I felt I had almost routine access to transcendent energy states."

About a year after the class at Half Moon Bay, I enrolled in the second part of Hammitt's Anatomy and Physiology course. I was drawn by the continuing promise of discovery, the lure that pulls the fly fisherman up the river from bend to bend. The course was held at a Holiday Inn about forty-five minutes north of Manhattan, on the far side of the Hudson. The parking lot was being repaved, and now and then, our meeting room reeked of fresh tar. I rented a car and zipped up against the tide of commuters each morning, and back home each night, late on the empty roads. In a few days, coached and checked and confirmed by Shelby, I was able to regain what seemed the level of sensitivity I had attained at Half Moon Bay. It was as if there were some muscle memory in my hands. I let them drop onto a fellow student's abdomen as gently as a pair of maple leaves descending to a pond, and then tried to sense down through the cotton jeans and through the body tissue to what seemed the distinct signal of the ovaries, a signal that emerged like a satellite transmission from a background of interstellar noise and formed the image of a fragile silk envelope full of caviar. I moved up to the adrenal glands and repeated the process and this time got a wiry, hyperactive sense that seemed to me like a mouse writhing in a sock. So I began to construct a primitive vocabulary: ovaries equal caviar, adrenals are ensocked mice. We were focused on the endocrine system, and we often worked in groups; one of my partners kept seeing flashes of lightning every time she made the connection with the target gland. I was astonished to discover that it was easier to pinpoint the energy of someone else's pituitary gland if I located the energy of my own first. All the while I had to rely on Shelby to confirm what was what—that's the pituitary you've got there, that's the thymus, and so forth. Learning these correlations that presumably related a gland to a signature of energy and sometimes even an image were part of learning the healer's language; they were the basic vocabulary and grammar of the hand, and the process seemed akin to the association Helen Keller made between the cool splashing wet stuff and the sign for *water* tapped out in her palm. Did I really have my hands energetically connected to the pituitary gland? I can't pretend to let on that I could detect the difference between the pituitary and the lateral geniculate nucleus, any more than a city person on the shore of the Bering Sea in winter can discriminate which of the two dozen kinds of snow he is standing on.

At the end of the last day, an evangelical group began to move in for a revival in the room behind the accordion wall of the space where we had been working all week. During Shelby's closing prayer—"Grandfather, Grandmother, Powers of the Four Directions . . ."—the piano player began rehearsing the hymn "How Great Thou Art." And at the stroke of four, the wall was retracted, shattering the feeling of sacred intimacy that had attended our room. A squadron of Christian frontmen descended with boxes of Bibles and tapes and began dismantling our circle of folding chairs and rearranging the seats into orderly rows. Some of the Christian workers looked uneasily at the little altar Shelby had maintained during the week, a table set with pictures of Sai Baba and Muktananada and, one of her teaching tools, a five-hundred-dollar plastic demo brain with seventeen ready-for-disassembling pieces. Were we satanists? Even the pianist rehearsing "How Great Thou Art" seemed leery, and pushed the hymn up a key.

A couple of months later, in December, Hammitt invited me to sit in on a day-long session of healing and teaching with three young healers, Mike, Susan, and Steve. They all were in training at the Brennan School; they had decided to pool their money to buy a day of Shelby's time for the chance to have her work on them and the chance to learn from watching her work on each of them. They were gracious enough to let me sit in. Shelby had set up her healing table in a large room at The Right Space (or TRS), a midtown Manhattan studio that rents space to a variety of alternative medical practitioners. On a shelf she had set up the same altar, minus the brain, that had weirded out the evangelical Christians.

The day began at midmorning and lasted nearly twelve hours. Mike was the first to lie down on the table. Susan went second; Steve last. All the healings were instructive, but Steve's was extraordinary—one of the most extraordinary sessions I have ever witnessed.

What I knew about him was what I had seen him do or heard him say. He was from a small rural town in New England. He had rough-textured skin and pale blue eyes like those of a Siberian husky. He was carrying too much weight and was in some emotional distress. He had been talking earlier about his ex-wife's taking his kids on a trip that he had wanted to take them on. He had a bad pain in his neck. He was constantly stretching his spine, trying to get comfortable.

He seemed to have a tremendous healing ability and to know his way around the subtle world. He could see and track energy as if it were child's play, as easy as riding a bike. But there was also a kind of obliviousness about him: he moved abruptly, and bustled around, and didn't attend as closely to the other people in the room as he might have. When Susan and Mike were trying to stay alert and "hold" the energy in the room, Steve closed his eyes. It looked as if he had nodded off. Understandable— Shelby's healing sessions sometimes lasted two or three hours, and to sit through three of them would exhaust anyone. When Susan was on the table, Steve did not wait to be invited to make an assessment, but put his hand into her field and briskly said, "C one is leaking," meaning the first chakra was losing energy.

His turn came. While Shelby was standing at one end of the table, Steve walked like an automaton to the other end and fluffed the pillow.

"Why did you do that?" she asked.

"I was just helping prepare the table," he said.

She didn't want to criticize him, but she did want him to be aware that she was trying to set the energy of the table and he had just disturbed it.

I was wondering what could be inferred from his style, which suggested that he was used to doing things without asking, used to taking action. I notice that when he scanned Mike's or Sue's energy field with his hand, he did not seem like a passive receiver, plucking what signals were in the air, but rather more like a radar dome, aggressively looking for the echoes of the blips he was broadcasting. Shelby had marked the same thing and gently suggested to him that there might be too much of his presence in his energy when he scanned. Too much "Steve" in Steve, she said. In some other setting, I suppose it would have sounded entirely paradoxical, but in this one it made sense.

Shelby wound a colored pillowcase around the face cradle (a part of all healing tables), and Steve climbed onto the table. He knew exactly what his problems were and reported them with a deft command of the energy lexicon.

"The bursa in the left foot is related to kundalini and self-development," he said. I wasn't exactly clear what this meant, but I'd read elsewhere that kundalini awakenings sometimes entailed discharges of energy that went rocketing not only up the spine but also down the legs, so much energy that sometimes the novice's big toenail turned black and fell off.

"The heart release point under the right scapula is connected to the pain in the occiput," Steve said. He couldn't put any weight on his left wrist either.

We had had to switch rooms, and the new room was much smaller than the one we'd been in for most of the day. I sat close by, near Steve's head. He joked that by sitting so close to him I might end up "plastered against the wall" by his energy. He was lying on his stomach, face planted in the padded cradle. Shelby placed her small hands on his heels, trying to soften the tissue. She could sense what was going on in his body; the heels, like the palms and the ears, were considered to contain a kind of holographic summary of the whole body's condition.

"There's part of you that's reached around the front and is down here watching what I'm doing," Shelby said.

"I can't fool you, can I?" said Steve, his voice somewhat muffled by the cradle. "That's exactly what I'm doing."

"See if you can watch from the inside," Shelby said. "You use your tracking ability to watch, but it's disconnected from your body. It's not that you leave your body, but that some part of you extends outward rather than remaining inside."

"Are you diagnosing, Shelby?" Susan asked.

"Healers aren't allowed to diagnose," she replied, laughing at the absurdity of it. At that moment, it seemed she could understand on a level unfathomably deeper than conventional medicine what illness was, could understand illness in a way that made conventional doctors seem like curators who couldn't figure how to get inside the museum. Susan asked about starting at the feet.

"The feet are a way of accessing the whole body," Shelby said.

"Do you read the person's connection to the earth?" Susan asked.

"I suppose—it's not something I generally focus on. You can be grounded in any position. We're on the eleventh floor."

Steve was sighing and breathing heavily.

I was thinking about Steve's way of running energy without running it through his body. I had given up trying to make rational sense of how you could be located energetically somewhere other than where you were located physically. It was boggling but no more so than how "I" was able to initiate the movements that produce this sentence on the keyboard of my laptop. The possibility that Steve could run energy outside his body lent credence to Cartesian dualism. Brain researchers maintained that consciousness comes from gray matter and is inseparably fused with it, but in the cosmology of healers, an encephalitic child born without a brain can have a spirit, a soul, even a consciousness, though obviously not the sort that can speculate on its own nature over a glass of pinot grigio.

"Your way of running energy feels like a way of developing a sense of safety without getting too close. When you get pain in your foot, where do you feel it?"

"The front of the joint," Steve said.

"I don't know if you're aware that it corresponds to the place on the back of your neck."

She shifted to his right heel.

"Hmmmmm, very different," she said.

"What?"

"Your heels."

She was palpating with energy, feeling her way from the heel up the back of Steve's calf.

"I just got an image of the whole back of your body. It's like part of your body is living in another time. Your right knee is in childhood around age four, your left hip is in some other lifetime—well, no, it isn't that." She concentrated, then took another crack at it. "You have put parts of yourself in other places. They're in other realms. They're not even here at all. Does that make sense?"

It made sense to Steve.

It made sense to me too, in that it seemed to explain Steve's mantle of self-absorption. When he made a connection, it was on his own terms; he seemed to forgo the subtle protocols that are usually negotiated and agreed upon before people, like telephone modems, will exchange information. Steve just dialed in and grabbed data without fussing with boundaries, protocols, the etiquette of the subtle world.

"Your heel is somewhere else too . . . southwest astral? That's the only way I can describe it."

She sounded apologetic for being so vague. I had never before heard points of the compass applied to the astral plane, that multilayered dimension of consciousness best (but inadequately) described as the state we experience during dreaming, especially during the kind of dreaming in which one is able to function with a measure of self-awareness inside the dream—"lucid dreaming" it's called. It goes without saying that astral-plane reality must be experienced to be known, and that any exegesis that tries to make sense of it according to the terms of the ordinary waking mind misunderstands its properties. In the astral world, the energy of thoughts create structures known as thought-forms. Phobias assume the shape of demons, and battles are waged between the forces of light and the forces of evil, or negativity. Or so it's said. I learned later that at a young age Steve had been sworn into a mystical brotherhood that considered itself thousands of years old, a brotherhood dedicated to helping people besieged by dark astral forces. His study of martial arts in the physical plane reflected his life as a warrior on the astral one, a warrior who had taken a brotherhood oath to fight the various demons and malevolent bodies that dwelled in certain parts of the astral world. He'd been a warrior for years, and what was unfolding that evening in midtown Manhattan was not just an unusually conversational healing that provided a window into the energetic aspects of the transaction, but an initiation.

"I'm on the astral plane too much—every night," said Steve. His breathing was somewhat labored. He seemed to be struggling with something. "I get called every night to do stuff."

"If you go out of your body too often without sufficient grounding in this realm, over time there'll be a degradation of your field," Shelby said. She reached for another analogy and came up with one from the new *Star Trek* movie—she could thank her thirteen-year-old son, Josh, for analogies based on television shows and computer games. "If you beam someone through the transporter too many times, they'll degrade. You need to take more time between trips. It's important to say no—you may get called; you don't have to go."

"I took an oath," Steve said. "I'm supposed to."

"I don't believe there's an oath that requires someone to sacrifice himself for doing the work the way you are—at least not an oath that comes from the good guys. Maybe you could take a sabbatical."

She had moved up his leg and now had both hands on his sacrum. Her eyes were closed.

"I'm going back to my old life; I'm going to a place where I have respite from these duties," Steve said.

"Is there a reason why you can't do it now?"

"Yes."

"If you could, would you go there now?"

"Yes."

"Okay."

Shelby was silent for a moment—her emotional pitch had changed, and the mood in the little room had changed with it. I could see Susan and Mike sitting against the opposite wall. Steve had stopped sighing. A strange silence had settled over our *temenos*.

Shelby took a deep breath.

"There's someone here who'll take you there now if you want. He's a guide, I guess, or an acolyte. It's his job. He'll take you. I'm unclear where, it's a guy thing." Suddenly she laughed, a mix of amusement and helplessness. "I don't know where it is."

Shelby had a habit of saying "be in the place of" (as in, "it's about being in the place of that knowing . . ."), a turn of speech that always seemed needlessly wordy and clichéd to me. But I was realizing now it was simply the most direct way she could express what was a literal place, as actual as any location at any set of terrestrial coordinates. She was 42 degrees 14 minutes north, 102 degrees west.

And Steve seemed to know exactly what she was talking about.

"White world with a cow?" he said.

"Ah, yeah," Shelby said.

White world with a cow? Did I hear that right? What the hell was that? A bucolic winter scene from Currier and Ives? A lost manifesto of apartheid agriculture? Even stranger was how valuable Steve seemed all of a sudden, how richly, touchingly, importantly, fully human he seemed, moving in his hardship, his commitment to some occult nightly service unknown to the rest of us, and moving in his possible delusion, or was it his deep sanity . . . It occurred to me then that any account of what was happening could not do justice to the transaction. I was divided myself, the impulse to weep vying with the impulse to laugh for the joy surging again. Wanting to laugh perhaps because I felt so much. Oy, the waterworks. Send in the clowns! Steve seemed to be crying; I heard what I thought were tears dropping through the face cradle to the gray carpet.

"Shelby, can you talk about what's going on?" asked Susan.

"Ah . . . In a minute," she said.

More time passed. Her hands seemed unalterably fixed to the area of his sacrum, under the back of his gray elastic-waistband pants.

"His sacrum is one of the shields of the brotherhood he belongs to," she said at length. "It feels like it's being . . . 'reconsecrated' is the word that comes to mind."

"Can you see him or hear what he said, or was that just for me?" Steve said.

"That was just for you," Shelby said. "I can only stand at the gate in this place."

"When it started, women were not allowed or able," Steve said. "They had different work. After about nine hundred years, it's changing."

"It feels like the molecules are being reconfigured somehow," Shelby said.

It was 8:30 at night, about half an hour into the healing. Mike and Susan sat motionless with their eyes closed, tracking the developments with some inward sight or kinesthetic sense of the changes in the energy of the room. Steve was muttering into the face cradle, "Year of change." I kept my eyes open to take notes on what was being said; dialogue during a healing was rare; in terms of conversation, Shelby's work on Mike and Susan had been like watching grass grow. In the dim light, angling my eyes, looking with that sideways gaze that sees without try-ing to see, that allows sight simply to happen and so, in theory, impli-

cates some other way of knowing in the act of seeing, I could see the
air waver and whirl above his back—colorless energy, perhaps, traveling like spindrift on the Great Plains in winter. White world with many
cows.

"Can you tell me what you experienced?" Shelby asked.

"When?" asked Steve.

"Anytime you want to talk about it."

"I was getting images of my incarnations on the astral. Did you see
me? In Bedouin garb? As a chevalier of the rose cross, a templar?"

"It feels like a part of what was done—I don't have words for it—
it feels like your heart and your connection from there to other realms
was cushioned—not closed, but . . . It's like now there's those thick
heavy velvet curtains around the opening. It's a cushioned place, dark,
heavy, dense, very very quiet. At the same time, your sacrum feels like
it's on fire, but it's not like fire, it's a different kind of burning and light.
I know this is not the right way to describe it, it's like it was re-
ingrained, re-embossed . . . It's so white I can't look at it. It's a very
intense brightness. Purified."

"They told me I was going to change, they didn't tell me into what,"
Steve said. "They told me I was supposed to do healing instead of defend-
ing. The change was supposed to take place at the end of a cycle in
September, and I've been stuck in limbo for three months."

"Now it feels like the physical part of your sacrum is back around
that other part," Shelby said. "I can feel it glowing from inside. I can feel
the bone again; I couldn't feel the bone before, it went away altogether,
and I couldn't have moved my hand if I'd wanted to."

"That light is what I take with me on the astral," Steve said. "Some
places I go, there is no other light."

Shelby started to reply and then broke off, saying, "No, that's me,
that's my view of the universe." And then she explained, "I was going
to say it's a sidetrack to go there, but that's not true. But it does feel like
you are being transformed."

"I can agree to take the oath again. But when I'm called, I go whether
I want to or not."

"But there's something special you've come to me to learn," Shelby
said. "I don't know what it is yet, but there's a reason."

"I don't know either," said Steve. "I've a lot to learn and not much time."

"There's enough time."

Finally Shelby removed her hands from Steve's sacrum, squeezed around the end of the healing table, and placed them on his right leg.

"One piece of the puzzle is you have the ability to bypass your body and do whatever you feel like, and that's not okay this time. There's an access your body gives you that you can't do without. What I felt when I put my hands on your foot and sacrum was that energetically you made the connection instantly, but that the leg was not in on the deal. It's slower to take your leg along, to include the leg. There's a set of ethical structures that go along with being in a body that don't apply elsewhere. It has to do with the relationship of the self and others, and it applies only in the physical realm. The rules are different. They make you move slower and more carefully."

She worked her way up the right leg, and with her hands now at his mid-back asked, "What's that in back?"

"Something I'm reluctant to say," Steve said.

"Have you seen the new *Star Trek*? You know when they let the docking clamps go? Do that on your back."

One of the classes in the complex was letting out, and the gabble of conversation in the hall filtered through the walls. A man was saying, "Visualize a screen. Now visualize some time when you were happy and healthy. See it on the screen."

Shelby laughed. "Healing 101," she said to Mike and Susan.

"What's so funny?" Steve asked.

"Oh, just people talking outside. Where are you now?"

"I just cut the clamps loose."

It was now nine o'clock, an hour into the healing. Steve rolled over on his back. Shelby removed the face cradle and drew up a folding chair close to the head of the table. She sat in a chair and settled her hands under Steve's head.

"What's it feel like, your back?" she asked.

"Back's okay. I have the usual excruciating pain at the base of my head."

"There's a little bit of energy moving through there. You run the energy up your back and it jams because it's not inside you. It doesn't come out your crown, it comes out the back, here, through a suture. It's not coming out where there's a real space, it's getting detoured and all crammed together. I just have to rearrange your head is all. Just melt a few bones, is all."

"I was attacked back there," Steve said, "that's where the flat spot comes in."

"Not the first time you've been attacked," Shelby said.

"It feels like it's jammed on the occiput."

"The one thing I'm feeling—it's, well, it feels like an ax." An ax! Little did she know, and yet her intuition had seized the very thing itself. "Whatever lessons there were, they've been learned," she continued. "You're just carrying around the residue."

"From the time I was betrayed," Steve said.

"One of the many—you were not entirely blameless however."

Shelby sat there, her hands holding Steve's head motionless.

"I never get to be Ivanhoe," Steve said.

"That book tortured me," Shelby said. "Okay, let the wound drain too, it's kind of mucky in there."

Maybe ten more minutes passed in silence. The Healing 101 crowd had melted away. Shelby moved back to Steve's feet to make an assessment of what she had done at the back of his neck. At length she said, "What I'm feeling is the energy going over the crown. There's still a little resistance at the edge of the occiput, but nothing like it was. There is a whole group of membranes connected with your jaw and roof of your mouth pulling that in and keeping it from dropping."

She went to work on his torso, starting at the hips, then moving to the midline and the chakras. Steve could sense that his second chakra was not spinning clockwise as is apparently its normal direction (somewhat akin to the Coriolis force, which controls the direction of water draining from bathtubs and other moving objects).

"Am I putting energy out of C2 instead of taking it in?" he asked.

"What you've done—what we've done . . ." Shelby started to say. She stopped and started again. "Because I'm trying to shift the whole central core of your energy so it's further forward in a more core place, it was like some of what was in back was in front . . ."

"That's difficult; it feels like the energy has folded in on my back."

"It feels like it has much more room to move. We gave it a bigger apartment. Now the rent goes up."

"Am I going to get astral calls in the morning?"

"Not if you don't want to. You can call on help yourself; you don't have to go alone. This is a martyr thing, is what it feels like." Steve was breathing heavily, and seemed somewhat distressed. Shelby settled her hands over his heart, the healer's gateway to the astral realm. "Let the breath come up," she said. "As soon as you feel energy in there, there's a part of you that wants to shut it down."

"I feel trapped."

"Why are you trapped?"

Steve said nothing.

"What's the pain about?"

"It's gone," Steve insisted, but it seemed even to those of us in the room that his words were full of wishfulness and will. And then, cryptically, he said something that did not make sense until later: "I was supposed to be at that house . . ."

"You have a sacred lineage," Shelby said. "These energies are part of it, but there is a place where you disconnect from God, a place where you are not acknowledging your own divinity."

"It's real easy for that to happen when there's a lineage," Steve said.

"The only way you can be complete in the lineage you come from is to let it go, let the pain go."

Now there was no mistaking the tears in Steve's eyes, the sheen on his cheeks.

"Something terrible happened a long time ago, and I disconnected from the source," he said.

Shelby finished the healing with a routine side-to-side cross, which was sort of like lacing a shoe. She set her hands on diagonals up the length of the body, left ankle to right knee, right knee to left hip, and then the converse, right ankle to left knee, and so on. Eventually Steve sat up on the table, and the story that he was reluctant to tell came out.

"I finally understand what the ax was," he said. "When I was nineteen or twenty years old, I bought a house, and at the time, I couldn't understand why I could afford it, why it was so cheap. Eventually I learned that some women had been murdered there by the man who owned it before me. He came back to the house when I was there and killed my dog. I went after him; I found him in the woods, sitting by a fire with pieces of my dog burning in it, and I lost it—the things I did to that man were terrible!" he said. He began to weep. Shelby handed him a box of tissues. "When the sheriff came, I thought they would arrest me, but they thanked me," he said at last. The air in the room was a strange mix of deep compassion and stunned shock.

"Is this the first time you've told anybody this?" Shelby asked.

Steve nodded. He had been carrying it for a long time, he said. He would carry it the rest of his life.

We gathered up our things, exchanged addresses, and waited for the elevator in the lobby, where an ersatz fountain contrived of plastic pipes and fieldstones made a sound more like the maddening drip-drip of a leaky faucet than the soothing ostinato of a waterfall.

At the time I didn't know what to believe about Steve's story. It seemed so improbably fantastic. Could it be true? Had he killed a man? If so, it was no wonder he was displaced psychically and prone to bypassing his body with his energy. *I was supposed to be at that house.* But what about the ax, and what about the "flat spot" on his head where he had been "attacked"? We all listened to the confession without cross-examining him. Shelby said later she had worked on Steve once before—during one of her Anatomy and Physiology classes—and while demonstrating a technique designed to change the way his body relied on his adrenal glands, she had sensed some heavy history in his tissue.

Almost a year and a half later, I talked to him again by telephone. That night had begun the first of four major initiations, he said. Not long after the healing, his father had died, and he and his wife had divorced. "I'm no longer the same person," he said. He had lost weight; his diet had changed. In his voice I could hear a new lightness, as it were. He told me about the brotherhood he had been a part of since his early teens. He was an adopted child, the product of an abusive home, and the mystical sect was his true family. But now the oath he had taken no longer required him to engage in the battles he had been fighting. He had been graduated. White world with a cow, he said, was probably a way of combining the new luminousness he had entered with the Hindu symbolism for the flesh of the sacred animal. In any case, the warrior had metamorphosed into a healer. He was seeing upwards of thirty clients a week. He still had the shield on his sacrum that Shelby's hand had been fused to, but the healing I had witnessed had produced a set of wings, what a blinkered newspaper consciousness would want to qualify as symbolic wings, but which to him were none the less real for not being visible. The fact that I had been there was remarkable, he said, and indicated that I might have some part in this esoteric circle, which I might one day want to embrace. I told him it had been amazing to witness his initiation—to listen and feel even with my limited faculties.

And then I asked about the violent revelation at the end of the night. And at first he was confused and wondered if he had really confessed all that detail, and when I reminded him, he said yes, it was true, but it was a delicate story, and he didn't wish to "energize" its occult aspects: He said that when he was nineteen or twenty, he had moved into a house in rural New England, and, as he remembered it, three nurses had been murdered there by a man who had been sent to a hospital for the criminally insane. The man had escaped, or had somehow gotten out, and had returned to the house, and had cut up Steve's Afghan puppy and with the dog's blood had scrawled occult obscenities on the walls of the basement. When Steve found him in the woods and confronted him, the man swung at him with an ax. Trained in martial arts, Steve deflected the attacker's arm enough to turn the blade so that only the flat of the ax head hit him in the skull. He was staggered by the blow, and bleeding profusely, and when the man came at him again with the ax, Steve delivered to the man's chest a punch that pierced the flesh, broke the ribs, and reached into the heart. "I had no choice, it was self-defense," he said, "but it weighed on me for years—taking a human life . . ." And, as he had said, the authorities handled it quietly.

Before we concluded our conversation, Steve said that the confession of the guilt he felt, while important, was not the centerpiece of that night nearly a year and a half ago, not what the others remembered. What loomed as truly significant was his initiation into a new life. There was an inscription on the shield that protected his sacrum, and it had been changed that night; new sacred words had been laid down, and they had set him free. The hands of the warrior that had destroyed a heart were now the hands of a healer learning to cradle hearts.

When we hung up, I found myself remembering the aftermath of that healing. It seemed to take forever for the elevator to come. We rode down in silence, and stood quietly for a moment on the corner of Thirty-second Street and Madison Avenue—still bound as a group, the five of us, still awed by what had happened. And then we all scattered in the blaze of a cold Manhattan night.

CHAPTER FIVE

Healer and patient are destined actors with archetypally assigned roles in a "sacred performance." The healer's personality is overshadowed by the stage mask of the healer-god, which includes his potentially dark side, the divine intruder-destroyer; the patient's archetypal role is that of the supplicant but harbors also a healer-destroyer in its unconscious depths.

—EDWARD C. WHITMONT, M.D.

1. WHO HAVE YOU LOST?

Nothing happened to Rachel that she did not believe was ripe with fate. There were no accidents, no events that were not pregnant with lessons, no gestures bereft of spirit. She was counseled by unseen "guides." If you crossed her path you were someone she had chosen at some level to encounter. I raise this to suggest that I was an inevitable antagonist in her life, and to the extent that we shared the same moonstruck brand of personal creationism, she was an inevitable antagonist in mine. She said once that when she had first spotted me wandering around the Brennan School, where she was a student, she had known instantly we would work together someday. She was right about that.

We had a friend in common, a woman I ran into one night at a restaurant in downtown Manhattan. What was this healing business about? asked Rachel's friend. It had to be a big fraud, didn't it? A charade? Rachel's friend was upset, and it was clear her feelings were tied to the changes she had seen in Rachel. Rachel was one of the most brilliant people she had ever met. Rachel had perfect test scores, and degrees from the country's top colleges. But since she'd begun studying healing, Rachel had changed; she'd embraced cultist ideas and prattled on about spirit guides and energy bodies. She seemed to have lost the ability to think rationally. She just didn't make sense the way she used to, her friend said.

As the night wore on and the waiter brought more bottles of wine to the large table where we were sitting with a bunch of people, Rachel's friend was unable to conceal her anger and the hurt she felt. She and Rachel had fallen out, she said, and she blamed it all on Rachel's interest in this stupid healing stuff. How could a smart person get so bewitched?

She gave me Rachel's number, and when I telephoned her a few days later and described the article I had written and the book I was contemplating, Rachel agreed to sit for an interview. She offered to give me a healing too. On a Friday afternoon in late June, 1994, I knocked on the door of the apartment where she lived with her husband and her young daughter. I didn't recognize her face from the crowd of students I had seen at the Brennan School during my visits there. She had dark hair and deep-striking eyes that opened wide so that the white of the eyeball encircled the iris and gave her a willful look of fortitude-under-fire. She was pregnant with her second daughter. She offered me a cup of tea, and we sat down under the high ceilings of a large, well-lighted living room. We talked about the friend we had in common. When your energy changes, she said, sometimes your circle of friends changes too, and while she regretted the distance that had come between them, Rachel said she thought it was the inevitable outcome of their divergent spiritual paths. Rachel described a bit of her background. She had grown up as an army brat and had gone off to college on a scholarship; she had gotten a master's degree in fiction writing; she had two novels in her desk that were still looking for a publisher, and she was humming along on a third.

"I never have writer's block," she said.

I missed the note of the bluff, the whistling past the graveyard. It seemed a surprisingly egotistical thing to say, and the uncharitable thought flashed across my mind that maybe if she had more experience with writer's block, her novels would be published. I didn't say anything, of course. Even at the time, I was familiar enough with the appeal of create-your-own-reality thinking to wonder if my half-conscious axioms about writing as a struggle were only another means of handicapping myself, a useless set of self-fulfilling prophecies that could be shored up with high-flown testimony from the likes of Thomas Mann, who once wrote: "A writer is someone for whom writing is more difficult than it is for other people." If one person chooses to think that writing is wretched toil and another chooses to believe it's a cheery breeze, who is the bigger fool? But as I say, I missed the bluff and the infirmity behind it, and marked only her unwillingness to feign modesty and the breach of literary decorum. In writing, the rules of self-promotion are the same as in the rough-and-tumble of city basketball: When you aren't too good you tell the world how great you are; when you are good, the world tells you.

We talked about healing for a while. She was in her second year of study, and her clairvoyant sight, to judge from her reports, was unusually advanced. I watched her scanning my field as Joel Wallach and the others had done. She gazed at the space over my shoulder, and studied my legs and the area around my navel, and as before, with other healers, I was struck by the figure/ground inversion, that sudden shift in perspective which relocates the self so that it is no longer the aviation light on the top of the steeple but the vast night sky and skein of stars into which the steeple reaches. Physician and healer W. Brugh Joy put it beautifully in his book *Joy's Way*: "You are not in your body. Your body is in you."

In addition to her own guides, Rachel apparently had access to *mine*, one of them at least, who was with us in her living room. He wouldn't be a Chinese guy about five thousand years old, would he? No, the sex wasn't clear, she said. She could see the guide over my right shoulder, presenting itself simply as a cloudy pink shape.

At length, I got on the padded healing table Rachel had set up in her dining room. She turned on a tape of some soothingly ethereal synthesizer music. She had me lie facedown at first and began to "clean" my spine with blue light, or something she had learned to call blue light. After a while I rolled over, and she stood at my feet, running energy into my legs to help charge up my lower chakras. She told me that I spent most of my time hanging out in the sixth chakra, the brow chakra. Hence the purple light I often saw when I closed my eyes. She scaled the ladder of chakras with her hands. At my heart chakra, she stayed a long time. I confided that for a long time I'd had the feeling of not being able to get a deep breath, as if there were bands cinched across my chest.

"There are bands," she said. "Did they have a useful function?"

I said I guessed they did.

"Do you still need them?"

"No."

"Well, undo them."

So I pantomimed removing an invisible band from around my chest as if I were unbuckling a belt. It seemed a ludicrous bit of make-believe, but Rachel said, "No, you've got the outer one in your hands right now.

It's a leathery brown band of stagnant energy." I went on with the pantomime because in some tiny corner of my mind I found a place to suspend skepticism long enough to allow my hands to sense their way into the texture of the air above my heart. I opened the belt and let the two ends fall away. Rachel said she could see other bands—one was pink, some were other colors. She said she could see an area of my heart chakra where it joined the vertical power current. It was clean and bright, and she surmised that that was where Barbara Brennan had zapped it during the Goddess Healing six months before. I saw Rachel braiding the invisible filaments of energy three feet over my navel. At one point I was so relaxed, I stopped making the effort to see—the normally unconscious but nonetheless willful effort to assemble a coherent visual image—and the room went dark, and I no longer bothered to differentiate foreground from background. Bookshelves blended into walls, coffee tables merged with the floor. And then the habit of panicky self-consciousness came jumping back, and I felt my will asserting itself, determined to pop a comprehensible picture into the slide projector. It was as if I could perceive a pattern deeper than "my" intention, which was the struggle of "my" will to impose order and to keep order imposed on the stream of visual phenomena. It eased a bit, and I was glad, because it seemed to me the premium my will had placed on keeping the visual cues sensible and rational was keeping me from "seeing" other kinds of things. By the end, new colors were surfacing—a pale lavender entirely new to my palette, which Rachel said represented a level of the throat chakra, and a molten lava-esque red light interspersed with black patches, which she attributed to the much-bruited-about-but-never-seen "molten core of the earth."

She told me later she pulled out a long needlelike bone, and—yuck—some white beetles that had been ensconced in my back. Oh, they weren't *physical* beetles and bones, they were *energetic* beetles and bones, and in theory they weren't extricated from the physical back per se, but from the back that resided in the astral plane—one of the subtle backs, the back that most doctors would probably dismiss as "all in your head."

"I tried to remove some batwing-like things which didn't want to come off," Rachel said, "so I zapped them with rose light and they turned into tiny white angel wings fluttering on your shoulder." As in other healings, the most impressive bit of energy phenomenology was once again the distended sense of time. I thought I had been down for an hour, but when I swung my legs off the table, two and a quarter hours had passed.

Rachel invited me to return for a second healing in three weeks, and I agreed. I had received treatments from other healers without the urge to repeat the experience. The reasons ranged from such trivial ones as wishing the healers had a table and didn't make clients lie on their room-mates' beds, to the more substantial objection that nothing seemed to have happened, and the overall sense of the futility of the transaction evoked something like an earnest math professor's attempt to transmit the rules of algebra to a dog.

With Rachel, however, much seemed to have happened, and the dynamic portended more. She was willing to work for free, which was fine with me and which also mooted the common skeptical argument that healers were in it for the money. She was articulate, technically ori-ented, and devoted to the work. She'd certainly made a big effort on my behalf. She knew I wanted to write in depth about a series of healings, and she was amenable to being one of the subjects. Looking back, I can see that my role as a journalist may have induced her to redouble her efforts on my behalf. I can also see my own motives better, the ways in which, even as I fenced with her and wrestled with the boundaries of writer and subject, I soaked up the attention she was paying me and felt the effects as she furbished up the flow in my energy. Even beyond that, I can see that part of the reason I returned for a second time, and a third, was that Rachel was learning on the job, a student healer, and thus was easier to spar with, less threatening. Her proclamations were easier to debate. As a student, didn't she expect to be questioned and challenged and even corrected? A more established healer might have taken offense. All of which is to say that the unreconstructed part of my psyche, which was battling the reality of the subtle world, figured, *Here's a healer who's easier not to take seriously.* Or more darkly, from the not-so-funny bully clown: *Here's a healer who's easier to push around.*

When I returned again, in July, Rachel had prepared my astrological chart—full of squares, trines, and a distribution of planets all pointing, she said, to the general theme of "mystery." Was that a polite word for incoherence, I asked, making a joke to see if she shared my paradoxical prejudice that astrology could be used in those desperate moments when you were trying to sustain conversations with fashion models or screening blind dates, but that ultimately it had to be disowned as the bastard fruit of an intellectually illegitimate romance, especially when star charts described the chief characteristic of the male Pisces as "feckless diffidence." No, we were not going to enjoy a good laugh about our mutual interest in astrology. "I use it because it works," she said, very seriously. She prepared astrological charts on her computer for all her clients and had found they yielded many useful clues and insights about patterns in her clients' lives. She explained the significance of my rising sign and the planets clustered in various houses. By the by, she said, my chart indicated healing ability; it wasn't something I had to use, but there it was.

I was very tired that day, at a low ebb, and after the initial sugar rush of learning the secrets of my stars, I slipped into that hypoglycemic swoon that always accompanies a surfeit of suspect divination. When I got on the table, I lay facedown, drained and sleepy. Rachel clamped her fingers around my lower vertebrae. After about ten minutes, the strangest thing happened: I was jolted awake by a surge of energy. It was as if someone had snapped on a light switch. All at once, I had three times the juice in my body. Whereas the instant before, I hardly had the strength to get on the healing table, now I could have run up ten flights of stairs with it under my arm. The speed and power of the transition were astonishing.

As she had the first time, after about ten minutes Rachel asked me to roll over onto my back, and she began running energy into my ankles and knees—the field-clearing and field-charging process known as chelating. The kundalini energy in my first chakra was ready to pop, she said. She could see the two little snakes, one red, one blue, peeping at her from their nest at the base of the spine. From books, I knew that people worked for years to awaken the two Pisas of the kundalini from their briefcase at the base of the spine, so this was exciting news. Too good to be true, in fact; it aroused my suspicions. I found that I was watching myself as Rachel worked, separated from the experience of what she was doing by the act of observing. But when she finished and left me alone "to integrate" the work, as she put it, the old car that had been revved up once already blasted off again like some sort of flame-throwing nitro-fueled dragster, hauling me with it as if I were a hapless bystander whose coat had got caught on the door handle.

After enough spiritual experiences, you start to believe not only that spiritual experiences are real but that they have some bearing on the health of the body, a palpable biochemical impact. I had been discounting spiritual experiences for so long. I had been staving them off, belittling them, interposing the clown to shut up the monk. What's that you say, you overweight cleric, the Virgin Mary was feeding you the host of Christ for nine hours? Cool. Did the Yankees win? But now, as I lay there on Rachel's table, in the strangeness and serenity of my robes, new-made, profoundly refreshed, I was ashamed to have dismissed the domain of the spirit so glibly. Did a clown's disdain come from some intuitive sense of one's capacities for mystical contemplation? You know what you can handle—what overloads your circuits, what burns you out. And yet here again, experience building on experience, I wondered how I could have overlooked the miracle of being, how could I have failed to reflect even for a second on the dreamy immensity of being . . .

I was thoroughly immobilized on Rachel's table. She said my guides and hers as well had taken over and were at work, continuing the renovation she had initiated. My own guides were plainly visible to her now. She could see two of them. A man on my right with blond hair. A woman on my left, also with blond hair. Blonds abounding. My spiritual epiphany was turning into a shampoo commercial.

Three weeks later, on a sweltering August afternoon, I knocked on Rachel's door for the third time. She had been meditating. Fortified light was pouring out of her eyes. Her first words struck me to the quick: "Who have you lost?"

2. SUFFERIN' SUCCOTASH

In the murky, maddening literature of chakras, the diseases that afflict the area of the neck and jaw—thyroid problems, gum difficulties, temporomandibular joint syndrome, sore throats—are attributed to malfunctions of Vishuddha, the throat chakra. The throat chakra is said to embody a raft of principles loosely organized around the themes of faith and expression—faith in the form of surrender to some larger mind or presence, ostensibly divine, and expression in the sense of creating one's story, shaping the script of one's life without excuses, judgments, or blame. Surrender and faith and expression and creation all converge at the throat in the idea of confession. Literal-minded science can scarcely address the subtleties of confession or discern its vital components, such as truth, integrity, meaning—all fundamental constituents of symbolic-minded art. Science understands language mainly as a means by which the species helps ensure security and find food. Chakra doctrine has a grander and perhaps more pretentious view, which understands language as a means of spiritual generation. As somebody once said in one translation: In the beginning was the Word. Elsewhere it came out as: In the beginning were the fifty sacred syllables of Sanskrit. And by the power of the word, the energy of sacred utterance, the verve of canonical vibration, the immaterial spirit shall be shifted into flesh, and the stain of sin shall be absolved, and the vigor of life shall be recreated. And any ailing zoo leopards shall be granted reprieves from inflammatory bowel disease.

So let the throat sing out what the heart has taken in, no? Let it speak plainly and not sidestep its own story, not answer Who have you lost? with What's it to you? Let it speak without irony, or fear of sentiment, or a lot of lip.

Who have you lost?

The straight answer that summer afternoon in 1994 was a woman to whom I had once been engaged, a woman I had known for five years, whom I had met on a blind date, in Central Park, by the boat pond, on a May evening. When she was thirty. When I was thirty-five. She was an only child, stoical, reserved, more than a little repressed—it's rare to find a native New Yorker who uses the word "intercourse." But she laughed when I said that with her blue eyes and yellow shoes she looked like the Swedish flag. I liked how the effect I had on her affected me. She wore dresses that covered her throat and complained that she could never say what she wanted to say with words. She was too shy to act out a role, assume any sort of persona, which is why I have never forgotten the time she said "sufferin' succotash" in the lisping voice of Sylvester, the long-necked cartoon cat with a body like a wine decanter. (Or am I thinking of Snagglepuss? She would know. She loved cats.)

From where we sat that first evening in the park, we could see boys sailing toy boats on the pond. A dog named Rosie waded into the pond in vain pursuit of some ducks. "Rosie, Rosie," the dog's owner cried. Evening stole in among the branches of the new-leafed oaks. Sometimes you know right away. You know when someone tells you a story, and you can see the face of a girl shining in the face of a woman. You know when a cartoon cat suddenly becomes a tender conjunction, a code word, a secret name. Hey, Sylvester!

We went back to her apartment. She fixed me spaghetti in a white enamel pot. Like waking up after a long sleep, we fell in love. A year later, sitting in a restaurant off Times Square, I asked her to marry me. On the trip home that evening, I lost my glasses and thought it was pointless to look for them, but she wasn't going to let any omen ruin the night, and dragged me off the subway and retraced the way we had come. When she saw the glasses lying intact by the Broadway curb, she snatched them up and put them on and danced around triumphantly. Sufferin' succotash! The double dream of union broke over me like grace.

Why did I turn away? Fly in the other direction? My reasons seem so paltry now. As the years went by, I came to feel I had made a bad mistake; that I had been frightened and heedless, and too stupid to know it. Kierkegaard, who jettisoned his fiancée, once said people lived life forwards, but they understood it backwards. I confess I was ashamed—of being afraid, of my piker's heart, of feeling overmatched and small and doomed to drift with no sense of dominion over life. I suppose I was ashamed to face the evidence that I did not know how to love someone for herself, only for her reflection on me . . .

Here is the part that took me years to understand. During the final months that we were together, she got pregnant. With precious little discussion or deliberation, we agreed that it was too soon to be parents. Bad timing. Not the way the story should unfold. When I look back at that day we walked up Fifth Avenue to a doctor's office, I see two people bent on not understanding themselves, two people with almost no grasp of the enormity of the undertaking, two automatons acting out a scenario devised to teach them some excruciating lesson. You stand beside yourself, you watch your hand strike the match that kindles the karmic fire . . . In the waiting room, I remember staring at some Hawaiian sunset travel poster, and half an hour later, how sad and shaky and lost my poor soul mate looked when she came out. Hadn't it been a very reasonable decision, a very prudent piece of family planning? Oh sure, we reassured ourselves. We'd done the right thing. That we were blind and terrified and drifting toward oblivion—it took me years to see that. And to understand how high the stakes were, how we had turned away from the offering of that pregnancy, from that token of our utmost complicity. We had refused fate's entreaty. Some other pair might have married after that—married in innocence, married happily—but we could not. Three months later when we broke up, it was almost a formality, the anticlimactic outcome of a fruitless union. We had unravelled our shared history.

What I learned was that you live with the life you don't choose, as well as with the life you do; the choices you make are like stones that cause ripples in the lake for years. Not being born did not stop the child we didn't have from growing. It grew in the shadows, and after five years it was strong enough to pull us back toward each other. Or pull me, at least. It kept some wound open that seemed like intimacy, some business unfinished that had the texture of love. Or perhaps it was only the texture of unconfessed guilt. I had never been ashamed of voting to terminate a pregnancy before. Now, older, in the hard light of isolation and selfishness, I wondered who could be so shut up inside himself that he would never say anything but "No, no."

I tried to make amends. Three years after we broke up, I tried to resurrect Sylvester. I tell myself I loved her as much, or more, as I had the first time, but I am not sure about that. For she was not the same person. She did not need me to be the light of her life, to finish her sentences and say what she couldn't say. The trust she had extended once was not something she could extend in innocence again. My desertion had hurt her badly. But where it had weakened me in some ways, it had made her stronger. And early that year, in February of 1994, she decided our reunion was not going to work. We had come full circle: She broke things off with me.

As the news sank in, my sense of loss grew, and by the summer, when I presented myself at Rachel's apartment for healing sessions, the grief seemed absurdly bottomless and apocalyptic. It was as if I had not simply lost her heart but my own as well. Lose heart, lose love itself or the hope of love, love's redemptive possibilities . . . Was that it—the redemption of love? Did I want to be saved? Was that ever love's job—to save any of us?

The loss of love is often described as a little death, a kind of rehearsal for the more catastrophic death of the body, but they are not the same. In some ways, the loss of love is harder to come to terms with. There isn't a body to grieve over, only an open-ended absence, the bodiless body of memory. The oblivion that one submits to when a person dies must, when love dies, be created or imposed or attained in some other, artificial way. It's as if the person were lost at sea and presumed dead, and you were required by effort of will to make that presumption of death, and to make it over and over again, day after day, banishing memory by force of will, so that your vain and dogged hopes were not reignited, and the hauntingly bodiless body could not suddenly unbury itself when a photograph tumbled out of a book; so the body would not wash up unexpectedly in a snatch of song, perfume, the voice of a cat. To keep a lover dead takes strength of will and a kind of faith—faith all the bleaker for coming full circle. Once, you had faith that she would never leave. Then you learned to trust that she was never coming back.

Yet we also take on faith that some stronger and truer self emerges from the little death. As if the only real insight into one's nature arises from the shipwreck of communion. In loss, we find who we are, what we require to be whole. But in a secular world, where spiritual rituals are discredited or in disrepair, we linger over troubles, helpless to move on. Where is it taught that grieving is a practice, something to be plied and completed? I was trying to speak a language without a vocabulary. Why did I want to retreat to the past? Why was I so afraid to press forward? What was I so determined to hold on to that I had made a fetish of mourning?

"Who have you lost?" Rachel asked at the start of that third healing. Gratefully I poured out the story of my stillborn campaign, the heart-crossed summer. I didn't think to mention the child aborted almost five years earlier; I didn't see the link then. It seemed enough to me that Rachel could read the emotion in my field and describe its depth. "This woman is lodged in your soul seat," she said, touching the area between my heart and neck. "She's associated with your soul's longing—maybe inseparable from it."

Well, I confess I took great comfort in that phrase "your soul's long-ing" with its connotations of a bond beyond love, a bond that rose from a stardust story much older than the heartache of a particular self. No, it wasn't on a par with that long-ago clairvoyant vision of the lily; it lacked particularity, but then if she told me that she had been prompted by her guides to say the phrase "sufferin' succotash" I might have had to hospi-talize myself. Soul's longing. Soul seat. Such solemn, earnest phrases! They reminded me of the high school poetry that you badly want to disown after your hormones cool.

Rachel began as she had begun the previous two healings, running energy into my legs. As I lay there feeling her hands on my socks, I was struck by my habit of disowning the high school poetry writer who had once in tremulous purple prose celebrated the yellow, orange, and red leaf pigments masked by chlorophyll. Him and most of the other mortifying geeks in my closet: personalities too tender for the world, too innocent, too delusional. The sentimentalist, the baby-talker, the victim of poignancy attacks; the old-letter saver, the melancholic, the hearer of lost voices. Hey, Sylvester! What did they have in common? They were clowns, they lived in their own stories, they made no accommodation to the world outside them, they paid no tithe to reality. It was the reality principle they ran afoul of, chasing butterflies over the cliff, stopping to pick the daisy on the train tracks with the express bearing down. They began with their dignity, and suffered the privation of it. "Fate's pawns," Henry Miller called them in *The Smile at the Foot of the Ladder.* You could laugh at them, but then you were flattering yourself that you no longer had anything in common with them, that you were somehow exempt from the folly of their circumstances . . .

Halfway through, when Rachel's hands were floating in the air above my chest, I had the eerie sensation that they were making a cut, like a surgical incision. But with what? And, good grief, *in* what? Not in my flesh per se, but in something I certainly would include as part of my juris-diction, part of the domain I was capable of sensing incursions into. A less material part of my being. And what would that be, exactly? It was a dis-tinct sensation in the area between the sternum and the solar plexus. It felt as if I were being opened up. I say "I," but at that moment the concept of "I" suddenly seemed like a bald plot device in a beach novel. Given a hard look, the substance of "I" often seems to evaporate. University of Maryland philosophy professor Steven Braude in his book *First Person Plural* tells the story of a Zen nun who was so disinclined to identify with her body that she would acknowledge that she was hungry only by saying "There is hunger here."

Put it this way: The locus of my identity seemed to have been expanded, and with it, my range of sensitivity. I—ha!—could feel things shifting around inside my body. (My body?) And then after some minutes, this "I" fellow could feel the edges of his "wound"—if "one" can call it that without shredding what remains of "one's" credibility—being gathered and sewn together. After the procedure, I felt a little nauseous, unsure whether to attribute it to the violation of my body or to the violation of my worldview.

"Was that some kind of psychic surgery?" I asked when the healing was over.

Rachel nodded and set a glass of water on a stool by the healing table. She seemed keyed up. "I wasn't doing it; my guides were," she said. "I was just hanging out, and they were working. We're not supposed to do surgery until junior year, but we're supposed to follow our guides." And her guides had their scalpels out. She said she had stumbled across a big block between my third and fourth chakras. She tried to move it, but couldn't; it wasn't ripe enough.

"She's near you, at least psychically," Rachel said. "I pulled out the cord that connected you, but there were still some energetic filaments linking you."

My head was swimming with the topsy-turvy metaphors of energy medicine. Guides, souls, cords, strands of energy that linked people across time and space. The bottom line was that I felt some relief from the congestion in my chest, but as I sat up and sipped from the glass of water and collected myself, the tightness, the impacted, heavy feeling, crept back. Half the struggle of learning a new way of being is unlearning the old one—the old language, the old patterns, the old assumptions. And to learn and unlearn simultaneously, to swear some allegiance to the authenticity of feeling while holding on to some measure of critical thinking—

this was no simple task. No simple task: It was at the heart of my adventure in the chakras. The notion that people were energetically connected by cords, for example—was it simply another way of describing the consequences of that impractical dream-drunk hope that is always countermanding orders from the captain, subverting will and reason? But then, didn't the heart have its reasons? I wanted to change course but did not have—well, what else can you call it?—the energy to change course. The question now was not Who have you lost, but Who were you trying to lose? Who couldn't you shake? The fire of hope would flare up on the oxygen of a postcard. Sylvester had written to confess the hardship of the withdrawal on her. Oh bittersweet pleasure to know that she suffered too! Then I looked closely at her card. She had transposed the numbers in my street address, and the card had arrived only by the grace of an alert mailman. And yet, for a moment, when I looked at the number scribbled in her hand, I wasn't sure where I lived.

3. THE DHARMA OF NARCISSISM

As part of her course work at the Brennan School, Rachel was required to present a paper detailing energy healing in one client over many sessions. At the time—September 1994—she was seeing only a handful of people, some of them other healers; she was doing one to three healings a week, working in her living room while a nanny took her daughter to the park. She was seven months pregnant. Her junior year was about to begin. She asked if I would undergo periodic healings and serve as the subject of the case study she would present during her senior year. She wouldn't charge me for the sessions and would give me copies of the write-ups she had to prepare every two months or so— status reports that would describe her observations of my energy field and chakras, her perceptions of my physical and emotional weather, changes she observed in the course of the healing, what had been easy to do, what had been hard, and so forth. The paucity of scientific evidence for hands-on healing had not prevented the deans of the Brennan School from devising a stringent program of testing and evaluation. Working on the assumption that energy existed and could be perceived, Rachel was required to analyze how I used mine, and—in the school's phrase— misused it. She had to assess my main energy blocks and the energetic strategies I mustered in self-defense, and then "psychically read any information" about my main "issues." This seemed like a pretty tall order, in that it presumed a high degree of psychological expertise over and above the clairvoyant ability necessary to perceive energy defenses. The idea of an energy defense had come from Wilhelm Reich, and had been further elaborated by Alexander Lowan and John Pierrakos, founders of Core Energetics therapy. Core Energetics proposes a number of common defenses as ways of coping with aggression or making unconscious bids for attention. Rachel was looking for ones that had been described in Barbara Brennan's textbook *Hands of Light*. They had bad–night–on–*Sesame-Street* names such as: Porcupine, Oral Sucking, Mental Grasp, Beside Himself, Withdrawal, and Boundary Containment.

Rachel was required to make sketches of my energy flow and to speculate on the initiating cause of my illness, such as it was or might be construed. Some of the questions she had to answer reached far beyond conventional medical considerations: for example, "Did you reach the person's inner light?" and "What higher qualities did you need to appeal to in order to help the person heal himself?" She also had to review the emotions she experienced in herself during her work on me, and assess her own strengths and weaknesses as a healer.

For my part, I saw the arrangement as a way of diving deeper into the question of how far energy healing could go—diving with what I thought was the safety rope of prudent reservations about the powers and limitations of a student. I was proceeding not on faith but under the license of suspended disbelief, in the manner of doubting Thomas, willing to believe but unwilling not to verify. And, sad to say, that is another way of saying that I really did not want miracles to occur; I wanted to experience only the phenomena my cosmology had room for.

And so that September we started a sort of partnership that spanned sixteen healings over the remainder of that year and most of the next. Rachel observed that it might have been called "an investigation of grief." It had many of the emotional dynamics of psychotherapy but few of the conventions. I went for a healing every three or four weeks, and for a period of a couple of months, I saw Rachel once a week. The benefits of cathartic chitchat were conjoined to the deep-diving intimacies of touch. Rachel was not constrained by the fifty-minute-hour or the protocols of the professional therapist, or psychotherapeutic assumptions that held that the psyche's patterns and secrets could be ferreted out only over months of conversation. Patterns were immediately accessible to her as energy; secrets were registered in the body. Emotions could be felt or seen or otherwise tracked energetically in the tissues—tracked, if need be, across dimensions of time and space outrageous to science. Healers did not have to wait for the unconscious to betray its hidden intent in dreams and Freudian slips, or projections and sublimations. The unconscious was constantly broadcasting. Energy was thought made visible. If you lied, if you were jealous, if you were attracted to someone, it was all right there in your field, spelled out and lit up like a billboard in Times Square.

Such was the theory at least, the faith and ground on which healers worked. In the creed of energy medicine, an illness could be approached anywhere along the mind-body continuum—as a physical, mental, emotional, or spiritual condition. Where they were not physically measurable, the benefits could not be easily quantified. They belonged mostly to the intangible, unscientific world of subjective experience.

And so in her young healership, Rachel was of necessity a jack-of-all-trades. She combined the roles of masseuse, physical therapist, shrink, counselor, and amateur ontologist. She even advised me on the health effects of fluorescent lightbulbs. Fluorescent bulbs disrupted the coherence of the human energy field, she said. I brought her one of the new electricity-conserving compact versions I had installed in my desk lamp to save the planet and lower my Con Ed bill. Rachel screwed it in, switched it on. She studied it for a while. She sketched its energetic silhouette, drawing a ring of spikes that resembled the Porcupine energy defense. Subtly speaking, the bulb wasn't too bad, she said.

In late September, when I boarded her table for the first time as CB, the case subject (my fourth session overall), it had been little more than a month since she had posed the question "Who have you lost?" Sylvester was still parked in my soul seat, but I had started the work of getting her out, imposing unilateral radio silence. No phone calls, no letters, no nothing. Just the work of letting go. And it was work. It was as if each day I had to snip a patch of canvas off a giant white tent with a pair of tiny scissors. The ghost in my soul would be dislodged only when all the cloth was cut away.

On the first report she prepared, Rachel included a brief description of my condition: CB was "a forty-one-year-old man who suffers from temporomandibular joint syndrome and has a kink in the central vertical power current. Because of the kink, his left side receives less energy than his right side." That was a start, a clear physical problem, hardly earth-shattering, but true enough. I had developed temporomandibular joint syndrome (TMJ) in my early twenties. Had, over the years, ground the points off my bicuspids. Had, over the years, worn a plastic mouthguard at night, but chucked it finally because it hardly went to the source of the problem, and it wasn't the prophylactic you were expected to produce if you were getting into bed with someone new . . .

I still didn't fully understand the stress that was making my jaw crackle like a bowl of Rice Krispies, but I was intrigued to learn from Rachel's vantage that TMJ implied some dysfunction in the throat's ability to gather and distribute the chimeras of vital force. Difficulty speaking from the heart was classically implied in "C5," or fifth chakra, tribulations, she said. She noticed that I tended to "clutch in" on the throat chakra and hold my jaws rigid, which signaled to her that I had some serious issues around the idea of receiving nurturance.

Was I choked up at the throat? Did I have a hard time talking? Was I blocked as a writer? She had observed I would rather talk about feelings than feel them, that I used "will" and "reason" to rationalize away my emotional needs. "See how your posture pulls back when the subject of feelings comes up," she said. My major defense was Oral Sucking, she noted. I tended to talk and ask a lot of questions, and drain energy from other people on the grounds that a good interviewer was like those beetles that sucked the brains out of certain frogs. I liked to argue, she said (and I would only be underlining her point if I were here and now to demur that arguing is an occupational liability of journalism). She noted that sometimes I could be "charmingly psychopathic," which was the Core Energetics description for the energy defenses of people skewered on issues of trust and betrayal. She'd seen me "leave my body" in a very "schizoid" manner, what shrinks might call "dissociation" and civilians who wandered into some of the weirder corners of health expos would describe as "lights on, nobody home." Whatever insights they offered, the character structures she cited seemed demoralizingly prefabricated. That Rachel had already donned the ones she thought fit her and now wanted me to try on the ones that I thought suited me was as depressing as the prospect of a trip to a men's store in Beijing during the heyday of communist uniformity, when your jacket choices were limited to the Mao style in four or five shades of dung brown and drab green.

Nurturance, had there been any available, would have been a lot easier to swallow than what Rachel was offering. And how could it be otherwise? My defenses were busy defending. Reason's pride of place was under siege. My reason had, in essence, been diagnosed as a disease. "Wait a minute," it said, "why are you buying this stuff; this woman could be a nut! You've been writing all your life! You've always made a living as a writer! If your throat chakra were b-b-blocked and *p-p-prana* were being diverted or backed up, how could you have ever paid the rent?" Then again, it didn't take much to entertain the idea that one could gravitate to a profession as a way of compensating. Suddenly I recalled my eighth-grade chorus audition, the strangled song of the pathetic young candidate and the awkward silence before the teacher gently said, "I'm sorry, maybe next year." Recalled this old belief that I couldn't sing, shouldn't sing, must not ever sing. Might not the faculty that you found hard, or challenging, or problematic, or impossible to exercise be the very faculty that you were driven to develop in one form or other? Poor chorus boy fleeing from the foot of the piano into the hope that he could make music by hand, with words.

But it struck me, during the conversation that Rachel prompted as she worked, that in my family words weren't ways of speaking heartfelt truths or even of making music but ways of asserting identity; they were instruments of self-definition and aggression. The struggle for adolescent autonomy had been waged over Anagram trays and Scrabble boards, with verbal broadsides; it had been contested with sarcasm and wit, or what passed for wit in suburban Connecticut. What introduction to the power of *logos* could be more intoxicating than when a whey-faced smarty-pants grasped that he could preempt or defuse criticism from Mom by the simple expedient of daring her to produce an on-the-spot definition of "virago," "termagant," or "Xanthippe." It was a power of a magic bordering on divinity to go from the frustration of flinging bottles of acne scrub at the bedroom wall to venting the lava of feeling in language. Never mind that *logos* was being pressed into service of execrably bad poems based on the still-incomprehensible symbolism of lemonade and occult plant pigments; the wonder then, as now, was that words could compel attention: could build fences, set boundaries, and stake the claims of the nascent self.

And didn't it follow that if you had cultivated a vocabulary to circumvent energy blocks in the chakra of expression, and had learned to write the better to dodge the emotional difficulty of speaking heartfelt truths, that maybe your so-called problems were actually gifts of fate? Maybe I owed my identity, my freedom, my sole proprietorship, the laptop hack's unfettered life, to a squirrelly, undercharged throat chakra. Wasn't that worth a Rice Krispies jaw?

We would see.

What was clear soon enough was how much I had invested in staying the way I was, in defending the style and strategies I had evolved and continued to justify even when it was obvious they were getting in the way. When I look back at that litany of healings conducted by Rachel, some were unremarkable, but others inspired long journal entries. After that first September session as CB, I made a lot of notes, particularly about Rachel's work on my right foot, which in a portentous, Freud-was-right sort of way, I recorded as my "write" foot. It had been bruised in a pick-up basketball game. Rachel looked past the immediate circumstances of the injury to say she thought it had been badly mangled two centuries ago under a wagon wheel. *Oy!* But my boggle threshold had been raised enough that I did not bound up in protest or yield to the impulse to ridicule her for *meshuggenah* ideas. I was tired of my opinions. And who knew for sure? Maybe when people got spaced out they really were somewhere else in space. The self was such a shifty proposition to begin with. Spaced out, timed out: Maybe you had to fight to stay anchored in the body; maybe you had to work to cultivate the nuances of consciousness. Otherwise, as Allen Ginsberg once wrote, you had no option but to get your emotional life from *Time* magazine. Maybe people who had that "lights on, nobody home" look in their eyes had vacated their bodies. Who knew what the lack of consciousness in someone really meant? If there were an infinite number of degrees of vagueness, perhaps there were as many degrees of awareness, planes of reality where the metaphors of past lives or entities or UFOs did not outrage the conventions of science. Reason was simply a mode of the intellect, and in one sense I was lying on Rachel's healing table because I was no longer satisfied with reason's discourse. It had begun to seem like a guest who monopolized the conversation at a dinner party, eclipsing other voices, drowning out the silence. I wanted to listen for new sounds, to find new forms of being; I warmed myself on the heretical fire in Heidegger's observation that "thinking only begins at the point where we have come to know that Reason, glorified for centuries, is the most obstinate adversary of thinking." Having to fret about whether you were one of Mesmer's suggestible dupes was no excuse not to do what seemed the real empirical work of refining somatic sensations and learning to discriminate among the manifold subtleties of being.

Some shift in my attitude must have been evident, because I started to hear back from people who wondered if I had "crossed the line." *What line? Who'd drawn it?* My monk's emergence provoked a fire-alarm response in some friends; their clowns stumbled over one another rushing to the trucks and getting the hoses going, desperate to extinguish any sparks of spiritual sincerity lest the fire spread and burn down all the comedy clubs. "How goes the journey?" they inquired, with heavy irony. "Are you actually buying this stuff?" they wondered. My father pointedly asked: "Is your book going to be *objective?*" "God, I hope not," I said. I was getting defensive. Early on in my work with Rachel, a woman I had dated for a month said pointedly as we were breaking up that she was only going to give me one piece of advice and that was to knock off the healing stuff and find a really good therapist, "a *regular* therapist."

The point was that if Rachel were picking up some kind of two-hundred-year-old proto-cowboy mishap involving my Write Foot, I was now willing to give it at least a little credence. If it was necessary that I be seen as a dupe to learn this stuff, so be it. Rachel's hands were twitching in the air above my Write Foot. I asked her what she was doing.

"I'm rebuilding the lines of light," she said.

After five or ten minutes, the Write Foot felt better.

"Now it feels as if there's a wedge in the left one," I said.

"Why don't you try pulling it out?" she asked.

"How?"

"Grab it with your hands, energetically."

I did, or pretended to, as I had done the first time with the belts of energy across my chest. It still seemed a piece of pantomime, not a "real" operation. Rachel could see more of those "astral critters" that she had seen in the previous healings. A few looked like big daddy longlegs, she said. I couldn't see them, or feel them either, perhaps because the concept was still weird and I was scared to . . . what, exactly? Accept the idea that spiders were embedded in my energy? Do the debugging myself? Act as if I had sufficient evidence to admit the reality of the whole astral construct itself?

Maybe I was putting a lot more energy than I thought into repressing the idea that Rachel's friend was right and Rachel had gone off the deep end. I was lost, and the maps of the territory were no help. One was a four-color, topographically reliable, measurement-based version of the mind-body landscape as mapped by cartographers from the scientific academy. The other was a vague, error-riddled treasure map drawn on the back of a palm leaf by a few Hindu seers and subsequently amended by some screwball Theosophists and a motley assortment of modern mystics . . .

"Hold the fourth level!" Rachel said sternly.

"The fourth level?"

"A loving state!"

The thoughts I was having were apparently compromising the opening through which the daddy longlegs could emerge. My fingers unfurled, moving like iron filings toward a magnet. I felt as if I were reaching for a bristly hairbrush and about to grab a tarantula instead . . .

"Hold the fourth level," Rachel said again.

She subscribed not only to the theory of the seven chakras but to her teacher's map of the body energy, which held that each chakra was identified with one of seven levels—sometimes the word "frequency" was used—and that these levels, these energy bodies within bodies, comprised a person's total energy field. A quick way to a loving state was to concentrate on the heart. As I put my attention on the heart, I had the sensation that something was crawling onto my extended fingers and then onto my palm. The feeling was too curiously vivid to be frightening.

"Hold it up into the light," Rachel said. "Send it love."

Act as if. Could thinking fondly amount to sending love? Could love vaporize an astral insect? Apparently so, for when I did, it vaporized. Allegedly vaporized, I should say.

In her first report, Rachel had attributed my physical ailments to "that twist in his central vertical power current." By the second CB healing, in October, she had divined the emotional causes that presumably had generated the physical condition: "The initiating cause of his illness has to do with deep, old feelings of being unworthy of unconditional love, love given to him just because he exists." These, she wrote, arose from "his feelings of not being able to trust his mother, and by extension, the universe, to meet his needs."

It was my mother's fault—I could swallow that.

When I went in for that October session, Rachel was determined to, as she put it later, "hold the ground of unconditional love." She told me she saw a sharp division between the high level of energy in my upper chakras and the low amount of juice in the lower ones.

"How do you deal with anger?" she asked.

I laughed and then realized that I often laugh when I'm uncomfortable. "Perhaps you deal with anger by masking it with laughter," she said. As if laughter could transmute anger into something palatable, something easier to swallow.

She asked me to extend my arms and imagine I was receiving a dose of that great clichéd desideratum of the New Age—unconditional love—and suddenly I was riven by shyness and slumped over on her healing table, wishing I could cover my face, which felt like the face of an eight-year-old boy. The mask of laughing-at-foolish-needs was suddenly transparent and hid nothing. Who but a dog, I thought bitterly, could ever give unconditional love, and who but a fool would want or expect it? Love from adults was necessarily adulterated. Can't find a dog? Get a healer.

To be loved for the sake of one's existence, what a novel absurdity! To live in the world was to learn not to need or want love of that ilk. After a while, the very idea of it was almost horrific—the horror of unearned regard, the horror of undeserved esteem. Love had to be won, earned, deserved. Unconditional love was infantilizing and claustrophobic; it was like being congratulated for burping and spitting up milk.

As for laughing to cover anger, where was the harm in masking feelings if such emotions could not otherwise be *handled* or expressed without making a situation worse? . . . Didn't you learn to work around strong emotions as you learned not to expect love without conditions? Didn't the family collude in this education, offering laughter as a way of dissolving what was dangerous, proposing achievement as a basis of love, crafting its uneasy truces and blind spots? Somewhere along the road that traveled from the primal scene and choral auditions to cracked bottles of acne scrub and inscrutable poems about the chemical companions of chlorophyll, I acquired a deep prejudice against the expression of emotion—I mean, against what I considered the banal expression of emotion. Simple honest statements about feelings had no weight or credibility. It was axiomatic that the legitimacy of feelings—their ability to be registered, to be heard and attended to—depended largely on the persuasiveness and originality of the rhetoric in which they were expressed. At the heart of *logos* there was a kind of seduction. Seduction was the way to grab an ear. It also was central to the method of any journalism that was ambitious enough to delve into emotional intimacies.

I was overflowing with revelations as Rachel talked and worked during that afternoon on her table—principally the one that my blithe existence as a laptop hack seemed entirely motivated by the feeling that I hadn't been heard as a kid—*Children should be seen and not heard.* But I realized as well that I had been tutored in a kind of duplicity, the duplicity of a parent who would trouble to deny that she was angry even when the red light of rage was seething like fire in a boiler. The lesson, which was that some things can be expressed as subtext, was converted later into an aesthetic law—some things must only be expressed as subtext; the essence of art is saying one thing but meaning another, saying without saying.

"That's good for art, but bad for the soul," Rachel said.

She had been running energy into my legs, and then started up the ladder of chakras, making the usual accommodation at the first chakra by holding her hands away from my groin. Next she settled them onto my abdomen at the second chakra. As she completed her work there, she was astonished to see between my second and third chakra the utterly incongruous sight of a fetus. It hovered there on the fourth level. An astral fetus.

"When I first saw it," she wrote in her report, "I asked myself, Is this perception or projection? I am nine months pregnant, so this was an important question. I re-centered and re-grounded and became very still, and received guidance that it was, indeed, his fetus, and that it was time for it to be taken into the light. I have often met babies in the fields of women who have had abortions; this was the first time I ever found one in a man's field. Because of my own current queasiness around this issue, I couldn't get a clear read on what the baby was doing in CB's field. Was it an abortion from a past life, cannibalism, something else? After a moment of wondering, I decided simply to hold it to the light. As I did so, the baby was received with love—I was very moved by the power and beauty and tenderness of that moment."

Afterwards, I told her about the pregnancy that had been terminated in 1989. What I marked most about her discovery was not its outlandishness but my own absence of judgment. It was beginning to dawn on me that perhaps this whole project involved much more than the dharma of narcissism. I did not know how a memory I had carried half-consciously for five years could surface in the lambent curtains of light visible to a clairvoyant, but it had, and for the moment, I was obliged to acknowledge—and make room for in the house of beliefs—the pertinence and truth of what she had seen.

Over the months, the pace of the case study accelerated. Rachel did healings on me in November and December. I saw her three times in January, three more in February. The bizarre business steadily became more familiar but was never unsurprising, and was often very intense.

Before I was allowed to lie on the healing table, Rachel had me assume the "horse stance" of the martial artist and hold the bowlegged position until my thighs trembled and sweat beaded on my forehead. The energy rumbled in my legs like a Harley idling at a stoplight and seemed to pull my awareness, which tended to hover like a lenticular cloud over the crown of my head, down into the flesh and bone.

In the midst of one healing in January when she was running energy between my heart and my throat, Rachel said she could feel me making a connection between the fourth and fifth chakras for the first time. It was beautiful, she said. Could I feel it? I thought yes, thought how the intercourse of heart and throat had to do with moving grief up and out, with the willingness to move on not in terror but in eagerness for whatever was next. There were all kinds of guides in the room, Rachel said, some assigned to her, some to me. One of my guides began to press her to relay messages. She had never channeled during a healing before, but found she was able to listen to whoever was supervising my affairs on the subtle planes. The guide wanted to pass on the news that my kundalini energy was about to commence rising, and that months of work were being consolidated and I was about to enter a new phase of life in which I would be able to "speak my heart," voice feelings, express love. I have to say that at the time it didn't sound as banal as it does now, but even then I thought maybe my guides were less than fully informed. They seemed to have skipped the first step of journalism, which is: Check the clips. Voice feelings? Speak from the heart? Hadn't they seen CB's "What a Man Learns from a Broken Heart," that internationally acclaimed sob story in a recent issue of *Glamour* magazine? Maybe guides don't read women's magazines.

At the moment, I cared less about whether my heart could speak and more about the chronic weakness in my left shoulder, the one from which Joel Wallach said the arm had been lopped off. As Rachel's work progressed, the pain in the shoulder increased. It was as if, in an expanded state of consciousness, the energy in my arm was too big for the container. The unroomy arm was incapable of holding as much, well, life, as the rest of my body. It felt like a riverbed that was filled in with silt and rubble and could no longer convey a large volume of water. I asked Rachel if she could quiz the ethereal fellows about this acutely physical sensation.

Rachel noted later that she looked at the shoulder and saw an energetic wound like a red mouth with "astral blood" oozing from it. When she went to fix it, my guides told her no. Then her guides and my guides got into some kind of an argument. My troops emerged with the last word, which was to have CB do it, have CB put some temporary astral stitches in the shoulder gash. Why? Because he would soon be working through the issues connected to the wound, and the wound would heal of itself. Was this a story a pattern-making mind concocted around the inspiration of some incipient arthritis, the pearl of a tale conjured around the irritation of a sand grain? Or was it just plainly and structurally true?

"Just use your intent to make the stitches," Rachel said.

As when I had unbuckled the heart bands, I found myself following her suggestion to work in a weird, criminally irrational realm while my law-abiding cop looked the other way. I imagined myself holding a pair of knitting needles and clicking them together to weave a chain of cross-stitches, like a seam on a softball. I said nothing to Rachel of what I was envisioning, but she said, "Oh good, I can see what you're doing," and then she drew out a chain of x'es: XXXXX. I patched another spot where there was a "rip" in my field. I could only feel it, not see it, but even so I was feeling positively gifted. Either I had suggested myself into a virtual healing practice, or there was more merit in astrology than met the eye. The arm felt better, but at the expense of my existing mind-body accord.

Oh please, the arm felt better.

No, it did.

Well, how?

Well, it's hard to describe. The life wasn't leaking out of it. I don't know how else to describe it.

What you're saying, in effect, is that in the body there are levels of life, degrees of liveliness. Some areas are more alive, more aware, than others.

I am. And I wonder if maybe death creeps in through those places where we are unaware, where there isn't life to oppose it.

If you go on like this, you'll be climbing in a baquet with Mesmer. I don't suppose you think he could have eased the pain of your sore arm.

I think he could have, but if you're implying that the panacea here was simply my imagination, don't you think you might at least credit me with a measure of authenticity, given that I was both receiving the treatment and conducting it? I was actively involved . . .

There are no limits to the dharma of narcissism . . .

So it went. Sometimes I resisted the dive into the pool at the start of each healing session, averse not to the encounter with energy so much as the encounter with therapeutic dialogue. Now it seems nothing more than contrariness on my part, for I can see the value in Rachel's ability to combine energetic insights with psychological observation. My very resistance was a measure of her acuity. At the time, the pairing of energetic and psychological descriptions often left me embarrassed or irked. I had a hard time getting around the feeling that Rachel was asking me play the stock roles of Angry Son or Aggrieved Ex-Boyfriend in yet another jargon-riddled production from the Inner Child Playhouse. Perhaps the issue here was nothing but a disagreement over style. I know the scripts as directed by Rachel were efforts to cut through my layers of reasonableness and circumvent the passive-aggressive strategies I used to stifle anger. As laudable and liberating as that goal may have been, I had to wonder at the time, as I wonder now, if maybe there were some virtues in not expressing anger, but in suppressing it. Maybe anger was meant to be used, harnessed, mastered, even bottled up; not dumped, vented, or confessed. Certainly it could provide the impetus to create, the impetus to change. It seemed to me—was I rationalizing furiously?—that putting a premium on making bald declarations of anger was contrary to an important, albeit much-maligned, masculine standard. There is a warrior spirit that inner-child monologues can only make a mockery of. There is a dignity in stoicism, in shutting-up-already in the face of pain, and the cult of broadcasted feeling could only diminish it. The early years of the New Age movement helped foment American talk-show ethics and the culture of fulsome disclosure. But tricky gender issues and a number of dangerous unproven assumptions about the nature of disease cropped up whenever New Age ideas were applied to alternative healing. For instance, some exponents of visualization viewed the conventional approach to cancer as hopelessly masculine, an outmoded example of mindless male militancy. They proposed instead that people meet the adversity of runaway cell growth with sweetness and light, a benign attitude of loving acceptance. They advised patients to ask themselves: Why did you need to create this tumor? What emptiness do you think the tumor is trying to fill? They assumed that was a better reaction than simply zapping the bastard. But politically correct holistic responses were not necessarily medically more effective ones. In a community dominated by women, whose healing abilities had long been disparaged by science and mainstream medicine, it was tough to make the case that sometimes what was wanted in the fight against illness was a fighter, an angel with a sword and an attitude, not a soft touch.

But Rachel's intention obviously was to force me to engage emotions I'd chosen to handle at a safe remove. She wasn't working on the Marlboro Man, but on a confrontation-phobic urbanite bent on saying things without saying them, if only to preserve a measure of deniability. She was sure she knew the madness of this character, because she could feel his method in his tissues. My legs were warehouses of anger, she said. Had I ever considered therapy?

Oh, therapy, New Yorkers' favorite sport.

No, really, she said.

Carlyle said self-contemplation is infallibly the symptom of disease.

No, really, she said.

I don't want to be wrenched into pre-fab schemes of human relations.

No, I really ought to try it, she said, if only to explore my antipathy to therapists.

How many therapists were there in Casper, Wyoming? Were high-strung Manhattan analysands any saner than unshrinked cowboys?

Whelping inner children is a thankless job. Rachel was good at making my resistance to therapy seem like grounds for therapy. She listened patiently as I flogged the theme of heroic stoicism and grimly protested the spiritual Stalinism that considered the refusal to submit to psychotherapy evidence of mental illness. I couldn't even get away with laughing at my own hyperbole. I'd laugh to disown everything I said; laugh with the subversive pleasure of volte-face, and she'd say, "Okay, where's the fuck-you?" As if there were never text without subtext, as if there were always more at stake than I was willing to acknowledge, as if I still had to learn to speak directly and truthfully, traveling the hard road from heart to throat, in sentences that did not contain outs, asides, escape hatches, parenthetical disclaimers. Perhaps there was more at stake—certainly there was more at stake. As Rachel put it later in one of her reports: "There are issues on which I could and should confront him, such as his refusal to enter therapy. But I don't want to displease CB, so I soft-pedal where I should confront. This results in CB's being mollified. Tacitly, I am condoning his behavior, and he is encouraged to continue it. I end up feeling bad about myself as a healer and doubting myself. I need to work on this need to mollify and placate men."

In February 1995, after talking the idea over with her own therapist and an older healer who was supervising her case study, Rachel announced that she would begin charging me for healings. She wanted forty dollars a healing, half her usual fee. It was hard for her to break the news. She was afraid I wouldn't come back if she charged me, but it was important to her that she clarify the nature of our relationship. My status had alternated between friend and client, as hers in my eyes had hovered somewhere at the intersection of friend, healer, and subject. I was never sure how to greet her that winter when she opened the door of her apartment, often holding her new baby girl. I had taken to bussing my healer on the cheek, but that's not how a client would have greeted a shrink or a physical therapist.

When she began what would be the last uncompensated healing, she found my legs were thick and unreceptive, and wondered if I was angry at her for changing the rules. I didn't think so. But the question of money did force me to weigh the value of the treatment and to ask not only whether each session was worth forty dollars but to reassess what my goals were, how progress was being measured. Was I really getting anywhere? What was it worth, this healing, this investigation into grief, whatever it was? I decided I would continue the work but would cut back my visits from three a month to one every three or four weeks.

During another healing, later in February, Rachel had her hands over my stomach and suddenly I flinched as if I'd been jabbed with a cattle prod. I asked her what she was doing.

"I'm upwelling your Core Star," she said.

Well, knock it off! I felt like saying. But didn't. And didn't press her for a definition of Core Star either. The phrase was one of her teacher Barbara

Brennan's less felicitous contributions to the lexicon of subtle energy. I understood it as a synonym for "soul," or whatever fragment or essence of the universe was pieced out in each of us. Core Stars, souls, essences: Who could be sure what any of these nebulous thingamajigs signified? More to the point, I wondered how my experience on the healing table was mediated by the terms in which it was presented. What if Rachel had said instead of Core Star that she was upwelling the Nebulous Thingamajig? Language denoted what was explicitly said in the lines, but it also upwelled whatever was between them. For me, Core Star had less tradition, less weight, less specificity and meaning than even a will-o-wisp word like "soul." I suppose I was annoyed at the vagueness of it, forgetting for a moment that all language is anchored in illusion. *One always perishes by the self one assumes: To bear a name is to claim an exact mode of collapse.* In the throes of my own confused apprenticeship, I was forgetting that Rachel also was a student, learning on the job, and it was to be expected she would operate on borrowed authority. Perhaps her healings could be considered the equivalent of the candy-striper practicing injections on oranges. Core Star was part of her vocabulary because it was part of the vocabulary of her school, a school breaking away from the traditional religious connotations of soul, seeking to bridge physics and metaphysics with the experience of energy.

I asked her how she managed to upwell whatever it was she was upwelling.

"First I upwell myself, and then I wait for you. See, here's me . . . And here's you."

I was suddenly overcome by embarrassment; the commingling of our presences generated an intimacy that seemed too large for the still-confused definitions of our relationship. It was as if we had wandered beyond the confines of the healer-client partnership into some profound existential affiliation. It didn't seem sexual in the least. Sex, at least of the mildly perverse, unenlightened sort I was familiar with, required some distance, a gap for a spark to jump across. Amid all the upwelling of Core Star soulfulness, there was no gap, no distance, only a kind of union, the union of agape, not eros.

"It's to know about yourself that you feel embarrassed at intimacy," Rachel said in what sounded like the archaic speech patterns of a spirit guide. It wasn't the intimacy per se that embarrassed me, it was wondering what to do with it, not knowing what to do. "The healing room is a laboratory where all your feelings in life are replicated," she said in a normal voice.

Maybe I was angry about being charged after all. I remembered the unexpected vehemence with which Dolores Krieger, the founder of Therapeutic Touch, had decried those healers who charged high fees to teach the laying on of hands and, in her view, put their own enrichment ahead of service to humanity. The professionalization of energy medicine abounded with contradictions. How could you presume to muster a flow of "unconditional love" when a check was a preliminary condition? Almost by definition, spiritual acts were impossible in a commercial context. Were healers any better than all the other barkers vending New Age fads? Forty bucks for something that might not even exist! It was enough to upwell your gorge.

But, in fact, I was relieved to start paying Rachel for healings. I felt obligated to her. She was doing so much work on my behalf, and I hadn't been able to reciprocate. As our work was unfolding, it was impossible to know how it would turn out or whether I would be able to feature it in my book, and anything that I might eventually write about it seemed too far off and speculative to be considered quid pro quo. My supposed "contribution" as her senior-project guinea pig seemed eclipsed by the benefit I was getting. Not sure what we were exchanging, I was glad to discharge the debt for the time she had put in, the sweat she had shed, standing with her legs bowed and her hands shaped over my head.

When I began meditating, in February, Rachel said she could see the effects on the fifth, sixth, and seventh levels of my field. These outermost subtle bodies were "enlivened," she said. She also detected an increase in my "hemispheric congruity" but worried that the energy systems associated with the emotions and the heart—the second- and fourth-level bodies and their corresponding chakras—seemed depleted. She was concerned that I was using meditation to sidestep feelings and avoid interacting with people. She noted in her report that I argued a lot. I made a case for sidestepping emotions. The serenity of meditation was a useful kind of relief, and wasn't chanting a mantra every morning a better way to cope with depression than Prozac? I liked to contest her authority. She was the clairvoyant, the energy expert; she was the person who knew the real story. Rachel noted in her reports that I needed to be right, I needed to annihilate opponents. She was generous and shrewd enough to observe that when she colluded with my tendency to argue, my need, as she put it, "to be special," she served me poorly as a healer.

I was never scared of what came up during healings—boggled often, dumbstruck with insights. In one healing I experienced a magnificent speed-of-light expansion of my ordinary boundaries so that it seemed I was both in the human-scale body and in a body vast enough to engulf the continent, a body growing more vast by the second until it seemed the earth was sitting in my palm like a sea-blue marble, and that I had some blood sense that completely contradicted the prevailing scientific equation of mind with brain: a sense of the vastness everywhere around us in even the smallest things, the universe in Blake's fabled grain of sand. Here was the Chhāndôgyas Upanishad that speaks of the "town of Spirit" wherein lie "heaven, earth, fire, wind, sun, moon, lightning, stars, whatever is and whatever is not . . ."

No, never scared, except once.

Since meditating, I had noticed a cloudy, congested feeling in the area above my right eye. It felt as if there was something under the upper eyelid, in behind the eyeball, like when you're bicycling and you get a bug in your eye. I couldn't get it out. Could it be a cyst or some kind of growth or a lost eyelash? Some stress thing—not that defining the cause as stress would explain the particularity and location of the feeling. Sometimes the right eye muscles would convulse.

When I asked Rachel about it in the middle of March, she said, "Let me connect with it." She held her hands at my temples, then without a moment's hesitation said, "It's an implant."

"An implant?"

"An implant."

An implant that existed on the astral plane, she said, a structure of energy that seemed to have been on site since I was eleven. She thought the reason I hadn't noticed it before was I hadn't been sensitive enough. She could see a reddish irritation around it. It looked like a computer chip, she said. Implants were generally ways for disembodied beings to keep an eye on the material world.

Oh, that's just great. Disembodied beings. Implants. Great. The idea that disembodied beings had the capacity to install nonphysical computer chips in my body, and were thus able to join me in reviewing say, my tax returns, was still on the far side of my distended boggle threshold. But I was too creeped out to scorn the proposition. At some level, we all feel the superstitions of the culture. You can laugh at the UFO-ologists and dismiss as perfectly ludicrous the whole tribe of aliens from Little Grays to Big Pinks or whatever, but there is a part of the brain that was formed in the thrall of superstition, and suddenly it's got you, and a shiver runs through you.

Rachel said she could take it out. She tried to hook on to it energetically, but the thing, whatever it was, slipped away. She made a number of attempts but couldn't get a purchase on it, and finally she quit trying. Hoping to reduce the irritating effect of the implant on my eye, she said, she wrapped it in a sheath of platinum light. The irritation in the eye was appreciably less.

4. GOOD-BYE

Three days later, the ghost in my soul seat called to say she was leaving the country at the end of the week. Moving abroad to live with a man she met, the man whom, as it turned out, she would marry before the year was out. She wanted to say good-bye in person. No good could come of that. I could only think of saying, Go, go, go, get on with your life. But it was hard to reject her overture, to swim against the current of sentiment. We exchanged some dolorous promises to keep each other abreast of major news in our lives, and then hung up. And I got through the next few days fine—felt okay, not bad, upwelled, excruciatingly sincere. Lived in my body.

And then on the night of her departure, the phone rang. She was calling from the first-class lounge at the airport, weepy and sad and overwhelmed. But the reason was not that our long strange march was ending, our ways finally diverging. She was having a hard time leaving everybody—her office mates, her parents, her therapy group, her dry cleaners. I was astonished—and yes, angry—at her self-absorption; angry, really, at my own absurd willingness to make myself available. But wasn't it the oldest story in the world? One person's open-heart surgery is another's paper cut. And in a matter of moments, the condemnation melted out, and in its place came a hot stab of feeling, the long-fended-off grief, the pain of desertion, loneliness, and finally some new devil, the sense of life-killing repetitiousness. The needle had been stuck in the groove of the record, and everyone who ever had anything to do with us was sick to death of hearing the same snippet of music over and over again. To run in the space of a few seconds from numbness to feeling, from cold to hot, was utterly exhausting. By the end of the conversation, I was too tired to be sad, or to feel anything but the improbable fondness that wells up when people are grateful for their history.

"Good-bye," I heard her say in a strangely breathy voice. She sounded forlorn, a little girl on the brink of an unknown life.

Sufferin' succotash! I could hear my body, mute for so many years! The machine had words for the ghost. This is what it said: We were comfortable in the world when you were not. We felt things when you were oblivious. We were dense, but never dumb. You thought of us as a basement, a vessel, a wilderness, a swamp, a prison, a death sentence, a home you did not want, something to flee, sometimes a source of pleasure and hunger and thirst, but never a story, never A becoming B becoming C. For so long, we were your steadfast silent companion. But now we are betraying you; as we change, we mark your time. We have become a box of frailties, a set of limits, a list of symptoms, deficits you record: weak ankles, lost speed, stiff joints, trail-away hair, crow's-feet, cuts patched with melanin-less collagen so that in summer the repair work from a thorn-bush wound blazes up as a white claw mark in a sea of sun-darkened flesh. We are the memory of mountain summers when it was no trouble to sleep on the ground and bound down talus fields and launch backwards into space on rappel. Our complaints now define us as a perfection you no longer have, a perfection you did not know was missing until you came up short. The story of your life is imperceptibly merging with ours. You are beginning to understand that the way beyond the world is through the world, through us. Where we go, you go. What we are, you will become . . .

"Good-bye," I said, suddenly awash in sadness again. I wanted to go on now, if only to move the dust around in my apartment or chart the ascent of my health-insurance premiums. Something, anything, was better than being perpetually suspended in hellish irons. Go go go, go on. When I hung up, it was like cutting a jammed rope.

5. SHADOW BOOKS

I did not schedule an appointment with Rachel in the next four months. Spring came, and summer, and I realized my life was no longer organized around an absence. The mountains of that country receded in the rearview mirror, and the change seemed the consequence of the energy work I had done with Rachel, the fruit of the hard heart lessons in opening and letting go. I fell in love with a willowy hazel-eyed woman whom it seemed possible to love as deeply as I had ever loved anyone, and to sustain that love endlessly, without reservation. I applied my healing budget to flowers and restaurants and plays. I learned later that Rachel thought I had stayed away, angry at her for imposing a fee, but I think it was rather a combination of factors, the foremost being the pleasure of spending time as a moronically happy, love-struck extrovert on holiday from scrutiny and angst. I was also sobered by the business about my eye and needed some time away from delving healers and wild extraterrestrial theories to get my bearings—to get "grounded," in Rachel's terms. Grounding and the kindred notion of "centering" were not just physical states. They could be extended to cover the psychological agenda of reclaiming boundaries, of restoring emotional and mental balance. I was wanting homeostasis on many levels, time to weigh and integrate or reject the heretical ideas, to make whatever modifications I had to in a system of beliefs that had never been so deeply challenged.

Drawn one way by intellectual arguments, another by emotional currents, I was struck by the artifice of my categories, the seemingly arbitrary partitions that social convention imposed on the spectrum of personal consciousness. To grant that psychic reality had as much substance as physical reality and that it was no less real, no less actual, was to deny one's self the relief of waking up from a nightmare and saying, "Oh, it was all just a dream." In the realm of the healer, the boundary between dreamed and lived events was not so clear; nightmares couldn't be glibly dismissed as fantasies, because all consciousness was actual, all awareness was real. Dreams were simply a form of experience, perhaps that very form which people were afraid to face without the state-of-mind distinctions of sleep and waking. There were levels and levels and levels at which—and of which—we could become conscious. Each awakening in the chain of revelations recast the one before it, changing the definitions of sleep and waking.

I suppose Rachel had come to personify my struggle with authority, not just with her authority but with the authority of my own awareness and the roles faith and science played in fashioning it. She had surely put a face on some of the more outlandish aspects of hands-on healing, brashly mixing medicine and religion. She told me once of a night when she had woken on the astral plane and found a wolf in the corner of her bedroom. (There is apparently no shortage of large-carnivore habitat on the astral plane.) She had a rule—no spooks in the bedroom. She tried to shoo the wolf out, but it sprang and bit her in the throat. In the morning, when she rejoined the day-side horde of sleepwalkers gulping down coffee and assembling at train stations, she discovered she had a terrible sore throat.

I was vexed and not just because I was having trouble with the concept of an astral wolf attack as being anything more than a melodramatic story generated by the unconscious around the inspiration of a throat infection. I was having my usual trouble because it was all, well, so *vexing*: astral wolves, untestable claims and premises, confabulated tales offered in defiance of seemingly more "reasonable" explanations. How was one to receive such stories? How did you analyze the question of priority—did the wolf attack cause the sore throat or vice versa? Or the fuzziness in the definition of waking—was "waking on the astral plane" akin to lucid dreaming in which one is conscious inside a dream?

It was easy to forget that for all its apparent privileges, clairvoyant perception was as subjective as ordinary vision—as much an act of a mind constructing a visual experience. There is imagination in all kinds of sight. In normal sight, the banana and the crucifix and the computer all appear *out there*, in the external world, and not in the brain, where the information is actually registered, and where the illusion of three-dimensional space is projected. So couldn't high sense percepts of "implants" reflect the preoccupations and interpretations of the perceiver?

I was further exasperated because even to myself I was beginning to seem like a tower of hypochondria. The muscles clutching my right eye were still throbbing weirdly, and I couldn't put to rest the conviction that something on the backside of the eyeball needed to come out. The eye exams I had been given while getting glasses had unearthed nothing untoward, and when I casually mentioned the sensation in my eye to an ophthalmologist I met at a party, she said that "foreign body sensation" was one of the most common eye complaints. *Foreign body sensation*: You don't know the half of it . . . I had begun waking up—in my actual bed on an actual patch of the actual Upper West Side—with my elbow crooked across my forehead. Give the domain of the symbolic an inch and it takes a mile: I wondered what this unprecedented configuration implied. Was I protecting my sixth chakra, the third eye and center of psychic sight? Or employing the ostrich defense against another member of Rachel's astral wolf pack? Or trying to soothe a head wound inflicted after some unauthorized psychic surgery?

Later that spring, with the eye-implant theory much on my mind, I drove up to Litchfield, Connecticut, to sit in on a group-healing circle led by Elizabeth Stratton, a well-known hands-on healer who was working on a book and whose press kit included a number of newspaper clippings and a videotape of a TV appearance. I asked her to have a look at my eye but didn't say anything about implants. Stratton worked with two assistants. She went around a circle of eight people, spending about six or seven minutes with each person. When the program was finished, she took me aside. She had a stricken look on her face.

"I don't know what was in there," she said. "It was so intense I couldn't even get in. When I went to connect with it, I felt something trying to choke me—hands around my throat. And I got a very loud crackling in my right ear." She asked if I had any problems with my lymph glands, my ears. "It was so intense I had to back off," she said. "I tried to release some of the energy around it. That was all I could do." I told her about Rachel's implant diagnosis. She shook her head, not to dismiss it but to say she hadn't heard of such things. She said she'd always discounted the possibility of extraterrestrial phenomena, but lately she was beginning to wonder.

In August, four months having passed since our last healing, I called Rachel. In the interim I had spent some time with a group of healers in New Hampshire, one of whom had concurred with Rachel's diagnosis. When I called Rachel to pass along this confirmation, she said she was surprised to hear from me. She confessed that she had felt abandoned, sad, and guilty for charging me. "We entered into a process, and I feel it needs closure," she said.

I told her I hadn't thought our work was over. And so we arranged a day and time to resume it. I returned to her table later that summer. It was more than a year after our first encounter. I thought I was comfortable enough that I didn't have to try to charm my way into her confidence, but she marked what she later noted was my old pattern of "seductiveness," surmising that it had to do with my need to reestablish our connection. In four subsequent visits, she was happy to find that quality had waned, and that I was able to be present and connected "without the slightest whiff of flirtatiousness."

"I perceived this as growth on his part," she wrote. "I felt proud of him."

Perhaps all that time—August, September, October, November— we were hunting for the resolution of our experiment. How does an investigation of grief end when the grief has cleared? With what ceremonies? If you found yourself moving from physical problems to psychological problems to existential and spiritual concerns with the ultimate goal being, what?—some variant of God-drunk guide-tended super-bliss?—well there was no end to the number of sessions you might require. Perhaps whether one was a healer or a client, part of an apprenticeship was learning not only how to engage the intense intimacies of the healing table but how to undo them. Terminating what was theoretically interminable.

I told Rachel in October that she had helped me get my hands around my anger. Passed it on very calmly. My body was sweating from the horse-stance warm-up, but my throat was cold, the fifth chakra suspiciously inactive. And then I saw her staring at my right eye, looking through me and saying "Hello? Hello?" And then to me: "There are two ET's peeping out of your eye." And suddenly I was in a rage—*not these things again!*

"I think they're just curious," she said, "they come in when no one's home."

I was pissed, and resolved to snip the sinewy little link I could suddenly feel at the back of my eye where the creepy dealy-bobs were fastened on. Snip it with my intention, my will, that mysterious enactor of choices. It was my idea, not Rachel's, and I said nothing to indicate my plan, but once again, she startled me with her ability to read the not-readily-apparent with her apparent clairvoyance. "Good," she said, "you're using your anger to cut the connection—the anger's giving you energy." She watched for a minute. "You've got most of it," she said. In this act of ministering to myself, I realized I drew on anger to extricate myself from sloughs of incapacity and fear. Anger spurred the desire to excel. It enabled me to shuck off the paralysis of stage fright. I was now suddenly quite generally pissed. Angry at little nonEarthly opportunistic eye leeches, at the New Age fruitcakes who identified them as such. Oh, why draw the line there? Why even draw it at Miss Soul Seat or my saintly mother? Wasn't the real villain here the wayward desultory authority overhead, the Absent Divine, the Omnipotent Slacker? I felt angry enough that if God had stood in front of me, I didn't know if I would fall on my knees or slap His or Her face. I was mad enough to rip a phone book in half—and yet not for a moment undelimited by a reality principle. So please, not the Manhattan directory, let me have a phone book from a very small town.

When the spasm passed, I told Rachel that she had helped me understand the difference between an identity based on achievement and one based on the love of being. I told her I was thinking of proposing to the woman I had been seeing since the spring. How did that play with the guides? The guides were very excited, Rachel said, especially the female with the curly blond hair. Rachel relayed their counsel: "They say the angels of marriage will be blessing this. They say this is a woman who will flow with you. There is lot of pink and rose light around the idea."

When the healing was over and I was putting on my shoes and sipping from the glass of water she had brought me, Rachel said she also had some news. She had finished her latest book, a novella.

Would I read it? she asked.

I said I would be happy to.

The manuscript arrived in the mail along with copies of her semimonthly healing reports about her subject, CB, and the sixteen-page paper she had prepared for her senior case presentation. She enclosed a cover letter, asking me to keep confidential certain autobiographical facts about her. She also requested: "In the light of the truth, please tell me honestly what you think of [the manuscript]. I remember that someone gave you a novel to read and you didn't think it was very good but you didn't say so. I hope you will be more candid with me."

Much too late I came across something Somerset Maugham once said, which I wish I had taken to heart. "People ask you for criticism," he wrote, "but they only want praise."

But then, by her own logic, wasn't I an actor in Rachel's play? The question goes to the heart of the issue of conjoint reality. "Conjoint reality"—how many times had I heard that phrase from the mouths of healers, yet never once was certain what it meant. Was it to say that people imposed their realities on one another or that they fabricated reality together? Both propositions begged the question of whether people created reality at all. Wasn't it more true to say that most of the time they simply found themselves in the thick of it, and that whatever it was, the psyche didn't have much to do with it, any more than it had to do with Jupiter spinning in the firmament. Ayurvedic philosophers might argue that reality is manufactured in the act of human perception, but then they sometimes treated rabies with only a poultice.

I say that Rachel asked me to read her book, but in fact I'm not certain that's true. If she were creating her own reality, it would make sense that she had asked me. But if I were creating mine, then it would make sense that I had volunteered to read it. Or perhaps we were operating in tandem, and had conjointly seized on the issue of her novella to end the business between us.

I read the case reports first and then her senior presentation paper. I was impressed and moved by the attention she had given my energy field and by her insights into my patterns and nature, her sense that at base what I lacked was the ability to trust and to connect, and that these short-comings stemmed from an inability to divine my connection to the Divine. It was, she noted, CB's "image of his own unacceptableness and undeservingness [that] led him to reject God as a defense for feeling rejected." The reports and the presentation were clearly and directly writ-ten, if somewhat jargony.

Rachel said that she was sometimes so happy working on CB that she had no trouble staying present, but when we argued, when something came up that provoked "her abandonment issues" she would leave, exit energetically. She had spent time in therapy dealing with her "counter-transference" and found the self-examination painful. I evoked many of her own issues—almost every issue she had. Her professional boundaries were weak around me. Her evaluation of me was that I wanted to seduce and she wanted to be seduced, that I needed to feel special and she needed to make me, and men in general, feel special. I operated on charm, and charm operated on her. Thus, she wrote, I was a "sublime mirror" for her, and she was proud that she had not let her issues collude with mine, she had not succumbed to my seductiveness, or fed my need to be spe-cial, or capitulated to my charm. She resisted the temptation to fence with me when I was in argument mode, even though she was shocked during one of our debates when I punched her in the solar plexus with a fistlike "pseudopod" of energy. "My diligent work to understand my counter-transference gave me a wonderful gift: self-respect. In this way, CB has healed me."

As depicted, we were two people who couldn't be more healthy or insightful. How wishful this seems in retrospect, a false summit that marked the advent of the real ordeal. Some other healing loomed that had nothing to do with the curriculum of subtle energy or discerning hands. Reading her autobiographical sketch, I was struck by the under-current of egotism. It seems poignant now; at the time, it seemed boastful and off-putting, and when I began to page through her novella, the claim that I had healed her seemed to speak to a capacity for delusion. Rachel had laid it on the line that what she wanted most was to succeed not as a healer but as a novelist. In her eyes, fiction writing was her true gift, and she insisted she had a knack for creating characters and stories, and that her prose was clear and accessible. Her ambition was to use her literary talents to teach people about "regulating energy" and "the plenitude of guidance and love." But with unpublished novels piling up, she confessed that she had often wondered what was blocking her success, what "negative limiting core belief" she needed to upwell and release.

Had I been brought in to tell her? Had she conjured Chorus Boy who couldn't sing to break the painful news? And not just to break it gently and let it go at that, or even to pursue the job with the clinical impersonality of a dentist looking for cavities in a tooth, but to funnel all the energy of his own transference into the mission? Which is to say, all the anger I could or would not direct at the real targets, anger now doubling back on Rachel for her inexperienced decision to put me in the position of becoming her critic, a position I wasn't smart enough to turn down, a position I must have secretly cultivated for the promised opportunity to reassert my authority in a field where I wasn't an apprentice but a member of the guild. Had my doubts about Rachel been waiting for just such a chance to plot some kind of vengeance? I fear if she was not engrossed in fantasies then she was merely naive, wrenchingly naive enough to think that the spirit of loving compassion with which healers approach a client was also the spirit with which critics approached a text. What was my role in reading her manuscript and rendering the "candid" opinion she desired? A fellow writer? A friend? A healing client?

I opened the novella hoping to be entranced by a story, and by the end of the first page, I had become a dentist. Beyond the fixable technical problems—fluctuations in tone and point of view, jarring diction, confused or sketchy motivation, superfluous characters, a tensionless structure, scenes that pivoted on coincidence—lay the shadow of aesthetic and moral defects. She had the germ of a good story, but the characters weren't sympathetic; the narrator had no perspective on her own obsession, and thus could give the reader none. After a while, I stopped marking the text. I wondered if the novella was a kind of shadow book where Rachel had stashed all her unangelic, impermissible feelings and thoughts. Did she need the outlet of fiction for all the stuff she was duty-bound to keep out of her work as a healer? If being a healer was a way of cultivating an inner light, maybe fiction afforded her a way of wallowing in darkness. It had to be a strain always being the angel in the church play, especially given that the psyche was a complement of angel and devil, monk and clown. If Rachel could not love her characters and esteem their flaws as deeply as she loved and esteemed her clients, it would be hard for them not to come across as shadow puppets enacting the drama of forbidden feelings.

People ask for criticism, but what they really want is praise. I should have been wise enough to refuse the role she had offered me. I should have said, "Well, Rachel, the book's not bad, there's a good idea here, here are the strengths, here's what you might want to think about in another draft." Short and sweet. But I didn't, and the reason will become apparent if it is not already. I composed a four-page memo, taking pains to note the odd reversal of our roles, how I now awkwardly found myself standing over her as a critic as she had once stood over me as a healer. I laid out my views in detail, alas, and spoke bluntly, leaning on the drill: "I think your ego is getting in your way and is kind of a blind spot for you. I would meditate on why it is so important to you that you be a writer. What is the big deal about it? Do you think you will be somebody if you're a writer? That you'll have an identity? I raise these questions because I was surprised that the therapeutic insight you show in healing sessions seemed to be missing from your manuscript." And because I took it upon myself to teach her the so-called truth, to get her to see things as they are, the right way, which was my way, and because I exhorted her to undertake the very self-examination she had pressed me to undertake and which I had resisted as surely as she would resist my exhortations, I have to acknowledge now that her shadow book had become a part of mine.

Even in less-fraught circumstances, it's not easy to strike a balance between imparting the hard-to-swallow facts and being a compassionate, supportive, uncompetitive critic. But I was guilty. I spelled out my views more vehemently than was warranted, not only in the black-and-white of a memo but more damagingly in the face-to-face conversation when we met for what turned out to be our final healing together.

We had planned to go over my notes afterwards, but the topic would not be delayed. When I launched into the spiel, it was immediately apparent that presenting the critique in person was a mistake. The tension escalated. Rachel sat rigidly on a chair, eyes wide, jaw tight, and in her resistance, her effort to appear composed, her reassurances that she was fine with what she was hearing, I could sense that she did not accept my points—that she believed my view was compromised by our therapeutic relationship, which is to say the transference issues that had arisen during the healing work. Since I was unable to vent my anger on her, she figured I was dumping it on her book instead. If you can't hit the therapist, you might as well hit the therapist's prose—hit what you perceive from your discredited perspective to be the author's shortcomings. Rachel endured this assault as if it were the difficult but heroic sacrifice a healer had to make.

In hindsight, I should have stopped when I saw her back go up. But the fact that she thought my perspective was discredited by our healing relationship and my insights had no merit really pissed me off and raised the stakes even higher. I had to make her see my points, and see that my points were not subjective opinions, not wild clairvoyant perceptions of pseudopods and astral fetuses; this was writing; assessments could be made based on relatively objective, even quasi-scientific facts. To hold that opinions about writing couldn't be separated from personal feelings—or that objective judgments were inevitably compromised by personal feelings—was to reject the idea that writing was a profession with standards. Yes, art was never right or wrong like science, but there were rules that went back to Aristotle, and writers violated them at the risk of their readers' wrath.

Why so emotional, CB? It's not as if there weren't failed novels or sheaves of dismal poetry in my desk drawer, or that I was immune to book-writing anxieties. Why—unless I was angry at her—did I care so much that I had to do her the big favor of stripping her of her illusions? I think it had to do with the relation of her writing to her healing. The failure to perform as advertised as a writer inflamed my doubts as to the extent to which she had incorporated a reality principle in her work as a healer. What seemed a lack of insight in one realm raised the possibility of a lack of insight in the other. All along, I was wanting to have faith in the authenticity of her incredible descriptions of astral wolves and fetuses and guides with curly blond hair. Even when I could confirm some uncanny parallels between her visions and my biography, it was hard to embrace her work simply as unalloyed truth. Now more than a year's worth of doubts about the reality of healing were suddenly aggravated by what seemed her inability to appraise her writing realistically. If she was mired in illusions as a scribbler, God knows what fantasies she was unwinding on the table. Who was this person who was leading me into outer space, extracting old sorrows and bedrock fears? What sort of reality principle had she established for herself, for us both?

I felt deceived in some way, confronting the de-idealization of my vaunted clairvoyant. Why had I entrusted my psyche to someone whose ideation seemed as fractured as mine, as drunk-on-dreams as mine, as full of unprocessed material from Repression 101 as mine? In short, as human as mine. I was angry at myself for forgetting what I always knew and for employing a method of learning that seemed to entail having to abandon myself in order to recover a new self.

There is no way to pretty this up: Whatever its merits, the vehemence of my critique was monstrous. It was all the more cruel because I knew from her autobiographical sketch that her literary aspirations were at the center of her identity. It didn't take clairvoyance to see that the harder I argued the prosecution's case, the more defensive she became, the more vulnerable. She seemed younger and younger, and strangely, she also seemed braver, like a little put-upon girl backed into a corner with only a teddy bear between her and the killer.

So, in the space of an hour in November 1995, I composed my own shadow book. In one fell swoop, Rachel had haplessly come to embody my darkest suspicion that I had been wasting my time with this healing business, that it wasn't real, that only a monk who was in fact a delusional clown would get involved in it, and only a bigger and more delusional clown would try writing a book about it. In some ways, I had addressed that memo to the wrong person, and Rachel and her poor beleaguered book had paid the price. The litany of questions I had invited her to contemplate were mine to ponder as well, perhaps even mine alone:

I think your ego is getting in your way and is kind of a blind spot for you.

I would meditate on why is it so important to you that you be a writer.

What is the big deal about it?

Do you think you'll be somebody?

Incredibly, she went on to perform the healing we had scheduled. I don't remember anything about it. I'm not sure I was even there, energetically speaking. Or if she was either. We were two shadows passing through each other. And then I got up, and reached the door, and made an awkward good-bye.

Not long afterwards, I came across physician and Jungian analyst Edward C. Whitmont's 1993 book *The Alchemy of Healing* with its resonant passage about healers and patients. Let me quote it again: "Healer and patient are destined actors with archetypally assigned roles in a 'sacred performance.' The healer's personality is overshadowed by the stage mask of the healer-god, which includes [her] potentially dark side, the divine intruder-destroyer; the patient's archetypal role is that of the supplicant but harbors also a healer-destroyer in its unconscious depths."

Those words came back to me one winter evening when I ran into Rachel on the Upper West Side. It was more than a year since our last encounter. We walked together for a dozen blocks. She was hurrying to get home to guests; I had my bicycle, and was hard-pressed to wheel it through the holiday crowds and keep up with her. On the fly, she said my sixth chakra looked good, more deeply seated and rife with fine new light—evidence, she said, of spiritual growth. Chakras two and three could use some energy, she added. I shook my head, amazed as ever at her ability to pick up the subtle world on the run, to see it silhouetted against the abstract expressionist backdrop of Broadway.

"How's the book?" I asked.

"Good," she said. "It's been through a million revisions."

We came to a corner. I was not ungrateful for our history together; truth to tell, I felt guilty for having never thanked her for all the work she had done on my behalf, work I was continuing with other healers, in other circumstances, work that in some sense was extending what I had learned in Rachel's hands. X becoming Y becoming Z . . . But the air between us was still tense, obscured by our history of shifting masks—healer, intruder, destroyer . . . She was late, and not disposed to reminisce.

CHAPTER SIX

Let us remind ourselves of what has happened in the wake of earlier demystifications. We find no diminution of wonder; on the contrary we find deeper beauties and more dazzling visions of the complexity of the universe than the protectors of mystery ever conceived. The "magic" of earlier visions was, for the most part, a cover-up for frank failures of imagination, a boring dodge enshrined in the concept of a deus ex machina. Fiery gods driving gold chariots across the skies are simpleminded comic-book fare compared to the ravishing strangeness of contemporary cosmology, and the recursive intricacies of the reproductive machinery of DNA make élan vital about as interesting as Superman's dread kryptonite. When we understand consciousness—when there is no more mystery—consciousness will be different, but there will still be beauty, and more room than ever for awe.

—Daniel Dennett

1. AJNA AND THE PURPLE CURSOR

By now, in theory, I should have known something. I should have been surfeited with insights. Priceless insights were promised as part of the process of cultivating energy; they were one of the rewards of imagining the body in terms of chakras. You scaled mountains in the subtle world; you expected the payoff of a panoramic view, an understanding of all creation and your part in it. The pattern was well established: In any series of healings, the focus would gradually shift, and the work you had probably begun in response to some specific physical condition, a concrete disease or obvious dysfunction, would turn to a more esoteric agenda. You were likely to find yourself engrossed not so much in the conversion of sickness to health per se, but in a more vast and subtle metamorphosis—the transformation of the bunkered, time-bound ego into the timeless, unbordered soul. In short: spiritual enlightenment, with its intimations of divinity and evidence for faith.

Theory's one thing, praxis another. The instrument of this spiritual alchemy has always been the sixth chakra, the forehead lotus known in Sanskrit as Ajna, which means "authority, command, unlimited power." These, I was discovering, were precisely the qualities I was losing (*as if you ever had them!*) during the months I found myself groping for insight into Ajna, reaching after its character like someone trying to find the last reflection in a hall of mirrors. The lower chakras seemed comprehensible in their way—engaging the energy of physical reality, emotional life, mental existence. Even the energetic principles that pertained to the double nature of the heart, and the necessity of speaking from it, seemed within a clown's grasp.

But Ajna! From the handful of books on the topic, I'd learned it was sometimes called the "purple ray" and that it often showed up in meditation as a pulsating little cursor of purple light on the screen of your mind, assuming your meditations included such homely, jury-rigged inventions as mind screens. Yoga scripture described Ajna as a two-petaled lotus housing the goddess Hakini Shakti, who had six red faces and held in four of her six arms a small drum, a skull, prayer beads, and a book. The so-called gateway of the spirit was rooted at the junction of three main subtle energy currents—the moon and sun currents (*ida* and *pingala*) and the main nervous current that paralleled the spinal cord, the *sushumna*. Ajna was said to govern all the chakras except the crown lotus above it. It was sometimes identified as the energy source of the pituitary gland, or the pineal gland, or both. It was said to nourish the lower part of the brain, the nervous system, and the left eye. (Energy for the right eye, according to clairvoyants who said they could track the flow, was provided by the crown chakra.)

What was especially paradoxical about my having so little insight into Ajna was that Ajna was the chakra of insight. It was linked to the development of wisdom, intuition, and clairvoyant perception, and was supposed to be the eye that saw the future. It was commonly depicted as a third eyeball gazing from the foreheads of gurus like a ghastly birth defect.

This was a metaphor, obviously; anyone born with an actual third eye would be dispatched to a plastic surgeon posthaste. But yoga practitioners, hands-on healers, and even a number of adventurous medical doctors insisted that Ajna itself had more than a figurative existence. They contended that Ajna, like the other chakras, was an actual, palpable formation that reflected the flow of the energy in the body as a standing wave or a whirlpool reflected the movement of water in a riverbed. Its function was to collect and distribute frequencies of energy vibrating in the range of the color purple, or somehow related to the color purple. Like all chakras, it could be shut down, opened, reset, charged, unblocked, and thus harnessed to treat disease that might be caused or exacerbated by defective distributions of energy—in this case, disorders of the eyes, throat, the upper endocrine glands.

The opening of Ajna was potentially dangerous and could cause a number of psychiatric problems in people who might be commencing their novitiates without sufficient preparation. (The dangers are illustrated in the story of Shiva, who raised the lid on his third eye—Shiva's Eye, as it is known—and reduced Kama, the god of desire, to a pile of ash.) G. A. Gaskell's reference book of sacred symbols, the *Dictionary of All Myths and Scriptures*, defined the third eye as "a symbol of the vague astral clairvoyant faculty of early humanity, which, as evolution proceeds, is exchanged for the physical organs of sight." Gaskell suggested the opening of Ajna was a primitive regression. Perhaps so: In less-complex reptilian brains, the pineal gland is often called a third eye because it shares some of the photoreceptivity of the regular eyes.

But generally speaking, the opening of Ajna signaled a propitious event, what mystics would call an illumination. If Ajna performed the function imputed to it, if it could stimulate "higher" states of consciousness, if it were, in fact, the gateway of the spirit, then it was a royal road of growth and transformation and ought to be embraced as such, as a rediscovered route to a spiritual domain all but lost to the secular mind. Ajna commentators claimed the chakra energized the ability to generate meaning and symbolic thought. It kindled the passion for spiritual knowledge, knowledge of what the Sufis called "the immensity" and the Quakers knew as the "inner light"; knowledge perhaps of what Alfred Lord Tennyson was able to discover in himself with the mantra-like expedient of chanting his name three or four times—*Alfred Lord, Alfred Lord, Alfred Lord* . . . "Individuality itself," he wrote in his memoirs, "seemed to dissolve and fade away into boundless being, and this not a confused state, but the clearest of the clearest, the surest of the surest, the weirdest of the weirdest, utterly beyond words, where death was an almost laughable impossibility, the loss of personality (if it were so) seeming no extinction but the only true life."

It was *toward* such rapture that hands-on healing was pointed. It was *for* such rapture that healers endeavored to improve the flow of energy through the sixth chakra, their own and their clients'. The time-tested way of opening Ajna on your own was to follow the example of the Buddha and meditate on your forehead lotus. With even a fraction of his success, you could expect to leave off the blind groping for insight and, in the words of Hiroshi Motoyama, a noted Japanese scientist and author of *Theories of the Chakras*, enjoy a rush of "important ideas and great visions." You would have achieved a significant milestone on the road to enlightenment with attendant powers and freedom from manic desires. As tantric healer Harish Johari put it: "When one establishes himself in the place between the eyebrows, he goes beyond all the kinds of desires that motivate life and impel one to move in many directions. . . . He is in a constant state of nondual consciousness. He can enter any other body at will. He is able to comprehend the inner meaning of cosmic knowledge and is able to generate scriptures."

If Ajna remained closed or blocked, or functioned improperly, well, forget about generating scriptures. Forget about a ticket to transcendence. While Ajna adepts settled down in "the abode of uninterrupted bliss," you had a season's pass to "cynical nihilism" and apparently nothing to look forward to beyond lusterless years of dating the wrong women and picking laggard mutual funds, and giving orders that subordinates felt free to ignore.

It was dawning on me that just as it would probably take what Saint Augustine called "the eye of the soul" to see such a thing as a soul, one could not understand the sixth chakra with anything less than a sixth chakra. Lacking one, or one that worked well, one that was busy taking in all the fine vitalizing stuff of *prana, chi,* orgone, and whatnot—maybe even taking in a few scientifically confirmable photons just for the hell of it—I would have only a limited understanding of the higher dimensions of energy healing. Eureka! I was conceptually fettered! I lacked cosmic knowledge and the knack of entering bodies at will. Without the privileges of nonordinary sight, I would never scrutinize vignettes from the future or see past the falsehoods of duality. Scripture? I would be lucky to scratch out a few pages of piebald journalism.

The strain was taking its toll. Luckily, you don't need a sixth chakra to complain. In those periods of cognitive dissonance when I felt more a casualty of energy healing than a beneficiary, when I was trapped in the infinite regress of knowing I needed faith to have the faith in the faith I needed to have, I griped to my friend Linda, who considered herself partly responsible for my welfare since it was her recommendation that had sent me to Joel Wallach in Los Angeles a few years before—the putative lark that begot this pilgrimage through the subtle world. The tricky part was that the higher you went on the ladder of the chakras, the larger and more rarefied the mysteries became, and the harder it was to maintain the footing Keats famously described as "negative capability," the ability to remain open in states of doubt and uncertainty "without any irritable reaching after fact and reason." Oh, what was this whole project if not one long, irritable reaching after fact and reason? What had I served up but a lot of whining and head-clutching and cuticle-biting about the reality of chakras and auras and light bodies? A lot of equivocal speculation as to whether our most glorious intuitions of divinity in ourselves were in fact a tribute to our delusion and grandiosity . . . Yet irritable reaching after fact and reason was irresistible, and in some way wasn't it the whole point?

The higher you went on the ladder, the harder it was to reason your way through or around the deepest questions, the questions that perhaps could only be faced silently with the fortitude of crazy, reasonless faith. Maybe I had it backwards. You couldn't reason your way into faith any more than you could reason your way into cosmic knowledge and the knack of entering bodies at will. "Understanding is the reward of faith," wrote Saint Augustine in the fifth century A.D. "Therefore do not seek to understand in order that you may believe, but make the act of faith in order that you may understand; for unless you make the act of faith, you will not understand."

As I struggled with the necessity of preconditions such as belief, the inner dialectic was growing shrill. My ideation was in the uninsightful position of contesting idealism itself, led by a distinguished philosopher clown, who was repulsed by any conceit that would accord as much *reality* to the unmeasurable phenomena of the mental realm as to the quantifiable facts of the material world, and who disdainfully asked: "How reliable are the mind's chimeras next to gravity or photosynthesis?" To which the Bishop of Ajna replied: "If you put the question that way, the answer is a forgone conclusion." The inner dialectic was giving me a headache.

I badgered Linda too. Just when I had finished hacking through a text by some Hindu jargon-master who described Ajna as having two petals, I found C. W. Leadbeater's turn-of-the-century classic *The Chakras,* which said no, no, no, the sixth chakra is really "a wheel of light with ninety-six spokes." Then the phone rang and it was some well-meaning ambassador from the planet Zork who "explained" that the disparity could be attributed to the fact that Leadbeater was reporting on the chakra from one plane of reality and the Hindu seer from another. *Linda, why can't these bozos get together on basic facts?*

Linda listened patiently and then said, "I would simply point out that when your heart chakra opened you got engaged. And when your throat chakra opened you started writing your book." Well, they were interesting coincidences, and I did get engaged, but more on that later. Maybe these Ajna troubles stemmed from the fact that my fiancée, Kate, was a quiet foe of Enlightenment Lite and one of the first things she had done after we got engaged was throw out all my purple clothes—sweatshirts, dress shirts, tee shirts all in various shades of purple, all amassed in some unconscious attraction to a color whose significance I was totally unaware of. Now I was stuck at the sixth chakra, and with nothing to wear! And my editor was asking where the rest of the manuscript was. And Linda was saying I would probably have to open the sixth chakra before I could write about it.

"It looks like Hakini Shakti has your book," she said.

"So what you're saying, in effect, is that my manuscript is being held hostage by a red-faced Hindu apparition with six arms?"

"Exactly that," she said. Well, that explained the book Hakini Shakti was holding. But what about the rosary and the drum, and, more ominously, the skull? I said if Hakini didn't fork over a manuscript soon, the publisher was going to break my legs.

"You can expedite new bone growth with low-voltage current," Linda said.

Easier to get somewhere on an M. C. Escher staircase than understand Ajna. Or seize the last image in the hall of mirrors . . . How could you stand outside yourself to study the instrument with which you were seeing? Was Ajna itself one of those phenomena that have to be taken on faith? If it functioned as the Vedic sages and sensitives proposed, it seemed the key to understanding the healer's progression from the physical to the mental to the spiritual—that shift in the focus from the dense, slow body of the flesh to bodies of increasingly higher frequencies, bodies formed of emotions, of mentation, of dream life, and ultimately of metaphysical issues related to notions such as karma. Ajna, the chakra of insight, apparently held the key to the mind-body problem and whatever causal role insight generated by consciousness might play in healing. It didn't seem to me there was much difference between understanding the chakra and solving the mind-body problem itself.

Hence my headache.

For much of the twentieth century, medical science accorded consciousness virtually no role in healing, and even today it can be reasonably proposed that "will" and "intention" have little to do with the capacity of living organisms to repair and regulate themselves. Bacteria patch cell walls; fresh skin closes over bears' wounds; broken arm bones knit together in chimpanzees. No mind, no *intention*, no tricky-to-define *consciousness* is required. It happens as a matter of course, in utter ignorance of the Upanishads or the God-drunk prayers of Mary Baker Eddy. You don't have to believe anything to heal. Atheists heal. Mice heal. Most healing occurs when organisms are left to their own devices; the healing is automatic, a property of being, a function of that "peculiar stimulated condition of organized matter." Conscious intervention of the mind, or the self, or the soul, or any other grandstanding artifact of Cartesian duality, is not necessary.

Is not necessary, but not, therefore, irrelevant or without effect. The fundamental axiom of the sixth chakra is that the energy of the mind *is* causal; the energy of insight *can* heal, with authority, command, and unlimited power. And increasingly, science has begun to verify the folk wisdom of the mind's role in illness. Research in the last twenty-five years has established that emotions and intentions and visualizations—healing energy, if you will, energy mustered by an act of will—can have some positive bearing on the outcome of the body's response to illness. Consciousness can affect how the body mends and may even affect the merriment of bacteria, as we have seen from those experiments that entranced Larry Dossey and Oprah Winfrey. It seems increasingly evident that the ghost, if it is a ghost, has some hand in the operations of the machine, if it is a machine. The beliefs we generate and embrace can sometimes influence the rate and success of recovery.

By the purple light of Ajna doctrine, even to raise the question of how healing is bound up in consciousness is a sign of an activated sixth chakra. There is doubtless much scientific ground to be gained on the nature of awareness and how our consciousness bears on healing and health, but there may never be much insight into any problem that includes the quandary of consciousness in the equation. Ajna, by definition, is more mysterious than any of the chakras below it, because it lies at precisely that point where the conundrum of healing flows into the conundrum of consciousness, where healing gets tangled in the dualistic paradoxes of the mind-body problem and the way in which we seem to shuttle in and out of ourselves, the object of our lives one moment, the subject of them the next. Inside, outside; matter, mind: physiological robots obeying the mechanical laws of Newton's physics one moment, disembodied minds sorting through illusions by the light of Bishop Berkeley's idealism the next. I suppose in the long run you either break your head on such conundrums or learn to suffer them in silence, following the advice of Wittgenstein, arch-foe of senseless questions, who wrote insightfully of the futility of insight: "We feel that even when all possible scientific questions have been answered, the problems of life remain completely untouched. Of course there are then no questions left, and this itself is the answer."

But I don't want to get ahead of myself. In the midst of all this metaphysical speculation, I flew to Tucson, where the mind tribes were gathering to move their purple cursors over these very matters.

2. THE CONSCIOUSNESS BAZAAR

Rounding up a bunch of scientists for the purpose of poring over the quandaries of consciousness was such a radical idea in 1994 that the landmark mind-brain bash organized by the University of Arizona in

Tucson was dubbed "Woodstock." Two years later, in the spring of 1996, when an even larger cast of physicists, philosophers, biologists, neuroscientists, medical doctors, ethnologists, cognitive psychologists, and other authorities from various corners of academia had assembled for "Tucson/Woodstock II," you could still hear a lot of nervous bourgeois jokes about how it might not be a good career move to get too wrapped up in such a hippy-dippy subject. "You can study consciousness," warned the noted philosopher John Searle, "but get tenure first."

But in what seemed the blink of a third eye, the enigma of mind, long considered too soft and unquantifiable for measure-minded researchers, long thought something better left to fiendishly brilliant pseudoscientists like Freud, had become a legitimate topic for scientific investigation. Exploring the subjective world of interior experience with the objective methodology of science had acquired more than a veneer of academic respectability. It had kicked off a landrush. There was the parallel drive for new territory, part of the colonizing march of materialism that, to take one example from medicine, had wrested the treatment of depression from witch doctors, priests, and shrinks and had given it to biopsychiatrists equipped with serotonin re-uptake inhibitors. But there was also the drive to reclaim the mind territory forfeited in the 1940s and '50s during the heyday of behaviorism, which had dealt with mental complexities by pretending mind didn't matter—by decreeing that what mattered wasn't what people thought or felt but what they did, how they behaved.

So "hard science" researchers aimed to conquer new ground and recoup old. To track the work, the *Journal of Consciousness Studies* had been organized. Representatives from prominent university presses were carting in boxes of fresh books on a welter of mind-body themes, healing among them. Foundations were finding money for conferences and grants. "Consciousness," said the philosopher Michael Lockwood at the start of the conference, "is the piece left in the box when the jigsaw puzzle is completed."

That first morning, more than a thousand people packed the Music Hall in downtown Tucson's Convention Center. All week, the crowd never dwindled. The debates stirred up at the plenary lectures often continued into tea and coffee breaks; people milled about in the lobby or wandered around the Convention Center plaza outside, where pigeons fussed in the trees and mild desert winds herded last year's leaves into a dry fountain. In the afternoon, the crowd dispersed to standing-room-only meetings in smaller rooms at the adjacent Holiday Inn, where experimental work and theories were presented in more detail. At night, they gathered in the Convention Center to browse through tables of books and wander around the "poster sessions," where it seemed anybody with a zany idea about consciousness and access to a copying machine could show his stuff on a wall of bulletin boards.

Deciding what to attend at Tucson II was like picking a route through the omnium-gatherum of a great bazaar, a kind of Brainiac Expo where the shelves were bursting with a catholic mishmash of studies, theories, and problems. You could go from lectures on "the chemistry of conscious states," and "the neuroanatomy of the intralaminar nuclei," to talks about "the molecular mechanisms of general anesthesia," "communication and cognition in dolphins," and "three ways of being a zombie." If you missed the presentation on "color perception in goldfish" there was a trenchant discussion about a parrot with a better vocabulary than most action heroes. I ruined my eyes staring at diagrams of the visual cortex that made oil-refinery flowcharts look simple. I heard some of the shop jokes: working with one neuron was neuroscience, working with two was psychology.

The variety of disciplines and the kaleidoscopic array of papers and presentations at Tucson II reflected the many ways of approaching the problems of consciousness, problems that began with the definition of the phenomenon itself. Was consciousness a kind of "informational sensitivity"? Or "sensory awareness"? Was consciousness, as many people treated it, the equivalent of "the mind"? Was it something that pervaded and unified all living beings, as religious and spiritual traditions asserted? In what sense were dreams and the activity of the unconscious part of "consciousness"?

Much work had been done where consciousness seemed to be absent or attenuated, as in sleep and anesthesia. The surreality of the brain's state in sleep cast a strange backward light on the seemingly privileged place of wakefulness, leading New York University medical researcher Rodolfo Llinas to speculate that "what we are staging when we are awake is a dreamlike state modulated by the senses." Conversely, the studies in "lucid dreaming," in which people are able to signal by blinking their eyelids that they are "conscious" inside a dream, led researcher Stephen LaBerge to plead for the reality of the nightside mind, accentuating the reality of dreaming rather than the unreality of waking. "Dreaming," he said, "is perception unconstrained by sensory input."

Some of the most interesting discussions were based on research into the phenomenon of "blindsight," in which people with lesions in the visual cortex are still able to make accurate guesses about the color and orientation of objects they cannot "consciously" see. Blindsight demonstrated the paradox of "awareness" without consciousness.

Consciousness could also be approached as a question of sentience. And because feeling and suffering are not confined to human beings, this tack raised the philosophical issues of the animal rights movement. Arguing in his opening talk that consciousness and sentience are synonymous, Michael Lockwood cited a twenty-year-old Society for the Prevention of Cruelty to Animals case in which a woman was prosecuted for tossing live prawns onto a griddle. "Is it possible to torture a prawn?" he asked. "There is not a single person who has a way of finding out."

Taking a different angle on the same theme, Victor Norris of the University of Leicester made a case for what might well be the "mindfulness" of *E. coli* bacteria. While *E. coli* might not be conscious in the way we suppose Marcel Proust was conscious, the bacteria had noradrenalin receptors and thus could sense when their human hosts were stressed out, and they exhibited an awareness of some sort—when they "felt" crowded, they released an antibiotic that killed off competitors.

But did they *know* what they were doing? Weren't they just reacting to *information*, and not *intending* to take life with their toxic exudations? Did their behavior generate something we would call *experience*? Were they self-conscious in the sense that they knew and intended and were aware of themselves as the subjects of their own experience?

Or were they perhaps only a body of information that for purely mechanical reasons would prefer their usual environment to, say, the heat of a griddle? Short of querying prawns, it seemed impossible to characterize their reactions as "conscious" or not. It was this epistemological problem that had led to the debate about intelligent-and-therefore-possibly-conscious machines, and to the discussion of zombies, hypothetical human automatons that did everything conscious people could do but had no subjectivity, no awareness of themselves as somebody doing something.

It was obvious that the harder you look at consciousness the more elusive it becomes. It seemed obvious that as there are two ways of knowing (the objective and the subjective), and two ways of speaking about what you know (the first-person language of the "I" and the third-person language of "it"), a divide was running down the middle of the consciousness bazaar, sharp as the sulcus that splits the brain into right and left hemispheres. Disregarding Blake's warning that "to generalize is to be an idiot," I found myself making quick assessments of speakers as either Obs or Subs. At a conference dedicated to the "science" of consciousness, the Obs ruled, of course. They comprised the majority of the speakers. Theirs was the camp with "real" data; theirs were the assumptions about consciousness and the methods of investigating it that had the prestige of science.

For all nuances among the Obs—and truly, you needed a field guide and the eyes of birdwatcher to tell a computational functionalist from a monistic materialist or an epiphenomenal eliminativist—most of them subscribed to the view that the mind was in the body. As neurophilosopher Patricia Churchland put it, "Consciousness is almost certainly a property of the physical brain." That eminently reasonable assumption—consciousness emerges from matter—formed the cornerstone of scientific materialism. It was axiomatic among Obs that mind could be reduced to matter. Mind was what emerged from the zip-zip-buzz of neurons and neurotransmitters.

Obs were certain that mind was not dropped on the brain by supernatural wizard gods or that consciousness in the form of a soul or spirit preceded the instantiation of organic tissue. Much of their confidence stemmed from the fact that ideas about self, soul, and spirit emerged from an era that had no understanding of how the human brain worked, an era when the brain was viewed as a kind of radiator that cooled the blood. Ironically, the superstitions about a self hovering in the brain were fueled by Descartes, whose objectification of the body helped stake out the philosophical ground for the medical and physiological investigations of modern science, but whose postulate of a detached thinking subject promoted the very mind-body dualism many scientists now considered logically absurd. As Searle put it, sophisticated Obs were loath "to get into bed with Descartes." It was their conviction that most people who had religious intimations of a soul or even psychological intimations of a Cartesian self simply could not appreciate the computing power of a neural network conservatively estimated to consist of one hundred billion neurons, several hundred thousand miles of axons, and so many synapses that if you counted them at the rate of one a second it would take thirty-two million years to total them up.

The prospects of facing life without the "fiction" of an immortal soul might not alarm people raised in a secularized society. But what can scientists mean when they say there is no self? Who falls in love? Who cashes Social Security checks? Who trips off to healers on a ruinous caprice? Who sickens and dies?

Brain scientists reply that they are simply following the signposts of experimental evidence. Consider a piece of famous research by neuroscientist Benjamin Libet that seems to argue not against the idea of personality or even something that might be called a self, but against the idea that the conscious self is the agent that makes decisions and acts on its intentions—that consciousness functions as what Daniel Dennett calls in his book *Consciousness Explained* "the Cartesian homunculus." The little man inside the brain. By means of a clever series of experiments, Libet found that activity in the part of the cortex associated with hand movement begins three hundred milliseconds before people consciously decide to flex their right hand. In other words, "they" (such as "they" are) do not consciously initiate the movement. Experiments with the reaction times of professional tennis players have shown that consciousness of the incoming serve occurs after the player has already moved to return it.

The implication in this case is that the unconscious processes of visual awareness and motor responses combine in such a way to bypass the "intending self-aware actor." The decision-making "I" becomes an afterthought, an irrelevancy. There is no decision-making "I." No little man deciding to move his racket arm or flex his hand. Rather, there are faceless committees of neurons acting in concert. Decisions are what the brain *does*, not what it *makes*; they are performed by neural networks, and seem to be credited after the fact to a manufactured "self" for the sake of convenience or social convention. The self is a kind of spectator auditing a story narrated by brain processes. Ostensibly in charge, the protagonist is actually a figurehead, like a television anchorman learning about a story as it unfolds in news-feeds.

Dennett termed this endlessly shifting and provisional self the "center of narrative gravity" and made the analogy to the "user illusion" of the computer screen, which displays the magnetic status of the hard drive for the operator's convenience. If you accept the self as cognitive psychology construes it, the concept of "free will" begins to seem illusory as well, no more than a brain state determined by other brain states. In fact, many of the Obs at the conference viewed free will, and its sister concepts such as intention and moral responsibility, as conceits from the outmoded realm of what they called "folk psychology." Free will, they thought, would eventually be dissolved by a more complete understanding of the brain.

And why not? The trend in the evidence was strong. What does the reality of the self, not to say its dignity, amount to if the construct of one's personal identity can be wiped out with a burst of electrical activity in the thalamic cells? What is special, not to say immortal, about the human soul if happiness is contingent on neurotransmitter levels? Whither religion, whither the Flemish mystic John Ruysbroeck's "Incomprehensible Light" and "Intuition of Eternity" when the phenomena of such divine ecstasy could be induced by LSD? All people who doubt the utter dependency of mind on brain have to do is hold their breath for two minutes and the oxygen-starved tissue will make the connection emphatically palpable. The mind, and by extension everything in it, does indeed seem to dangle from the brain as perilously as a silent-film star from a clock tower.

While absurd to neuroscientists, Descartes' separation of mind and body is ingrained in custom and language. The presupposition of duality where it seems more natural to say that none exists, causes more confusion in medicine than any other science. The very word "psychosomatic" is an awkward attempt to bridge the mind-body rift—an effort to solve a problem in therapeutics that wasn't a problem until people began to view the world and themselves as subjects and objects.

Cartesian dualism, in essence, was a compromise between Ob and Sub knowledge, and if you rejected it, you were forced to consider either of two extremes: The materialist position that the mind was subordinate to the brain, or the more hair-raising position of the idealists that the brain was subordinate to the mind. To an Ob, mind and consciousness were simply the sum of the processes of being conscious, the operation of turning the world into data and distributing it about a neural net; of integrating bits of incoming information with memory and out-putting behavior. As the fact of digestion didn't have to be distinguished from a functional demonstration of digestion, so consciousness in the materialist view was nothing mystically set apart from the processes of awareness. During his talk at the end of the week, John Searle argued that consciousness could indeed be studied according to the objective principles of science. Contrary to idealism, there were always distinctions that could be made between those features of reality which depended on observers and those which did not. The existence of subjective aspects of phenomena did not rule out scientific evaluation. "The fact that a dollar is money is not intrinsic to the paper," Searle said. And then he turned to the cultural divide in the room.

"At these conferences," he said, "there's always an undercurrent of opposition between hard-nosed scientists and people interested in mysticism, trance, and transpersonal experience. It doesn't matter. The real transformation for us, the one that changed the world, began in the seventeenth century. The world has become demystified. If God exists, that's just another fact of physics. There will be five forces instead of four. The important thing is not whether paranormal events are possible or we can have out-of-body experiences. The important thing is that we have demystified nature. We regard it as intelligible in principle, even if we don't understand all of it. There is no inherent mystery."

Consciousness stripped of mystery! It was choicest of all scientific conceits. It was the very theme Dan Dennett had sounded with an almost scriptural intensity in his Ob masterpiece, *Consciousness Explained*, when he spoke of the "ravishing strangeness of contemporary cosmology." Dennett was a professor of cognitive science at Tufts University. Subs often wisecracked that his book ought to be called *Consciousness Explained Away*. Early in the week, during a presentation by the physicist and author

Roger Penrose, Dennett had gotten into a Dadaesque exchange on the subject of zombies, which many Subs took to be a perfect demonstration of the perils of the reductive view of consciousness. After all, it would seem you would indeed have to be a zombie to make the argument that unself-aware zombies who possessed the functional aspects of consciousness but had no knowledge of experience per se, could decide to risk their reps at Tucson/Woodstock II, make airline reservations, check into the Holiday Inn, listen attentively to lectures, respond to questions, and propose their theories of consciousness.

"As for the point about my being a zombie," Dennett said, "yes, I am a zombie, but I'm not an ordinary zombie. I do believe I am a zimbo. [A zimbo is just a zombie that is behaviorally complex, thanks to a control system that permits recursive self-representation.] The question if you're a zimbo is: How might you prove it to yourself? We cannot evade our responsibility to tell what we think the truth is about evolution. Brains are what we've got. If people are worried about the fact that they don't have an immortal soul, then we should address it. There is a very big conflict between science and traditional beliefs. But we know a lot of things to a moral certainty that we should not keep quiet about."

"I think you are a fine zombie," said Roger Penrose.

As the week wore on, that waterless fountain in the center of the Tucson Convention Center plaza began to seem an ever more apt symbol of the aridity—if not the barrenness—of studying consciousness scientifically. There was, it seemed, a desert out there, and it did not lie simply in the antiquated views of folk psychologists bent on defending their beleaguered conceits about immortal souls.

"There is a gross misconception of what consciousness is—witness the last five or six days," said Amit Goswami, the author of *The Self-Aware Universe*. "Consciousness doesn't mind that you don't believe in consciousness."

The essence of Sub dissent was that science could categorize and predict and even make interesting correlations between mental experiences and physiological states, but it nevertheless missed something crucial. It missed the essence of mind. Science had lost its mind. It missed the pungent doubleness of puns, the depth of jokes, the savory redness of a red-red rose—it missed the self-conscious heft and feel of knowing things poetically, the conundrum of experiences, the conundrum of having the *experience* of having experiences, of being able to say *what it was like to have been there and done that*. It discounted to the point of missing altogether the subjective mode of knowing—of knowing from within, not without.

Take Searle's analogy about money, which seemed better suited to the Subs' argument. Sure, you could study money scientifically, but would you learn anything significant about it? It could be analyzed from the point of view of chemistry and physics, but it has no real meaning outside the realm of culture. Its crucial attribute is not the objective reality of wood pulp and ink and spooky eyes floating atop Masonic pyramids on the backs of dollar bills, but the intangible value attached to it by two or more people.

In just this way, it seemed essence was doomed to elude scientific methodology. The effort to understand consciousness under the present metaphysics of science would always come up short, or seem absurd and beside the point—as futile, one speaker said, as "trying to study electricity by putting lesions in a toaster." Subjectivity could never be captured in objectivist nets. Something vanished in the reductionist approach—intention, meaning, value—all the mental qualities that distinguish a human being from a zombie. The question was whether the brain's relation to consciousness was like a radio's relation to music. You certainly wouldn't find the music if you opened the receiver and rooted around in the wires. Neither could the aesthetic beauty and meaning of the adagio passage in Beethoven's Eighth String Quartet be found in a printout of binary number sequences; without the CD player, without someone who understood what was being communicated, they were just pits in a disk.

Well, wait a minute, the Obs would reply. Wasn't this just a question of the form of the language? Couldn't you could learn to read the "music" in a sequence of ones and zeroes, and savor the beauty of what was encoded there? We hadn't forgotten the sonic beauty of English when the format of the language which once exclusively relied on the medium of the ear was enlarged to include the medium of the eye. Written language struck as deeply, and perhaps in new and unexpected directions, as the spoken word.

In an eloquent Sub rebuttal to the whole reductionist drive of modern neuroscience, David Hodgson, a philosopher and judge on the supreme court of Australia, made the case for free will and the other tattered standards of folk psychology. He pointed out that voluntary action, intent, and moral responsibility were the basis of virtually all legal systems and crucial to principles of justice and human rights. "There is no proof that they're myth or fictions," he said. "The mechanistic view of the mind is no more than a hypothesis, and yet the hypothesis is treated as if it were established fact by scientists and philosophers. The emphasis is on discrediting folk psychology." What, he asked, do you say to a woman who has been forced to have sex without her consent? That people cannot make choices? That free will and consent are illusions and she has simply been victimized by someone else's brain state?

Ultimately, as plausible as it might seem, the gospel of consciousness science which says that the mind is in the brain is only an assumption. A shared view that bound the community of scientists together, part of the consensus that helped them establish research procedures and terms with which to communicate. But no one had any way of knowing for sure, any more than they had a chance of getting an opinion from a prawn about the agony of the griddle. To hold that consciousness was contained in, or emerged from, or was limited to its physical referents, was at base a belief. As the transpersonal psychologist Charles Tart, one of the Sub graybeards, pointed out: "Science has become a priesthood defining what's real and what's not. It takes a certain view of the physical universe and regards it as revealed truth instead of regarding it as a certain set of theories. Saying mind equals brain ignores data about consciousness. Lots of data is the data of experience."

Of course you can ask, How does anyone trust the data of experience when so much misapprehension and bias and even outright delusion are built into the mind's instrumentation? We could ask just as easily how we know the sun goes around the Earth, short of taking someone's word for it or doing the astronomy and the math for ourselves. The fact that the Earth orbits the sun, however, is a different class of fact than the epistemological questions about what we believe about how we come to believe what is real or true.

For some reason, brain scientists are sure of the brain but not sure of the mind, even though it is the mind they use to develop their convictions about the brain. The brain, in the mind of Marvin Minsky, who produced this inimitable phrase, is a "computer made of meat." It is weighable, anatomizable, ineluctable tissue, whereas the mind is—what? A house of qualities, unquantifiable. An abode of uninterrupted bliss. A nightmare factory. A fount of pretensions. The warehouse of the noosphere, with premiums on beauty, value, depth, elegance, symmetry, rhythm, justice, humor, and truth. Easier to call the self a user illusion and to say the mind is a property of the brain. But is there really any insight in that?

The mind is a property of the peculiar stimulated condition of organized matter. The quandary of consciousness is only the quandary of life, more narrowly framed. Consciousness is what seems to disappear from the brain when life stops. Subs will say the mind is not in the body, the body is in the mind. The mind—consciousness—is not a property of the brain; the brain, rather, is a property of the mind. And all you have from them is their word on it . . .

Which is all you have from me too, all any of us has from each other, words and the senses. One night toward the end of the week, I staggered back to my hotel, fell on the bed, and flipped on the television. Bill Moyers was interviewing the famous religion scholar Huston Smith on the nature of spirit and divinity. In the wake of all the science that had been churning for days, the long discussions of neurological correlates of consciousness, the severe views of consciousness, Bill Moyers and Huston Smith seemed as insane as any pair of donkey-headed stockbrokers. What asylum had released them to prattle on deludedly about figments and Sub shadows on the big user-illusion screen of culture itself? They were like imaginary toads in a real garden, or maybe it was the other way around, real toads in an imaginary garden.

But at least there was something honorable about their conversation, something not entirely witless. It was filled with figurative truth, and what seemed to me then to be that oxymoronic stuff known as symbolic reality. Yes, I knew at heart—I lived by the fact, as I'm sure every scientist at Tucson II did—that lots of important things couldn't be measured. Aesthetic beauty, emotional meaning, love, values, justice—they all weren't any less important for being unquantifiable. I hit the remote. Over on CNN, two true jackasses were arguing on *Crossfire* whether America was too secular or too godly, in a fundamentalist Christian way, a debate (if you could call it that) brought on by a recent speech by the Supreme Court justice Antonin Scalia. Scalia had professed belief in the literal truth of the Bible. So on one hand you had Tucson's brilliant doubters led by hawkeyed science to conclude they didn't have free will or immortal souls, and on the other hand you had X million true believers led by blind religious faith to conclude that they did. The exponents of enlightened reason were persuaded they might be zombies, and the people who seemed to better fit the description, given their slavish devotion to dogma and religious fables, were convinced they had the full measure of human freedom and dignity. Even with three eyes wide open, this was not a conundrum that could be resolved in a night.

3. WISHING MAKES IT SO

As scientists explored consciousness from the outside in, other investigators tackled the problem from the inside out, less interested in unraveling mind-body interactions than in putting them to work. Unconventional healers often turned the neuroscientific view upside down: It was not the health of the mind that hung on the operations of the body, but the health of the body that depended on the action of the mind—on its wisdom and insights, its inner divination of spiritual forces and beliefs. Healers worked under the assumption there *was* a mindful ghost, who from the lectern of Ajna could address and shape the destiny of its own flesh.

As it had been at the outset, I think the core of my struggle was still the effort to find a path between these physicalist-materialist and idealist-transcendentalist positions. In runaway form, mind-over-body idealism had spawned untold harm and folly over the centuries. You had to pity the patients treated under the Augustinian doctrine that "all diseases of Christians are to be ascribed to demons." Even in our own time,

Christian Scientist parents have been prosecuted for medicating their diabetic children with prayer instead of insulin. Most Westerners are too practical, or too insufficiently devout, to take the look-Ma-no-doctor strictures of Mary Baker Eddy seriously. But even so, the idea that mind can make the body well by fiat had a subtle grip on the imagination of even the most inveterate materialist. Science had dented but not dispatched the belief that the right doctrine or fervent prayer could influence health. Science had to contend with all the centuries in which belief had been the drug of drugs. Belief, expressed as the placebo effect, had been the only useful ingredient in millions of worthless prescriptions.

Even in contemporary times, belief is still working some of the weirdest voodoo in the healing world. I had put a toe into the large lake of literature on the placebo effect, or what the medical anthropologist Daniel E. Moerman called "general medical therapy," as opposed to the therapy of "specific" effects. General medical therapy comprised the effects that were not attributable to the specific corrective measures of a surgeon or the specific pharmacological actions of a drug, but stemmed rather from the symbolic dimensions of the treatment, the rituals and forms of the therapy, the doctor's white coat, or perhaps even the hospital admittance procedures or the insurance reimbursement forms. Experiments had shown that placebo belief could give plain saltwater the analgesic power of morphine. Placebo belief could make drugs that normally induced nausea settle an upset stomach. It could melt warts, relax bronchial spasms, and quell seasickness. It could make sugarless but sweet-tasting saccharin raise glucose levels in the blood of diabetics. It could neutralize the skin-rash-inducing toxins in poisonous leaves and turn innocuous leaves toxic. In an age in which pharmacological effects were carefully calibrated in double-blind placebo-controlled experiments, studies had shown that for some diseases placebo-healed patients were less likely to relapse than patients healed by drugs. For all the prowess of biomedicine, belief—that is to say yet another facet of consciousness—was still one of the most powerful potions on hand.

Nevertheless, the placebo response varied greatly from person to person. Henry Beecher in his famous 1955 survey set the rate of placebo healing at around thirty-five percent, but in the case of acute ulcers, for example, the number of people healed by placebo treatment can range from five percent to ninety-five percent of the study group. It was a slippery business to tease out the extent to which beliefs were based on experience and the extent to which experience was determined by belief. The placebo effect seemed to draw not only on the idea of belief as "faith" but belief as "expectation," belief as a set of conditioned responses, habits, cultural assumptions. Placebo-healing rates were very high in Germany, for instance, and very low in Brazil. Why? Nobody knows. Rational, scientifically trained people, who often think of the placebo effect as a kind of trick and of themselves as too smart or skeptical to fall for it, were no more immune to placebos than any bunch of suggestible naifs.

One of the most dramatic examples of a placebo response was the case of "Mr. Wright," which was first published in December 1957 in the *Journal of Projective Techniques and Personality Assessment*, and has since become one of the most popular scriptures in mind-body medicine. According to the case report of his physician, Dr. Phillip West, Mr. Wright was suffering from advanced lymph cancer and had tumors the size of oranges in his neck, chest, abdomen, and groin. The medical team at the veterans hospital in Long Beach, California, had given up on him, convinced he had less than two weeks to live. In desperation, Mr. Wright seized on the idea that he could be cured by Krebiozen, one of the faddish wonder drugs of the early 1950s, which was produced by injecting horses with a tumor-causing mold and then extracting the antibody from the animals' blood. Krebiozen was being tested at the veterans hospital, and Mr. Wright begged Dr. West to let him have some, even though he was too far gone to qualify for the study. His persistence paid off, and he got his first shot on a Friday. Dr. West thought his patient might well be dead by Monday, but when he returned after the weekend, he was astonished to find Mr. Wright's tumors had "melted like snowballs on a hot stove." In a few days, they had shrunk to half their original size. Mr. Wright was breathing without oxygen and moving about the ward. Within ten days, he was well enough to be discharged, "all signs of the disease having vanished in this short time." Mr. Wright felt so well he was able to fly his own airplane up to twelve thousand feet. Eight weeks later, reports emerged questioning the efficacy of Krebiozen. Mr. Wright, whom Dr. West described as "reasonably logical and scientific in his thinking," was disturbed by the new reports casting doubt on the medicine that had saved him. His tumors returned. At that point, it was his belief in the reality of what healed him that began to melt like snowballs on a hot stove.

"Here," Dr. West wrote, "I saw an opportunity to double-check the drug and maybe, too, to find out how the quacks can accomplish the results that they claim (and many of their claims are well substantiated)." Dr. West decided to perform an experiment contemporary ethical standards would most likely disallow. "Knowing something of my patient's innate optimism by this time, I deliberately took advantage of him." Dr. West lied to Mr. Wright, telling him that a new double-strength, longer-lasting batch of Krebiozen had been developed, and that it would arrive in a few days. "When I announced that the new series of injections was about to begin, [Mr. Wright] was almost ecstatic and his faith was very strong." But what Dr. West injected into Mr. Wright was *fresh water*. Astonishingly, the tumors shrank even more dramatically than they had the first time. Mr. Wright's faith in a "drug" that was nothing more than sterile water drained the fluid in his chest. It shrank the neoplasms. Once again he was walking easily around the hospital. Once again he was well enough to be discharged and to take his plane up for a spin. "He was certainly the picture of health," Dr. West wrote. For two months Mr. Wright was symptom-free. Meanwhile, clinical tests had demonstrated that the wonder drug Krebiozen was ineffective. The verdict was announced by the American Medical Association, and the news came to Mr. Wright's attention. "Within a few days of this report Mr. Wright was readmitted to the hospital *in extremis*. His faith was now gone, his last hope vanished, and he succumbed in less than two days."

So much for life on the information superhighway.

In the 1991 anthology *The Anthropology of Medicine*, Daniel Moerman wrote that the failure of biomedicine to explain such phenomena arises "from the naive dualism of contemporary medical science, which characteristically assumes a fundamental mind-body dichotomy in its conceptualization of the human organism. And since disease is an affliction of the body, whereas perception (of treatment) is an aspect of the mind, and since the only available mediators of this dichotomy are as ineffable and 'unscientific' as the 'soul', biomedicine simply tends to ignore, even deny, the significance of general medical therapy."

In the mind-body models debated by most neuroscientists at Tucson II, the mind basically *was* the brain. Which is to say that nothing could happen in the mind that wasn't physical, that the mind was subordinate to the body. But the prestige enjoyed by modern drug therapies and many forms of biomedical treatment was based on making distinctions between psychological and physiological effects, distinctions that perpetuated what many scientists dismissed as Descartes' nonsensical division of mind and body. "Naive dualism" was naive because it split entities that could not be riven. But if there were only a unified body–mind, if modern science were striving to reunite what had never really been separate, how could the mind be ruled out in placebo-controlled experiments? If Descartes were wrong, why was medicine so invested in sustaining distinctions between physiological and psychological effects? Why the bias, the feeling that somatic diseases were "real" or "organic" and psychic diseases were just gossamer moods or something that could be changed with the will? If you could change the mind at will, with the will, why not the body? And conversely, what sort of coherence was there in the argument of quack-busters, who for years denounced procedures like acupuncture on the grounds that the effects were simply caused by suggestion? If body and mind were one and the same, why shouldn't the mind be as legitimate a gateway to healing? Distinguishing between specific and general effects might not be so urgent.

"The placebo idea contains a philosophical trap," wrote Anthony Campbell in a 1994 issue of the *Journal of Consciousness Studies*. "The modifier 'mere' frequently hovers invisibly in front of 'placebo' in medical texts. The ghost has not been fully exorcised from the machine; a shadowy vestige of it, at least, still haunts clinics and laboratories in which clinical trials are conducted."

So in some ways medical scientists were still bogged down in the dualistic folk psychology their peers in other disciplines had abandoned. Medicine was caught between the science of healing and the art of healing, unsure of the ultimate question. Was what mattered most the rationalist's longing to know why therapies worked, and whether effects were based on placebo beliefs or on factors defined as being more "real" under metaphysically suspect assumptions? Or was what mattered most simply the question of empirical outcome: Did the medicine work?

In his paper in *The Anthropology of Medicine,* Moerman envisioned "a kind of religiosity" emerging from the empirical emphasis of holistic therapies. Advocates, he wrote, "seem almost inevitably to begin speaking of archetypes, gods, or souls. Even the more scholarly of them, we feel, are straining against the temptation to break into song."

Still mired, obviously, in my Ajna muddle, I received a letter from a doctor and psychoanalyst in New York City named Gerald Epstein. He was an assistant professor of clinical psychiatry at Mt. Sinai Hospital, but a most unorthodox one, as I learned from reading his book *Healing into Immortality.* For two decades, he had been using imagery to treat conditions ranging from asthma to cancer to AIDS. That was nothing special; envisioning with the mind's eye has been a staple of alternative medicine for decades.

What made Epstein exceptional was his categorical advocacy of what he called "spiritual medicine" based on imagery. "The spiritual factor in health is the critical factor in all healing," he had written. He was a sort of Super Sub who had broken into song and couldn't stop singing. He viewed illness as a "deviation from the truth, presented in biological and emotional form." Diseases were "a display of the accumulated falsehoods we bear." The scientific insights of evidence-based medicine had no more validity than the emotional insights patients might glean for themselves with their intuition. For too long, people had been tyrannized by "false beliefs," medical and scientific presuppositions that wrongly decreed mind and body were split, that the world was meaningless, and that things just happened by chance. People let themselves be buffaloed into believing that "outside authorities know more about us than we know about ourselves." And the icing on this flamboyant cake: The "experiential world is the effect of our beliefs, not the cause."

So here was a doctor, a product of the American medical system, who was in essence saying water runs uphill and day is night. You didn't have to be a frothing logical positivist to wonder if he'd sung his way off the deep end of idealism and was now lost on Planet Zork, humming a Judaic version of Christian Science. Certainly, most psychotherapists would dismiss his unflinchingly contrary view of the relation of belief and experience; their therapies were based on the premise that experiences create belief, and traumas in childhood produce neurosis in adults. Epstein said they didn't look deeply enough at the problem. But set aside questions about the source of mental woes; there were even more compelling examples of physical disease that would seem to contradict Epstein's spiritual philosophy. How, for instance, was jaundice in a newborn the effect of an infant's beliefs?

I don't know whether I wanted some answers or just the pleasure of arguing with someone who had brazenly taken sixth-chakra tenets to their illogically logical extreme, but I telephoned Dr. Epstein. He invited me to stop by his apartment on Manhattan's Upper East Side. We sat by his living-room coffee table. He was about sixty, a little overweight, informally dressed. He had a plain, friendly face and a professional therapist's ferocious attention.

Imagery, he said, was the key to spiritually based healing; it was what he called "the true language of the mind." In his years of practice, Epstein had found only a small percentage of people who couldn't master the Esperanto of glyphs and pictures. I asked how he could tell, and he said, "I give them a little test. It takes a minute."

Could I take it?

"Sure," he said. He told me to sit back and close my eyes. "Now breathe in through your nose and out through your mouth three times."

When I had taken the breaths, he asked, "Can you see a table?"

Well . . . yes, in a manner of speaking. I could *imagine* I was seeing a table, but was that what he meant? Wasn't there a difference between imagining a table and actually seeing a table? My imaginary table compared poorly to the actual coffee table I had just been looking at. It wasn't even as detailed as a specific table I might fetch up from memory, say, the wicker and glass job in my parents' old kitchen. For that matter, it wasn't even as vivid as a table I might evoke with a few context-laden words—say, an oak-planked, sword-scored, mead-hall groaning board beset by warmongering Visigoths and breastplated, proto-lap-dancer comic book Valkyries . . .

Oy, a simple request and suddenly another Ajna muddle! Wouldn't it be nice to have a few minutes every day without an epistemological crisis? For fear of proving one of the visual dunces who can't see their way into the techniques of mental imagery healing, I said I could see a table. Who was going to know? The doctor would have to take my word for it. This was the kind of test where you could cheat and get away with it!

"Can you see a box on the table?"

Yes, in the same half-assed way.

"Can you see balloons in the box?"

Sure, why not?

"Can you see what colors the balloons are?"

Yellow, purple, blue . . .

"You can image," he said.

Well, so what? Well, here's what: The ability to envision images was the passkey to the idealist's castle. In theory, at least, I might glean knowledge of the invisible realm of the spirit via images. Spirit is what heals, and healing in Epstein's cosmology was a kind of reenactment of Genesis, the restoration or remembering of a lost Eden. As in the biblical tale, "doubt" was the snake in the Garden. Doubt, which Descartes had so famously embraced at the outset of the investigation that split mind and body, was in Epstein's view "the root cause of all illness."

"I'm proposing what I call a homecoming," he said. "It's an approach to health based on Western spiritual traditions." The Ten Commandments, he said, could be reinterpreted as a guide to all aspects of health—physical, emotional, mental, social, spiritual. It was a testament to his erudition and rhetoric that he could make such fundamentalism seem intriguing and almost reasonable. Let me give a few examples. He read the seventh commandment to be more than a proscription of sex outside of marriage; it forbid any act that weakened a commitment. The sixth, barring murder, could be extended to mean that one should not destroy one's self either—should not succumb to depression or turn away from the present to obsess about the past. The story of Lot's wife, who became a pillar of salt, stood in his view as a metaphor for the rigidity and hardening brought about by regrets and preoccupation with suffering. "Every story associated with depression is just a story, with no truth value, as illusory as a story about the future," he had written in *Healing into Immortality*. "We always seem to think that our circumstances determine our inner state. Yet we are in charge of our inner state and have the capacity to create our own circumstances."

You didn't have to buy the biblical health guidelines to profit from the imagery techniques, but Epstein argued that the spiritual traditions enhanced the power of imagery. Wasn't that to say nothing more than that you were better off with beliefs that gave you the security of believing rather than beliefs that obliged you to make a fetish of doubt? I daresay that for people who actually believe in the resurrection of Jesus there are untold dimensions to the White House Easter egg hunt.

I asked Epstein about a study he had completed on the use of imagery to treat asthma. In one of the visualizations, "Light in the Lake," he had directed patients to imagine themselves descending to the bottom of a lake, inhaling easily and exhaling slowly. They were to sit on the bottom for a while, enveloped in golden light, and then, rising out of the lake, they were to envision themselves sitting under a nearby maple tree, where they would pick up a leaf, note its texture and color, and then, in a move right out of improvisation class, enter the tissue of the leaf, merging their breath with its breath. Finally, they were to emerge from the breathing, lunglike leaves filled with the conviction that their own breath was smooth and regulated.

Was this any more sophisticated than the Healing 101 stuff that had amused Shelby Hammitt and her students?

"In the 'Lake of the Light,' you are immersing yourself in a situation where you can't breathe," Epstein explained. "The idea is to enter the feared event and go toward it, not away from it. In conventional medicine, you go away from pain and fear. In spiritual medicine, you go toward it. You see something healthy at the bottom of the lake—the golden light—something to give you hope. Then you leave the lake and enter the perfect breathing of the leaf."

"Aren't you in effect saying that wishing makes it so?"

"Wishing makes it so," he agreed. "It's the basis of all fairy tales."

In *Healing into Immortality*, an unequivocal manifesto of spiritual medicine, Epstein advocated the classic Sub idea that consciousness begets the body. But the mad rigors of that view don't hit home until you see the idea formulated as a stark and almost indefensible proposition about illness. Health, he had written, was not simply influenced by belief. It was a function of belief. Not a function of toxins in the environment, or of bacteria, or of genes, but a function of *belief*. I'd been grappling for months with this reading of reality, so dear to many in the consciousness-is-causal crowd. Certainly, it was easy to see what was seductive about the logic of fairy tales, but not what was compelling; weren't you much more likely to meet someone who thought he was the reincarnation of Jesus Christ than someone who could actually walk on water? I popped the jaundice-in-a-baby question, but I could have asked the same question about pediatric AIDS, or childhood leukemia, or Down's syndrome. What was on a newborn's mind that could cause it to arrive all yellow?

"A child comes in with its own belief system," Epstein replied evenly. "The jaundice didn't happen by chance." He had developed the point further in *Healing into Immortality*: "When an infant or young child becomes ill, the child is being given the opportunity to learn something that he or she needs to know at that time, just as an adult who becomes ill is being offered a similar opportunity. . . . In the case of childhood illness or even early death, it seems that the illness often brings some great transformation in the family dynamic. Families are brought together in a profoundly new way or are split apart by the event. The true relationships within the family come to light." So one reason children die is to uncover the true relationships within a family . . .

Epstein had billed himself as an exponent of Western spiritual traditions who didn't need to import Eastern concepts like karma or chakras, but this life-lesson rationale bore an uncanny likeness to the karma cop-out. Healers who found they were unable to help a sick person rescue himself from his illness often resorted to metaphysics. It was your soul's destiny to check out early. Epstein believed that everyone had a choice, infants included. They could choose to believe that life arose from a providential creator, or, constrained by science, they could choose to believe that life was the handiwork of randomly interacting molecules. Choose Providence and many benefits would accrue, foremost among them being the immersion into the eternal present, the sacred realm one attained in prayer, the realm from which healing was supposed to unfold. In short, the utopia of Perfect Health, where every experience was charged with meaning, and, ultimately, aspirants might achieve what most great spiritual traditions promised, which was the healing of all healings, the cure for death. Resurrection.

Certainly, the doctor's propositions lay outside the scope of the laboratory, and I never did understand how he thought infants who couldn't reflect on the merits of strained bananas versus puréed peas would be in a position to choose between Darwin and Yahweh. We talked again on several occasions, and I found that whenever it seemed I might have him cornered, he would moderate his views. No, he said, he would not argue that the "false premises" of modern medicine have not contributed to the betterment of humanity, that scientific medicine never eradicated a disease, that the discovery of antibiotics and painkillers was a step backwards. Would he forgo antibiotics to treat bacterial meningitis in a child with imagery or prayer? Of course not, he said. His argument was not that the useful parts of medicine should be discarded but that the imbalance should be redressed. Medicine had arrogated to itself powers that properly lay with God. "Medicine occupies too large a space in the pantheon of therapeutics," he said. "I come out of a visionary tradition that is trying to show people what's going on, what you're really here for, and to help them understand how they can choose life or death at any moment."

Who could argue with that? But why were metaphysical ideas required? For centuries doctors have crusaded to free people from the suffering created by errors in consciousness, belief in the guise of superstition, moral judgments, and religious stigma. It can't be said enough: Modern medicine counted the secularization of disease as one of its greatest victories. And the campaign is far from over, as the taint still attached to cancer and AIDS attests. The urge to impute meaning to illness often reflects nothing intrinsic to the disease, only cultural bigotry and fear. In her classic book *Illness as Metaphor*, Susan Sontag wrote that "Nothing is more punitive than to give a disease a meaning—that meaning being invariably a moralistic one. Any important disease whose causality is murky, and for which treatment is ineffectual, tends to be awash in significance."

"I don't think people should be blamed for being sick, or blame themselves for creating their sickness," Epstein replied. "But the cost of stripping illness of meaning is too high. We demean our own experience. You want to take the moralizing out of the meaning, but if you don't search for meaning, you don't become your own authority. And you are here to become your own authority."

As always, the line between extracting meaning and making moral judgments was very fine. Epstein would meet periodically with a group of psychologists and therapists and other healers interested in using imagery in their practices. They brought cases for discussion. One morning I sat in on a session. One of the therapists introduced the case of a woman with a thyroid condition. The woman had already consulted an herbalist and an acupuncturist, and had been given various interpretations of her medical problem by the other practitioners.

"They've been schmoozing with her about her life," Epstein said. "They've all been obliging her with commentary and penny-ante psychology about why she's ill."

"How is that different from what we're doing?" the therapist asked. It was a question I had too, for the answer seemed crucial to the worth of the technique. Epstein had said imagery therapists relied on clues to meaning that could be found in the roots of words and in the historical associations of disease. "Heartache" and "heartsick" and "heartthrob" all formed some nexus of meaning around the organ of the heart. "Thyroid" had roots in the Greek word *thyra*, for "door." "Pancreas" could be traced to the idea of bitterness. Another therapist in the session said that anger had been associated with the liver since the time of Hippocrates. Such associations were wonderfully poetic, but what did they prove? Greek medicine was as misinformed about the body as Chinese medicine, in which tradition held that the liver secreted tears. What was the difference between penny-ante psychology about illness and a phenomenological approach based on imagery?

Epstein replied without a moment's hesitation. "In our work, the person is finding out on their own. We're not adding a psychological presupposition about a feeling state. We're only making correlations and connections. Illness is the body's language. The body speaks by symptomology. The patients come to the meaning of their illness on their own, through their own inner process. We just help them read the glyphs."

Well, okay. I left supposing it was possible that everything Dr. Epstein believed about the relation of mind and body was founded on sand, and that spiritual medicine with lung-leaf visualizations and the guiding trellis of the Ten Commandments might be just another example not of specific or general medical effects but of the quackery that has been seducing people for centuries. But then—and here I am going to decisively assert the virtues of being wishy-washy—it was also possible that the good doctor had achieved just that level of insight one needed to mend the wound at the heart of modern medicine; he'd found an intellectual position that reconsecrated the profaned ground of being and resolved the medical contradictions of dualism with the soul-pervaded idealism of the spirit. When had there ever been anything reasonable about faith? If you were a zombie in want of a forehead lotus, maybe there was hope. Maybe wishing could make it so.

4. AFTERWARDS, YOU'RE A GENIUS

Extraordinary healings that seem to involve extraordinary psychical or spiritual energies are very similar to phenomena that have been studied much more thoroughly under the rubric of parapsychology. Not long after the consciousness conference in Tucson, I flew to Las Vegas to spend a few days at the University of Nevada's Consciousness Research Lab, an academic backwater where experiments were conducted according to the standard protocols of objective science but the hypotheses being tested were entirely heretical.

In the spring of 1996, the lab was one of two parapsychology labs in the country and, as such, was on the cutting edge of a debate that has raged for more than half a century among the scientific classes and healers as well: Is consciousness causal? Can mind exert an effect on matter? Can some psychic energy or information be transferred across space and time by an unknown process that confounds the laws of physics as they are presently understood?

Over the years, the controversy has illustrated nothing so much as the difficulty of using objective methods to explain or even verify accounts of subjective experiences. Confronted with the question of "Are psychic phenomena real?" many scientists roll their eyes and say, "No, no, no, a thousand times no." They reject psychic effects (or "psi" as they're called for short) as theoretically impossible. But a small iconoclastic band of tenure-averse parapsychologists insist that their research findings affirm the reality of *psi*. They argue that any guild of professionals truly dedicated to rational appraisals of data would not behave like the clerics who refused to look through Galileo's telescope.

When parapsychologists say "mind over matter," they do not mean mind over matter in the sense of your deciding to move your arm and then causing it to move. They mean it in the sense of your deciding to move someone else's arm and causing it to move, or otherwise affecting someone else's physical condition with your consciousness, your energy, your intention—and performing this bit of voodoo when your mojo is out of reach, removed to the next room or even, in the case of long-distance healings, comfortably reposed on planet Zork. While all transactions between the Sub world of mental intention and the Ob world of physical action are problematic, some are less obviously puzzling than others. However murky the transition from mind to matter, at least there's a pathway of nerves connecting brain to muscle; when the link is cut or blocked, the arm can't move.

But how to account for the thousands of reports of events in which it seems that some energy or bit of information has been transmitted without any intervening medium like nerves, phone wires, or microwaves? Consider the apparent transmission of information across space and time in a precognitive dream, one of the more dramatic "spontaneous cases" collected years ago by the well-known parapsychologist Louisa Rhine (and retold in Richard Broughton's 1991 book *Parapsychology: The Controversial Science*).

A streetcar operator in Los Angeles dreamed one night he was on duty running a southbound trolley on the W line. He passed a northbound streetcar. He greeted the other motorman with a wave. Suddenly a red truck made an illegal turn across the tracks and crashed into his streetcar. Two men in the truck were killed; a woman riding with them was thrown onto the pavement. When the motorman ran to where she lay screaming, he looked into the "largest, bluest eyes" he'd ever seen, and he heard the woman say, "You could have avoided this. You could have avoided this." He woke up. His pajamas were soaked in sweat, but he put the weird dream out of his mind and reported to work. His first run passed without incident, but on his second trip, he began to feel sick, and as he neared the same intersection he'd seen in the dream, he actually threw up. And yet he could not figure out what ailed him. He pressed ahead, keeping to the schedule. As in the dream, he saw the northbound train. As in the dream, he waved to the other motorman. All at once, he remembered the dress rehearsal of the nightmare. He slammed on the brakes, and the streetcar lurched to a violent stop just as a panel truck, with an ad-space blanked over in red paint, shot across the tracks. Two men and a woman were riding in the truck. The woman looked directly at the motorman. She had the same huge blue eyes he'd seen in the dream. She waved. She flashed him the gesture for "okay." The motorman was so flummoxed he had to be relieved of duty.

In the eyes of science this is just another anecdote; however intriguing, it has no objective credibility. Hard-headed parapsychologists know too well that astonishing experiences often can have mundane explanations. Precognition can be coincidence; chance has a flair for theatrics that is often unappreciated. Telepathy can be information gleaned via subtle cues, or by the gypsy fortune-teller's art of cold reading. Eyewitness reports are notoriously vulnerable to suggestion and unconscious influences. Studies have shown that therapists can implant bogus memories. Magicians bank on the limitations of the eye and the expectations of the mind. In an age when it seems that the tide of faddish belief is running in full flood—when Supreme Court justices proclaim their belief in the literal truth of the Bible, when the tenets of science are attacked by postmodern critics who insist that reality is a social construction, when frightened, disenchanted people entertain the idea that if "seeing is believing" then maybe "believing is seeing"—all psychic claims can seem suspiciously wet. "Parapsychology is a farce and a delusion along with other claims of wonders and powers that assail us every day of our lives," writes the magician James Randi, who has made a second career as a scourge of psychicism.

Even less-intemperate skeptics of psi argue that its proponents have cried wolf too many times. Psi researchers have trumpeted findings as proof that psi exists, only to see problems crop up—results tainted by fraud, flaws in research methods, data that can't be replicated. How can the field be taken seriously when it lacks a theory of how psi works, or even a good predictive hypothesis that can specify the conditions under which psi will appear? In what is probably the most commonly cited objection, skeptics point out that psi effects cannot be demonstrated each time an experiment is run. At best, researchers get significant results one time in three—a rate that would pass for Hall-of-Fame hitting in baseball but which does not satisfy the Ob criterion of "repetition on demand."

Perhaps the most withering dismissal of the field was the 1988 report by the National Research Council (NRC) of the National Academy of Sciences, which concluded that there was "no scientific justification from research conducted over a period of one hundred and thirty years for the existence of parapsychological phenomena." The report staked out the position of the extreme skeptic, for whom the failure of parapsychology to dry up and blow away is a continual affront to rationality, a testament to the persistence of superstition and humanity's incurable longing for indications of the soul. Parapsychology, it's said, is not a real science at all, but a pseudoscience, a form of "modern occultism."

Many psi researchers thought the NRC report was an example of a kind of fundamentalism antithetical to the ideals of science. The rhetoric of "one hundred and thirty years" misleadingly implied an enormous effort, when in fact parapsychology is a tiny field with only about forty active researchers. University of Utrecht psychologist Sybo Schouten calculated the amount of money and labor invested over the last century in quest of psi phenomena was equal to two *months'* worth of research in conventional psychology.

As for repetition on demand, parapsychologists argue that psi is a performance, like hitting a baseball, and even a skilled practitioner will not be successful every time at the plate. Moreover, demonstrations of psi effects are intrinsically more complex than showing how prisms break white light into rainbows. Psi effects in the lab are statistical phenomena. Researchers draw the analogy with medical science: In the study that showed the benefits of aspirin for cardiac patients, researchers had to screen twenty-two thousand people; if they had reviewed the impact of aspirin on the hearts of only two thousand people, the life-saving effect would not have shown up on their methodological radar.

For the most part, this debate between parapsychology and the rest of science has simmered in obscure professional journals and books. At Tucson II, it broke into the open late in the week at a plenary session on parapsychology and consciousness. It was mildly newsworthy that parapsychologists had even been invited to present work at Tucson II; the program committee had agreed, provided a skeptic—in this case, Susan Blackmore from the University of the West of England—was part of the panel. Among the psi proponents was the founder and director of the UNLV Consciousness Research Lab, Dean Radin.

That the suasions of rhetoric are part of making converts is something of a dirty secret in science, which has traditionally emphasized drama-free writing and monochromatic presentation on the grounds that arguments should be won on data, not on style, not with what Francis Bacon called "the romance of words." Radin had co-authored a paper that had been published in *Foundations of Physics*. It was a "meta-analysis" that combined data from many psi experiments in which people tried to influence mentally the output of random-number generators, a standard tool in psi research. At one time a professional violinist, Radin was much at home on stage, but he took a seat in the audience, agreeing it would be strategic in the credential-conscious forum of Tucson II to let his co-author, Roger Nelson of the Princeton Engineering Anomalies Research (PEAR) lab, present their work. But Nelson's talents in the lab withstanding, his case for psi suffered for want of some old-fashioned showmanship.

The contrast was all the more striking when Sue Blackmore offered her dissent. A lively speaker with a lemony English accent, Blackmore has been a thorn in the side of parapsychology for many years. She did two decades of her own psi research but unlike Radin and others, who because they get positive results are considered to have "golden hands," she never produced what she considered evidence of psi functioning. Having caught no fish in the river, she concluded the river had no fish, and at the 1987 meeting of the British Society for Psychical Research, she announced that "parapsychology has failed." Her apostasy included a dramatic defection to the Committee for the Scientific Investigation of

Claims for the Paranormal (CSICOP), a group of skeptics that might be described as religiously rational.

As Blackmore paced the stage, chopping the air with her hands, the audience snapped awake. Are there psi phenomena? she asked. Probably not. If there were, would they tell us anything about consciousness? In her opinion, no. She ridiculed the notion that some people have golden hands and others have personalities that inhibit the phenomena.

"My experience," Blackmore said, "has been that when I looked in detail to some claim, I have always come to the conclusion that there was not any psychic phenomena. But what if I'm wrong? What if there are? Would that tell us something interesting about consciousness? I'm not sure. The New Age view of why consciousness is interesting is that consciousness makes me what I am. It's what allows me to interact with the world and have experiences. But science—nasty, messy, reductionist science—says consciousness is just a lot of neurons messing about with other neurons. It's nothing spiritual. If we could show consciousness having a direct effect on the world, it would prove the power of the mind."

Parapsychologists, Blackmore observed, were headed in the opposite direction of neuroscientists. As she noted in the article from which her talk was drawn: "The more we look into the workings of the brain, the less it looks like a machine run by a conscious self. There is no place inside the brain where consciousness resides. . . . Indeed the brain seems to be a machine that runs itself very well and produces the illusion that there is someone in charge."

While Blackmore spoke, Radin was working up a slow boil. He annotated a copy of her article, scribbling in the margin: *This is nonsensical. . . . Her term, not ours . . . Misinterpretation of mystical view . . . i.e. Sue is a zombie . . .*

"I'm always upset when she talks," he said afterwards. "Her theatrical method is much more compelling than most talks about data by parapsychologists. The only thing we can do is demonstrate correlations. Something is going on in the head that is affecting something in the world."

A week after the conference, when I arrived in Las Vegas to visit the lab, I found Radin in his office straightening a line of rubber dinosaurs on the windowsill. At forty-four he had a thin, compact build, watchful brown eyes, and a severely receding hairline. He was brooding about an interview he'd given to a science journalist from England who had described one of his ideas—a switch that could be turned on with only the mind—as "wacky."

"The thing that gets me upset every so often is the word 'wacky' written in conjunction with what I do," he said. The idea of how to build a psychic switch had come to him in a blinding flash eleven years ago; he'd constructed and was testing a prototype. "You're wacky before you succeed," he said. "Afterwards, you're a genius."

Radin had worked almost everywhere a parapsychologist could collect a paycheck: a psi fellowship at the University of Edinburgh; stints at the PEAR lab and at SRI International, a private company in Menlo Park, California, that did the classified U.S. Army research on clairvoyance, or "remote viewing" as it had been termed. During his six years of industrial research at AT&T Bell Labs and four years at GTE, Radin had also been able to conduct psi experiments, and he'd twice served as president of the Parapsychology Association.

"This is the nerve center," he said as we entered the lab proper, which lay just down the hall from his office. The walls were decked with posters to make the place seem less clinical, and there was equipment scattered everywhere: Geiger counters, random-number generators, a pair of magnetometers sensitive enough to detect changes in the geomagnetic field when anyone summoned the building's elevator. Radin's assistant Jannine Rebman, a Ph.D. candidate in consciousness studies, was working on a computer. They had both recently returned from a New Age expo in Las Vegas, where they had been reminded of their relatively conservative place on the frontier of outlandish ideas.

"Somebody was selling a subtle energy generator," Radin recalled. "It was some kind of high frequency circuit board. You plug it in, and supposedly it bathes you in subtle energy. The boggle factor was very high."

"What do you mean?"

"There was nothing to base it on, no scientific data that showed it did anything!"

But the gizmo seemed harmless enough, unlike the blue-green algae cookies on sale at a nearby booth.

"I had assumed they wouldn't give away poison, but I was wrong," said Radin.

"They tasted like dirt," Rebman said.

Radin sighed. "I try to remember that people think what we do is boggling."

The work at the Consciousness Research Lab starts from the premise that psi experience is a mostly unconscious sensitivity or faculty that can be enhanced or inhibited by variables ranging from temperature and fluctuations in the earth's magnetic field to personal beliefs and character type.

"We're not trying to prove the existence of psi anymore," Radin said. "We're trying to understand the correlates under which the phenomena will appear." He showed me the prototype of his psychic switch, and I have a fuzzy, boggle-factored memory of his explaining how it was supposed to work, even though he said he was constrained by patent considerations and didn't want someone to swipe the idea and cash in on his invention. Of course, it was too soon to know whether the switch would end up at NASA, helping ground controllers reestablish telemetry links with wayward satellites, or at New Age health expos, where it might be marketed to decrepit hippies who wanted to switch off their lava lamps from bed. Or whether it would just fade away completely, the artifact of a bizarre pipe dream. On one of the shelves in Radin's lab were a couple of psi tchotchkes that served as tokens of the folly of premature excitement and unverified claims: a pair of vacuum-sealed glass vials containing perfectly round silver and brass rings. Never used, they had been fabricated years ago by some of Radin's colleagues to test the putative metal-bending or teleporting abilities of the controversial psychic and magician Uri Geller.

Radin had many experiments running at once. He sat down at the keyboard of a Dell computer, which was hooked to a Robix robotic arm whose lobsterlike claw dangled over a red peanut M&M.

"Okay," he said. "Press return."

I took a seat and hit return. Robix began to wheeze and twitch. At the back of the computer, millions of electrons were tunneling through two diodes, producing a random stream of ones and zeroes. The computer sampled strings of those numbers in order to create a Z score—a number representing a degree of deviation from chance. A low Z score—a low deviation from chance—caused the robot arm to stay where it was or reverse its progress. Middling Z scores produced only incremental progress. High ones inspired Robix to zip past all the intermediate physical positions and, like some overzealous new employee, snatch up the M&M and drop it into a little cup. (The M&M was meant to provide some motivation—people participating were promised they could eat the M&M after the experiment.) Radin's hypothesis was that a person's mental intention could speed up the delivery of the M&M by pushing the random output away from chance. One thousand baseline trials had established that, unobserved, Robix would complete the job in an average of twenty-five steps—that is, it would stop at twenty-five incrementally different positions before finishing. Radin told me it could be done, and had been done in a trial with a person trying to get the machine to speed up the delivery, in two steps.

Robix was a playful twist on an old format. Since the days of pioneering ESP researcher J. B. Rhine at Duke University, who in the 1930s moved the study of psychical phenomena from séance rooms to laboratories, parapsychologists have produced statistical evidence of what seems to be the mind's effect on matter. The assumption has been that, however slight, these deviations from expected outcomes are the evidentiary shadows of mind-matter interactions. Rhine worked with the simplest devices for generating statistical results: tumbling dice and specially designed cards. His results suggested that people could guess better than chance, but skeptics exposed flaws in his methods—subtle biases, "sensory leakage," and other limitations inherent in dice and cards. Many of these were overcome in the breakthrough work of the Boeing Laboratories physicist Helmut Schmidt, who in the 1960s had test subjects attempt to influence the random output of radioactive isotopes. Schmidt's studies were imaginatively expanded by Robert Jahn, the founder of the PEAR lab at Princeton University. Random-number generator experiments now make use of "electronic coin flippers" like the two diodes on the back of the computer I was sitting in front of.

Radin could hypothesize all day about the effect of mental intention on the computer diodes that would determine the rate of Robix's M&M drop-off, but how intention might interact with a flow of electrons to cause a nonrandom pattern, he didn't have the foggiest idea. Neither did anyone else in the field. As you quickly discover in a parapsychology lab, mental concepts such as intention, which seem so much a part of everyday life—inseparable from getting out of bed and making coffee and telephoning friends—become strangely chimerical under scientific scrutiny, which is so weighted toward the physical. Intention is as hard to measure, as tricky to define, as consciousness itself.

In another experiment, explicitly related to healing, Rens Wezelman, a visiting fellow at UNLV, and Radin's research associate Jannine Rebman devised a protocol that drew on the tradition of positive voodoo. They had subjects make dolls in their likeness out of Play-Doh and snippets of hair and other personal effects. They found a "patient's" blood flow and electrodermal activity increased during periods of time when another experimenter, acting in the role of a "healer" in another room one hundred meters away, massaged the patient's doll.

Those results were no more boggling than the data from a series of "mass consciousness" studies at the lab, which were designed to test the idea that millions of people focused on one event can affect physical systems. Radin correlated climactic moments in broadcasts of the Academy Awards and the O. J. Simpson trial with fluctuations in the output of random-number generators. In his view, the results suggested that large numbers of people concentrating on a common event or goal can increase the "coherence" and "order" in the world around them.

That may be, but it has to be said that any increase in the order and coherence of some hypothetical global mind field makes a royal mess of presently accepted scientific theories. What can these correlations mean? What is the connection between something happening in the head and something happening in the world? Correlation doesn't automatically imply causation. You can correlate the prevalence of smoking in the 1930s with church attendance and divorce rates and draw some patently stupid conclusions about cigarettes and family values. The sun doesn't rise because the rooster crows. Radin argues that correlations are part of the spectrum of causation. "Some are more or less self-evident, and some are more complex," he says. "The emerging view of complex ecosystems suggests that everything is constantly affecting everything else."

I began to think it wasn't just the foundation under parapsychology but the one under all psychology that was shaky, and maybe the one under the rest of science too. By Susan Blackmore's standards, parapsychology had failed, but it wasn't much of a leap to start wondering what had been "proved" forever in all the deluge of scientific formulations. All was maya, the Hindu philosophers would say, and at this rate I would soon lack epistemological confidence in my own name . . . Sure there were nerves that joined the arm and the brain, but did anybody really understand how the "will" sent impulses down the axons to make the muscles wave good-bye? The "act" of the mind that intended the arm to move seemed awfully close to "psychokinesis," in which matter was moved or transformed without any physical means such as nerves. How were subjective perceptions of pain formed independently of the objective sensation of pain? How did "ideas" emerge from tissue? Were there even such discrete things as "ideas"? Weren't they just "physical" states in the brain? I was teetering back toward the Ob line of materialist thinking that had led to the philosophy of epiphenomenalism, which handily solved the mind-over-matter problem by eliminating the mind. Was it inevitable that if you asked questions about consciousness the self started to seem like an afterthought? One would think that any theory of mental life that did away with mental life was fatally confused, but something about the study of consciousness brought out the zombie in people. Or maybe it was simply the premises of psi that at this moment were asking me to locate my nonmaterial being and register it on a piece of inscrutable computer equipment.

Picture it: There you are, an arguably more colorful zombie planted in front of a zombie with no visible illusions about itself, one of you trying to project intention onto the other. How? Well, any way you want, apparently, as long as you don't hit Robix, which, as I quickly discovered, is intensely tempting. Radin and Rebman encouraged participants to express emotion. It was kosher to shout or curse. I tried some hard frowning, as if Robix were a child cued to an authoritative face. Shazam! The obedient puppet plucked and delivered the M&M in seventeen steps.

"That's fast," Radin said.

Skeptics would say there was no way to tell whether my existence as a subject attempting to influence Robix could play any role in the M&M delivery. Radin, like most psi researchers, assumed my presence mattered, but he couldn't quantify the degree to which it did or what it was about my presence, my subjectivity, that produced a response in the objective physical system. If psi were independent of conscious intention—many parapsychologists suggested it was largely an *unconscious* human faculty—why did I have to try to do anything *consciously*? Come to think of it, why couldn't a mind-matter interaction be posited between a random-number generator and a disembodied kidney? Not too many people thought kidneys were the seat of consciousness, but weren't they full of spirit? Weren't they brilliantly intelligent in their ability to regulate acid-base balances and excrete urine? Could you speculate that a kidney could "desire" and "intend" to excrete urine? And if Robix was opening a locked bathroom door instead of delivering a red M&M, maybe the kidney's desire and intention to excrete urine might effect the flow of electrons in the computer diodes. But then you'd have to separate out the kidney's intentions and desires from the bladder's . . .

Maybe Robix was picking up my turmoil, because in the second round, it started to equivocate, hovering over the peanut like some parody Hamlet paralyzed by a bountiful candy rack. I tried yelling "Come on!" but that was as effective as giving orders to a cat. Gentle swearing didn't work either. Finally, a bit of truly profane language spurred on some desultory progress. The performance—Robix's? mine? ours?—was worse than chance: thirty-five steps. On top of that, Radin said I couldn't have the M&M; it was the last one in the lab.

As it turned out, everyone's scores on the robot experiment were not better than chance and did not indicate psi functioning. But the purpose was not simply to see whether a class of subjects could demonstrate significant above-chance results with Robix and two other random-number generator experiments on the computer. It was to correlate the performances of people in all three experiments with dozens of variables from geomagnetic field activity to the moods of the experimenters and subjects, to air quality and rates of domestic violence, and then to build a neural network using those correlations to see if an artificial intelligence system could predict their performances. Here, then, were the makings of a predictive model.

"We know psi performance varies wildly from one study to the next," he said. "The question is why. We wanted to test the idea that the environment modulates people's psi ability, just like any other ability. If psi had been shown, that would be great, but I did not expect to see significant results, because the subject population was so heterogeneous. If you're studying violin playing, and you pull twenty-five people off the street and ask them to play like Itzhak Perlman, you are going to be very disappointed, and will probably come to the conclusion that no one can play the violin very well. The point of this study was that everyone may show a little psi 'all of the time,' but you can detect it only if you take into account lots of external factors that modulate our ability to perform."

It's a puckish fate that would post a parapsychologist in Las Vegas, if only because those who argue that psi is bankrupt often cite Sin City as exhibit A. If psychokinesis were real, wouldn't roulette players be steering the ball to winning numbers? How can psi, which suggests that people can beat the laws of chance, exist in the same universe with a city built on the indomitability of chance?

Unlike most parapsychologists, Radin has actually studied what he thinks might be psi in the casinos and why there isn't more of it. The simple answer, he said, is that the state of mind most people attain in a casino isn't conducive to psi. Radin lucked into a heap of data in the spring of 1995, when Bernice Jaeger, the assistant general manager of the Continental Casino, called him up. She'd read an article about his work in the UNLV alumni magazine, and she was intrigued enough to let Radin have four years of daily payout data. Payout data is the percentage of each gambler's dollar that the Continental returns in winnings.

Radin decided to look at moon-behavior correlations, which are controversial—some researchers put stock in them and others don't. To his surprise, he found that four out of the five major slot-machine jackpots in the time-frame of the Continental data occurred on the full moon. While it's possible that's just an interesting coincidence, he also found that the daily payout rates over a four-year period correlated with lunar cycles. When the moon was full, gamblers got a little more of their money back—about two percent more. As Radin saw the correlations emerge from the compilations of data, he felt the blood rush to his face and a twinge of nausea. He was getting a new way of looking at the world. How could it be explained? Had he made some mistake? He started over again to see if he'd made some obvious error, but the second analysis confirmed the first. Was this psi-enhanced performance, a faculty of the mind enhanced by conditions in nature? He couldn't say. Whatever it was, it was subtle. And not that meaningful in practical terms: People weren't beating the house on the full moon, only having the pleasure of losing a little more slowly.

It was late in the day, and we had been talking in his office for hours. As we walked to the student center to get some iced tea, the ersatz pyramid of the Luxor casino and the skyline of the Vegas strip shimmered in the west over the playing fields and parking lots of the campus. Radin looked around bewilderedly.

"This is the last place in the world I thought I would end up," he said. He had been born in New York City and spent his early childhood in Atlanta. He started reading at three. He took up the violin, and by age eight, when the family moved to western Massachusetts, he was on the prodigy track, practicing three hours a day. "The single word of my childhood was 'creativity,' " he said. " 'Do something creative.' I heard that a hundred thousand times growing up. That and 'You're not living up to your potential.' Even today, I wonder how do I know when I can stop pushing?"

At nine, he built an abacus-like computer out of jelly beans; at twelve he built a TV and glued himself to *Love, American Style*. At thirteen, he stumbled on C.E.M. Hansel's book *ESP: A Scientific Evaluation* and was struck not by the dismissal of psychic phenomena but by the revelation that weird stuff could be scientifically studied. He played violin in high school with the Springfield Youth Symphony and won a major science prize ("Math Whiz, 17, Proves Textbooks Wrong"). He enrolled at the University of Massachusetts at Amherst and went on to the University of Illinois for his doctorate in educational psychology.

In the late seventies, a job on the technical staff at AT&T Bell Labs in Columbus, Ohio, was an experimentalist's dream. "Anybody who wanted could do stuff, whatever you liked," he recalled. "I wanted to focus on scientific anomalies, because that's where the history of science shows the breakthroughs occur. I guess I had a streak of rebellion. When it comes to something you can test yourself, I thought why not try it, why not set up an ESP experiment?"

He devised a pseudo-random-number-generator experiment on a computer, which posed the question: Could wishing influence the movement of a computer cursor? Apparently yes. He looked into applied kinesiology, a fringe diagnostic technique based on the theory that muscle strength reflects the body's sensitivity to various substances. Radin ran double-blind and triple-blind trials with fifty-eight adults using vials of sugar and sand and a dynamometer that measured gripping strength of the hand. The results startled him, and he noted in the report he published in *Perceptual and Motor Skills* in 1984 that indeed they seemed "preposterous." But data were data, and his data showed that people's muscle strength decreased significantly when they held vials of sugar. More surprising was the reaction of one of his colleagues at Bell Labs, who accused him of "doing the work of the devil."

"Parapsychology was the first thing I ever did that became more interesting the more I looked into it," Radin recalled. By 1985, he had been recruited to do classified work at SRI International as a visiting scientist. The background checkers from the FBI wanted to know about his life for the last fifteen years and whether he'd ever smoked marijuana.

The issue of belief crops up so frequently in parapsychology that it's fair to say a number of parapsychologists have had what could be called "conversion experiences." Radin is not one of them. "When I started at Bell Labs I was trying to prove to myself whether I could believe in psi phenomena. I spent five years doing experiments but that didn't really do it. What really did it was the meta-analysis I did at SRI of random-number generator experiments. I thought, 'Well somebody like Helmut Schmidt did this experiment and got this result, maybe I'll try it.' I did and got the same result. So I thought, 'Maybe we're both nuts.' But then there were half a dozen others. People at MIT and Bell Labs and Princeton and Stanford and the Lawrence Livermore Labs. Surprise! Maybe there were seventy-five people around the world, and they're all nuts! They were using different ways of looking at the same thing, different random-number generators, different protocols, different subjects. But one thing was the same. Somebody doing something in the head caused a generator to fluctuate and to establish a correlation between the mind and a physical system."

At SRI, Radin had access not only to classified U.S. research in remote viewing but to psi literature newly translated from Chinese and Soviet journals. The staff debriefed defectors and interviewed coopera-tive researchers. "I was blown away," he said. "There was a huge body of stuff, operational stuff. I had no idea that remote viewing could be that good, for real, on real-life important targets. I had no idea it was being used to hunt for Patty Hearst and other well-known missing people. And that it was useful in this regard. Mainly I was surprised to see a long list of Department of Defense and intelligence agencies that had been fund-ing the program for decades, with the highest level of support in the gov-ernment, and most importantly, the fact that within the agencies there was no question anymore that the basic phenomena were real. They weren't funding for the hell of it, they found the stuff pragmatically use-ful. This was an eye-opener, because at that time, 1985, there was still debate within parapsychology as to whether we were even working with genuine phenomena. The meta-analyses had yet to be done, so the degree of persuasiveness of the data was not yet clear."

Psychical research had received a tremendous impetus from cold-war paranoia about the Soviets' exploiting a supposed "psi gap" for military advantage. Stories about Soviet psychic prowess were going around in the 1960s and 1970s. "They were saying that by directing one's thought at a rabbit, you could stop its heart," Radin recalled. "Presto, psychic assas-sins! By killing a baby rabbit and monitoring its mother, you could get a big response in the mother even if she were isolated from the baby. Presto, psychic communication methods! The classified literature from the Soviet Union suggested that such experiments did take place. We know from our own open literature that thinking thoughts at someone at a dis-tance does influence their nervous system, so there is independent face validity suggesting that a properly talented individual with sufficient motivation may be able to do some serious damage to a human target. Of course, the reverse is also true, and serious healing can also be accom-plished."

The only time Radin ever personally experienced something that seemed like ESP was one night with his wife, Katy. They had met in college and married in 1981. They stayed together when Radin went off to SRI, and when he came east to New Jersey to direct psi research at Princeton under Robert Jahn, and when he returned to private industry to set up a psi research project in Waltham, Massachusetts. They tried for seven years to have a child, but the strain of fertility treatments and failed attempts at adoption, and the intensity of professional life crushed the relationship. They divorced in 1990.

But one night in 1983, when he was playing Trivial Pursuit with Katy and a bunch of friends, Radin had the uncanny feeling of knowing the answers when his wife looked at the cards. Even when he faced baffling questions, the right answers just popped into his head. When Katy didn't look at the card, he wouldn't have a clue; then she'd look and suddenly the answer would come out of his mouth. Again and again. Ten in a row he reeled off. In tandem, that night at least, they had all the answers, and the sort of communion you never forget.

However meaningful such an experience is to a husband, it could only frustrate a parapsychologist—more anecdotal evidence of a tantalizing phenomenon that so often slipped through the nets of science. Radin had collected enough data of his own and reviewed enough gathered by colleagues to convince himself that *something* was going on. Psi was real.

And after years of belligerent, often ignorant skepticism, some leading parapsychology critics were begrudging a little ground. In 1995, two consultants were hired to evaluate the U.S. government's two-decade-long remote-viewing research. One was University of California statistician Jessica Utts. She made no bones about the results: "Using the standards applied to any other area of science, the case for psychic functioning has been scientifically proven." The other was Ray Hyman, the dean of psi skeptics. He concluded that "the case for psychic functioning seems better than it has ever been. . . . I tend to agree with Professor Utts that real effects are occurring in these experiments. *Something* other than chance departures from the null hypothesis has occurred in these experiments." But, he added, "inexplicable statistical departures from chance . . . are a far cry from compelling evidence of anomalous cognition."

So it goes. You can understand wishy-washiness in a civilian when the technicians, despite new areas of agreement, are still disputing the issue. If psi effects are real but as weak and capricious as they seem, can they have any use? Psychic switches and applied psi technologies may well turn out to be commercial pipe dreams, and certainly it is hard to imagine a mind-to-mind communications device that surpasses the reliability of the telephone. To the question of why anyone should care about something whose nature is so shrouded in doubt—something that at times seems like a synonym for God—Radin's short answer (and this was an article of faith on his part and on the part of all parapsychologists) was that psi phenomena seem to extend what we can know about ourselves, our capabilities, what he called our "deep interconnectedness." Psi phenomena imply our notions of singularity and separation are blinders keeping us from seeing the extent to which we embody some deeper reality, the underlying unity celebrated by mystics, saints, and enchanted screwballs. But it would be nothing if not bathetic if the effort to realize that vision of deep interconnectedness, a vision that has inspired psychical research since the days of William James, had only the practical effect of sucking more zombies into Las Vegas on the nights of the full moon.

People do have extraordinary abilities; they do undergo unutterably weird experiences. The power and appeal of science is also its vexing limitation: It does not cater to belief. It refuses to accept reality as a social or personal construct; it insists that something that does not have to do with us exists *out there*, an objective universe with properties and laws independent of the minds describing them. Of course, the inescapable paradox is that science itself is an act of the mind. This Ajna problem of trying to stand outside of what we are ineluctably inside of is what makes mind-matter quandaries so labyrinthine. Time and again, philosophers and neuroscientists are compelled by the logic of materialism to refer to themselves as machines beset by some weird yearning to generate the illusion that they are really minds or souls or spirits having experiences— that they are, in fact, beings bowled over by the cards, or a run of luck, or a flood of incommunicable feeling in the heart.

5. SEVENTEEN RED

The revelation about revelation is that sometimes it finds you when you are least expecting it. It took me months to realize that I had already seen Hakini Shakti, goddess of the third eye. It was in Las Vegas, of all places, at the end of my visit to the Consciousness Research Lab, a visit in which my boggle threshold had been crossed more times than I could count. I had an early flight and I was tired, ready to go back to the motel and crash. But first I wanted to take a quick look at the Continental Casino, whose manager had given Dean Radin the data for his psi-in-the-casino study.

The Continental lay a mile or so back from the glitter of the Las Vegas strip, and, sad to say, the place seemed down on its luck, threadbare and thinly populated with people who looked as if their Prozac prescriptions had run out. I didn't stay long. I drove back to the motel, undressed, and climbed into bed.

And suddenly I couldn't close my eyes.

It was the night of the new moon, absolutely the worst time to go gambling, according to the data. But you can't keep a moth from the flame. I got up, got dressed again, and set out on foot with no clear destination. Las Vegas is a car culture; off the strip, hardly anybody uses the sidewalks, and it's no wonder, because when you walk you feel the tenuousness of the city, its doubtful purchase on the desert, and its desultory zombie heart, where tumbleweeds and vacant lots lurk like emblems of the oblivion that waits to return when the machinery has run its course. I went into a few casinos, not knowing what I was looking for, more to escape the feeling of mindlessness in the air than out of any desire to gamble.

I ended up finally at Bally's, where I ran aground on a roulette table and lost a hundred dollars in ten minutes. I went to a cash machine and floated myself another hundred, thinking this was folly, this could only put an ugly finish on an illuminating trip. But then I thought maybe I was like my father, who plays tennis better when he's got a bad wrist or a sprained knee, some handicap he can heroically overcome and thus sustain the vision of the greatness he might achieve if only he were at full strength. Maybe the strategic use of self-imposed adversity was the way he got himself into the Zone, and we were similar that way. Heart surgeons, clairvoyants, gamblers—all performers, really—acknowledge the concept of the Zone, of getting into a rhythm, of feeling that time can be slowed or speeded up as needed, that outcomes can be anticipated and failure is not possible. Zone consciousness is ingrained in the lore of athletic greatness. You have to get there and stay put as long as you can. But how? I remembered something I once heard about psychokinesis: Moving objects or imparting information might not be a matter of bending reality to your will but of participating in it, of meshing with it as you would flow along with a partner in a dance.

Alas, vigilant gorillas stand by at Bally's to prevent gamblers from hands-on dancing with the roulette wheel. And it was all too clear the rock-faced English croupier was sick of being asked to dance. Her beleaguered expression said she hated her job and would hasten back to London that night if she had her druthers.

Before I knew it, I was down another hundred.

It was at that nadir that merry, curly-haired Curtis took over the shift. It seemed to me certain numbers came up more frequently with Curtis than with Ms. Stonehenge. It seemed Curtis had a pattern, and I could tune in to it. Reason says this is superstition. Reason also says it's stupid to play roulette. But as Jung insisted, rational decision-making draws on the irrational-seeming states of feeling and intuition; human ratiocination is bigger than strict rationality. I bet on my unscientific hunches, and lo, a modest tower emerged from what had been a pitiful puddle of chips. Then Ms. Stonehenge returned, and my tower shrank. I had to play like a church mouse until Curtis came back. Sure enough, when he returned, "his" numbers started hitting: twenty-two, twenty-five, thirty-two.

Now it was after midnight. The group at the table had turned over several times, and the rail was crowded with conventioneers from the

National Association of Broadcasters. One guy from New York was betting seventeen and continually losing. His friends at the table said that with his bonus he could afford it. It was painful to listen to him try to get Ms. Stonehenge to crack a smile. But Curtis wasn't hitting seventeen for him either. Again and again, the guy would put three or four chips on the number only to see them raked away.

"I can't believe seventeen hasn't come up," he cried.

And then he did something dramatic. He moved a giant stack of chips onto seventeen.

"Seventeen has got to come up," he said.

Everyone at the table stared at the stack a moment, hesitating. And then they started leaping in, putting their color on top of his. The woman next to me put a chip on, the guy across the table laid on five. Another fellow put a few on, as did the woman next to him, and the man next to her. I laid two chips on seventeen and spread a bunch more around it. The corners and the sides of seventeen vanished under chips and the chip skyscraper directly on the number looked straight out of downtown Singapore.

Curtis gave the ball a whirl.

I don't know if time slowed down, but it didn't speed up. I can't say I had any precognitive aperçu of where the ball would land, but I can say that everyone at the table who had been pursuing separate strategies all night was suddenly bound together, pulling as one. We had one goal, one purpose; we were projecting our intention, our most ardent hopes, as a unified team. Perhaps at some level our consciousness was massed and struggling to declare itself, I don't know. But there was much more at stake than a red M&M. And it wasn't just the money. We were the put-upon losers, patronized by the gorillas in the monkey suits; we were the suckers being fleeced, the fools hungering for revolution in their secret hearts.

And there was a moment when I looked up from the spinning wheel and the whirling ball. I saw the faces of my fellow gamblers arrayed around the rail in a godawful light, six red-faced heads on a single body. Hakini Shakti! The ball scrabbled and hopped and settled, and then Curtis with astonishment flooding his voice called out, "Seventeen!" and a roar went up that rocked the far ends of the casino.

In truth, I don't know why the ball landed on seventeen red on that spin, on that night, in that casino. It would be nice to think a goddess that I helped constitute had made it happen. But, as Midas knew, if wishing made it so, the pleasure of winning would disappear. The game would have no meaning. There would be no game in the game. If I had to take an official position, I would say the number just came up; it was gorgeous dumb luck. Off the record, I like to think maybe not. I conceal the hope that something unexplained happened, and that we all contributed to it. Call it psi or luck or Spirit or the fruit of Ajna, whatever it was it had stepped from the flux of randomness to give us a waltz.

Something I do know for sure is that my moment in the abode of uninterrupted bliss abruptly ended when Curtis began to chatter about all the UFOs he'd seen in the Nevada desert over Area 51. There's nothing like extraterrestrial phenomena to bring you back to earth. My beliefs rebelled. The synchronicity was gone. It was time to cash out. My net for the night was thirty hard-won dollars. I walked back to the motel, drinking the cool night air and the smell of desert sage. The money in my pocket was a paltry sum, but it felt like more somehow, as if it had been stolen from the moon.

CHAPTER SEVEN

Metaphysics is not human knowledge. Thus, it is not in so far as he is man that man can attain it; it is the grasping in effective consciousness of supra-individual states.

—VALENTIN TOMBERG

1. MIDNIGHT ON THE PONT DES ARTS

What can I say: I'd run right off a cliff like the coyote in the cartoon, and now was scrabbling for traction midair in the abyss of mind and self and soul, those spectral constituents of my user illusion. A clown mishap, truly, and it couldn't have come at a worse time. If you've read this far, if you've persevered through chapter after chapter of exasperating equivocation, you're expecting some conclusions, some solid summing up that says "This is where we stand, this is the ground under our feet, etc. etc." And I agree, you *deserve* conclusions, real Earth-based ones that delve beyond what my user illusion is probably equipped for, which are basically pat lessons that wrap up essays in women's magazines, or maybe some gamely deployed Bartlett's pith of the sort that high school seniors are always posting under their yearbook pictures. Even now, the user illusion is tempted to wheel out a disingenuous bromide from Socrates ("I know that I know nothing") or maybe that pseudo-epigram from Oscar Wilde ("Nothing that is worth knowing can be taught"), which falls apart the moment you put it in the context of flying a plane or operating a heart-lung machine.

I know the last thing my user illusion wants to suggest is that developments in his personal life were the prize at the end of the chakras. I mean, bully for him if they were. Bully for him if his stocks were up and his cholesterol down. Bully for him if he'd learned to speak from his heart and was a better yuppie, and had developed the knack of chatting with his discarnate guides, the five-thousand-year-old Chinese adviser and the tag-team of towheads. Bully for him, and so what: The one enduring law of spiritual insight is that those who crow about their gains know nothing.

On the other hand, there was the lead I buried in the last chapter, a happiness so noteworthy that even the most circumspect user illusion had to throw caution to the wind and have out with the news. One night in Paris with Kate, on a bridge across the Seine—

Let's go back a paragraph.

I thought this was going okay.

It's fine. But you crossed out a line. In the paragraph that starts "I know the last thing my user illusion . . ." Could you read it back?

"Bully for him if he walked on air like Wile E. Coyote, or skipped across a river as confident of the lily pads of faith as of the stones of reason."

The question we have for you is: What happened to the monk? What happened to speaking from the heart?

What do you mean?

Here you are, faced with the task of writing about the greatest leap of faith in your life, and the possibilities of spiritual belief, of going beyond what you can know through the intellect, and how those possibilities bear on the communal and metaphysical aspects of healing—and the figure you come up with to draw it all together is Wile E. Coyote walking on air, or on lily pads, or whatever?

I cut the lines—

But you're still hiding behind the clown.

How could I argue with my own guides? It *was* a leap of faith that was at issue, and I *was* hiding behind my clown, not one clown but a thousand: warrior clowns with mocking comebacks, supercilious skeptic clowns, the know-it-all rationalist clown, the science-will-set-us-free clown, the jokey keep-it-light foe-of-sincerity clown, the cartoon clowns inspired by hepcats like Snagglepuss and Sylvester, and now, at the eleventh hour, Wile E. Coyote, who was always deliberating in the path of an oncoming truck or standing at the impact point of a plummeting anvil or charging off the precipice in pursuit of his quarry, and going great guns too, until he made the fatal mistake of looking down and discovering the mile of air beneath his paws. And don't forget the clown-with-a-quote-for-all-seasons, rifling Bartlett's for another *pensée* from Socrates about the futility of producing conclusions for his book. They were superimposed on one another like subtle bodies, and underneath them all, at the core, was the original clown, the tender, bumbling, credulous child clown.

Who is not a clown at all.

Who was not a clown at all, my guides were saying. Who was not a monk either, but what my monk and clown were before my psyche was fractured into monks and clowns, before the monk was drawn into dialectics with the white-faced genius from the commedia dell'arte: which is to say the unformed self that had to be protected and compensated for and hidden behind costumes, whether they were uniforms of some religious order, or rubber noses and layers of greasepaint. Clown and monk: They were the same, two faces of one nakedly innocent fool.

In *Meditations on the Tarot*, his remarkable book on Christian hermeticism, the French author Valentin Tomberg writes that the Fool represents the transition from ego consciousness to spiritual consciousness —the segue from the lesser knowledge of the intellect to the higher knowledge of love. The Fool unites "human wisdom, which is folly in the eyes of God, with divine wisdom, which is folly in the eyes of man, in such a way that the result is not a double folly but rather a single wisdom which understands both that which is above and that which is below." The Fool resolves the discord of head and heart, and so leads you into your first wholeness, an intimate and congenial sort of intrapsychic community. I would say it takes faith to relinquish the masks of personae and embrace the unity implicit in the figure of the Fool. But that is only the first step toward community. Further ones await, and each one requires in its way a more intricate leap of faith.

Wherever two or three are met.

Wherever two or three are met, my guides are saying, though in this case, if you were standing on a bridge with a proposal of marriage welling in your heart, two would be company enough. Three would be illegal, in fact. Some forms of community are explicitly forbidden by law.

The point being . . .

The point being, could I know whether the leap of faith I was preparing to make into the community of two—the leap of faith inherent whenever one person asks another for her hand in marriage—could I know whether it was emerging from the work I'd done in the subtle world, or was only the inevitable result of getting older, of growing up and finding fortune?

It's more important to witness faith than to analyze it.

Sure, but the distinction still seemed vital to any conclusions I could draw—a distinction as vital as it was hard to make, given that lives didn't unfold as placebo-controlled experiments; you couldn't plot the outcome of story A against story B. I was hard-pressed for conclusions because I had only a single set of events to work with; I couldn't tweak variables and tease out the active ingredient by which the user illusion arrived at what he knew and determined what he chose.

Some things you'll always know without knowing how you know them. It's the nature of inner voices—why we're called guides. We come from the metaphysics of silence.

Then why are you talking so much? I have to say I feel a little queasy about you all getting so chatty. Some people are considered nuts because of over-enthusiastic conversations with inner voices. I mean, what if I'm in the Food Emporium, and you all start jabbering . . .

We'll do our best not to compromise your facade of normality.

Can I turn you off if I want to?

Progress of this kind is hard to undo without medication. Remember, we're here to aid you. We can help form the conclusions you're hunting for. The onset of our voices, in context, might be one of those conclusions. You may find you'll turn to us when you confront the unresolved incidents in this book that are causing you difficulty precisely because they intimate the possibility of our existence.

You mean I'll ask you to help me get a grip on reality when your existence is the reason I'm doubting my grip on reality in the first place?

Paradox is the water you are learning to walk on. Our main aim, as ever, is to remind you that it's always been your nature to try to reason your way toward realities that are contingent on faith, and to point the way when you wander beyond the limits of your method.

Late in October 1995, when I had finished most of my remedial heart work and had roughed out the events of my shadow book with Rachel, and was just starting into the mine fields of the third eye—feeling at that point that I had crept far enough from the pale of the so-called hopelessly sane to know that some of the insanely wild country of the chakras might be a better place to settle down and build a house in—I went to Paris with Kate for four days. What bliss it was to be rid of clown metaphysics and whirl about the valentine heart in the capital of romantic communion, the lyric city that, except for that patch of revolutionary unpleasantness with the guillotine, had favored an integrative approach to the mind-body problem, prescribing love, food, and wine to mend what the philosophy of Monsieur Descartes had cleaved.

On our last night in Paris, it poured rain. We went to dinner at an out-of-the-way restaurant on the Right Bank, and when we got up to go, the place was empty; the proprietor stood at the door and shook our hands as if he'd had us to his house. It was half past eleven. The rain had let up. The streetlamps in the mist looked like small moons ringed with auras, auras anyone could see. We wandered down the rue de Mail like two fools for love. We passed by the colonnade of the Palais Royal, and then skirted the palisade of the Louvre, where ghostless stone personages eyed the night from their niches in the pantheon.

At the Quai du Louvre, we walked upriver and then onto the famous footbridge, the Pont des Arts.

One of the long boats that ply the Seine was returning to dock after a late-evening cruise. It was packed with tourists, and when it swept beneath us, visible through the planks, the Pont des Arts suddenly seemed suspended over a great height, like an aerialist's catwalk above a gallery of circus-goers. We found a bench halfway across and sat down in what seemed at that moment to be the heart of Paris: the Eiffel Tower bathed in light, the spires of Sainte Chapelle, the shadowy hulk of Notre Dame, the gilded domes, copper roofs, the labyrinth of boulevards and alleys— all of it set to the eternal murmur of the Seine. The river was alive with shattered light, coursing forward, pushing on; I felt its current in my hands as a kind of doubtlessness. Dare I now call it faith? All right, faith: faith that I could leap into the unknown, faith that all of life turned on such gambits. I had my grandmother's ring in my pocket, and conviction in my heart, and oh, don't you know, Kate said yes? She said yes, which for all my conviction was still so amazing that I asked again and she said yes again.

And in the sway of feeling we did not notice when the lights of the city went off for the night, or when the sparse crowd on the Pont des Arts dispersed, or by what art or blessing it was exactly that we came to find ourselves alone at midnight on the Bridge of Arts. But we were alone. We were alone, but not in a way we'd ever been alone before: which is to say that we were no longer alone; we were walking on the air of a double dream. And it seemed we lingered there a lifetime that night, in the heart of Paris—lingered in our newfound community so we might always remember the moment of our metamorphosis, the water we had crossed, the bridge we had dreamed into being.

2. THE EPIDEMIOLOGY OF FAITH

The illimitable whirlwind has ushered us up the body to the crown of the head and the threshold of Sahasrara, the lotus of a thousand petals. Here is the camp at the end of the mind from which mystics set out for the Realm of the One and some hoped-for rendezvous with that incommunicable essence, the Absolute, the Ineffable, the Profound Something that has to do with something profound. In its quiescent form, the crown chakra is said to have a shallow concave shape; but as the high-minded disciple navigates the knife-edge of the Mystic Way— proceeding under the guidance of a religious order or going it alone, unsponsored and unroped—the profile of the chakra expands. It brightens; its very luminosity becomes a measure of the pilgrim's progress. In the God-realized adepts who have reached the summit, it blazes with the thermonuclear light of "ten million suns." Of such radiance the halos of the saints are made and the mystic realm "replete with every form of bliss" is signified. And yet for all its glory, Sahasrara is infinitesimally subtle; the Sanskrit verses translated by Sir John Woodroffe in 1928 liken it "unto the ten-millionth part of the end of a hair."

Modern clairvoyants, untroubled by the scientific angst that surrounds the question of the soul's reality, generally agree that the seventh chakra is the soul's entrance at birth. Before the divine will-o'-the-wisp can occupy the finite space of an embodied existence and revel in the pleasures of blushing, allergies, taxes, and scientific arguments against dualism, it has to be shoe-horned in through the fontanel at the top of the infant's skull where the cranial bones are late to knit. The newborn is as diminutive as the soul is vast, and apparently karma can sometimes make the installation as awkward as getting a professional basketball player into the backseat of an economy car. Once it is situated, there is only the matter of extrication: The way in serves also as the way out. For a person on the verge of death, the scouts of the subtle world say Sahasrara is the final touch-point, the last button to be unbuttoned, the final anchor weighed before the soul casts itself free and drifts over the horizon like a shaman's canoe.

Some authorities do not group Sahasrara with the other six chakras, as the energy it supposedly transduces comes from outside the human ken. But then it's also said that the chakra can be activated when a person kneels: The nerves of the knees are represented in the sensory cortex near that point where the chakra initially enters the skull, and when you stimulate the knees, you buzz the brain and pique the chakra. Ergo the correspondence between kneeling and the transports of religious feeling. (An imprecise correspondence, perhaps: Neuroscientists suspect the temporal lobe is the wellspring of religious visual imagery.) Whatever the case, in its energetic reality and symbolic dimensions, Sahasrara expresses the paradoxical role, if not the chronic human delusion, of divine activity in human flesh. It is the bridge we dream into being that connects us to beings greater than ourselves, to Being itself. To open the crown—by kneeling, by meditating, by raising the kundalini up through the six lower chakras so that the two streams of energy converge at the top like the twin snakes of the caduceus—is to be engulfed in what the great German professor of religion Rudolf Otto called the *mysterium tremendum*. That is, the immensity of the superconscious mind, the "cosmic self," wherein all dualities are resolved.

The glory of an awakened crown chakra is this state of nonduality, the mystic's unitive consciousness where the Many are One, and nothing divides Ob from Sub, or mind from body, or (as the neo-Melanesians would say) *meat* from *think-think*. "All feelings, emotions, and desires, which are the activities of the mind, are dissolved into their primary cause," writes Tantric author Harish Johari. "The union is achieved. The yogi is sat-chit-ananada, truth-being-bliss. . . . As long as he stays in his physical body he retains nondual consciousness. . . . It is possible for anyone to feel the divine, and to realize divinity within himself."

So Sahasrara is the instrument of Gnostic revelation—what Jung had in mind when he made his famous remark, "I do not believe in God, I know God." As such, it often serves as the stage on which the dramas of miraculous healing unfold. Those overtly religious healers and charismatics who seek to perform "spiritual healings" through prayer and the laying-on of hands will harness the energy of the crown chakra much as secular energy healers employ the lower chakras. Assuming the spiritual healers aren't the cynical frauds who in some spectacular cases have been shown to be seeking only to capitalize on the desperation of the sick, the difference between the two groups often lies only in the terms and fine points of technique. In place of concepts such as energy and frequency, you hear "grace" and "holy spirit." Where a Chinese *chi gong* healer might try to "build a patient's *chi*," the spiritual healer will petition God for an infusion of strength. Where a lay healer trained to work with body energies might gingerly initiate the business of "restructuring" the etheric body, making acute distinctions between the frequencies of healthy and infected tissue, a spiritual healer in the Christian tradition might hope to open herself to an influx of divine power sufficient to drive out the demon of sickness with one cataclysmic jolt of energy, trusting that Providence will supply the right dose and distribution.

Mainline churches have long frowned on the idea of personally realized divinity, and seldom included the hands-on cultivation of body consciousness as part of their spiritual mission. Health was no longer a spiritual question, and whatever healing franchise they once might have had—the first hospitals were in monasteries—they had long since forfeited. Indeed, it seemed to many people of my generation, which came of age in the sixties and seventies, that organized religions were themselves a kind of illness, irrelevant anachronisms that viewed the body with suspicion and were more interested in repressing ecstatic experience than in nurturing it.

Rapture, not to say healing, was certainly not on the agenda of the church I was packed off to each Sunday morning. With its premium on rote observance and its obsession with the sinful appetites of the body, St. Clement's offered a typically lifeless brand of denatured suburban Catholicism. The mortification of the flesh that the monseigneur described as a virtue in his Sunday sermons was often actualized the following Tuesday afternoon at the catechism classes, where nuns would crack your knuckles with a ruler if you didn't know who was in the manger with the baby Jesus or what the term was for when the incorruptible body of the Virgin Mary was hoisted to heaven.

For this stint in purgatory, I have my parents to thank. They couldn't be bothered with church; they only shipped me off to placate my pious maternal grandparents. I was duly baptized, confessed, communed, and confirmed. Throughout, I was mostly bored, given to meditating not on the glory of presences unseen but on the pervasiveness of moralizers and hypocrites. The sacrament of "first confession" was supposed to introduce our cohort of seven-year-olds to the concepts of sin and absolution. In my case, it did in the sense that when it came time to confess, I couldn't think of any sins, and in a moment of maybe divine inspiration I invented some, and then realized that in lying I had sinned for real, and was torn between guilt and a paradoxical sense of pride and virtuousness for having an authentic crime to repent.

If the teachings at St. Clement's had been more interesting, more passionate, more hands-on, if the teachers had not been so fixated on a creation story as farfetched as any scenario of New Age cosmogony, something might have engaged my imagination and I might have stuck around. The proceedings at a Catholic institution were supposed to be much more vivid than the pastel show over at the Episcopal place, but you would not have guessed it from the droning Mass and the out-of-it Fathers who had a knack for trite homilies and apparently a grave aversion to the pressing secular and spiritual concerns of the time. Why was the church so congenial to the government's war in Vietnam? To the corporations pillaging the environment? Why did it subscribe to a view of humanity that seemed rooted in outright hatred of the body when St. Paul himself said the body was a sacred temple? The subtext was always "Don't ask questions." Where poetry was wanted, the spiritual masters of St. Clement's offered prose. It was as if Marx or Nietzsche or some other demon had kidnapped their rhetoric and they had never recovered from the scientific demystification of the body, the loss of their franchise as healers. They seemed dispiritedly content to let the observance of empty rituals stand in for the invocation of real gods; they promoted a soul that, to me at least, seemed mostly a bloodless abstraction divorced from any physical reality. Was this their fault? Probably not. They served an institution that didn't know how to summon divine energy from the sky, and trusted only one guy—the Pope—to serve as the pontifical man, the bridge between heaven and earth. And like so many Protestant denominations, the Catholic church had little talent for sacred theater. By the time I got to college and cottoned on to the scientific view of man and nature, I was an unqualified secular humanist. The party of the clown had beaten the monk's slate by a landslide, and it was easy to dismiss the whole business at St. Clement's as Freud dismissed religion in general—as a pathetic longing for a benevolent protector, an exercise in sublimation. The blanket you crawled under when you could not bear any more reality.

But what have we gained by attributing spiritual feeling to psychological theories whose only real advantage over religious fairy tales is a veneer of pseudoscientific respectability that makes them seem less transparently preposterous? I felt compelled to examine the consequences of my religious background because the tenets of hands-on healing couldn't be any plainer: The degree to which any religion accents abstract faith at the expense of engaging the palpable current of divinity is the degree to which it has lost touch with the instrumentality of the seventh chakra and the vital essence of spirituality itself. Once in my late teens, when I was in a monkish way, I asked my father what "spirituality" meant to him. "A dead word signifying nothing," he said. The starkness of his reply gave me to understand there were important questions here, that religion or the lack of it was still a live wire for me, and perhaps for my dad too. His contempt for the religious interpretation of spirituality had been shaped by the hypocrisy of organized churches and the long, dismal history of inquisitions, crusades, and various homicidal enthusiasms for one true deity or another. But in rejecting the spiritual aspect of man for the havoc spiritual institutions had caused, wasn't he throwing the baby Jesus out with the bathwater? For all the inspired atheism in his voice, I thought I could see wistfulness in his eyes, as if he longed to be reconnected to something he had lost. He was an exile, like Shin the snow leopard, barred from the country she was born for. And I suspect in his heart of hearts he understood the spiritual nature of the impulse toward religion, the longing to "re-connect" embedded in the etymology of the word—which is perhaps to say the work of mending, healing, inspiriting; of finding the energy to lift the self above the illusion of its separateness.

I suppose we shared the tacit understanding that religion no longer worked or was even relevant in a world where the soul had been eclipsed by the ravishing strangeness of scientific discovery. I suppose we were also both afflicted with a kind of spiritual poverty, which the remnants of our defeated religions were powerless to relieve. Maybe science had not destroyed religion. Maybe religion had destroyed itself.

Certainly it was in response to the sense that spirituality had become a dead word signifying nothing that new religions and new forms of spirituality emerged, especially in the United States. Many, such as Zen Buddhism and Transcendental Meditation, came from the East. They could be practiced outside a community. God was not to be found wherever two or three were met, as Reverend Diane and millions of Christians believed, but wherever *you* were met when you looked within yourself. "The modern religious quest is largely an inward search for the psychological foundations upon which faith might rest," historian Robert C. Fuller wrote in his 1982 book *Mesmerism and the American Cure of Souls.* Many of the new faiths were native to the U.S., and whether they took up positions on the far left or the far right, whether they were based on the inspiration of John Coltrane's saxophone music or belief in the literal truth of the Bible, they shared an emphasis on the subjective experience of God; they swayed to the holy impetus of unmediated divinity. Practices popularly known as New Age faiths often embraced the Hindu concept of the subtle body and used the techniques of yoga to help cultivate spiritual consciousness; they viewed the crown chakra not as a nice shiny headpiece exclusive to saints but a power outlet that anyone could access. And lo! in poured God-to-godhead voltage, the wild neuronal jazz of Dionysian excess, the abstract god of the mind trembling in the body, the room enlivened as in any Pentecostal invocation or session of orgiastic Baptist pulpit-pounding.

This accent on the authority of personal spiritual experience and the accent on healing go hand in hand, writes Damian Thompson in his study of millennialism, *The End of Time*. "They reflect the preoccupations of societies in which traditional social and religious structures have been failing or even disappearing." As the Islamic scholar Seyyed Nasr noted in *Religion and the Order of Nature*, "Almost all New Age religions emphasized the significance of the body, the cosmic correspondences between microcosm and macrocosm, the holistic attitude toward mind-body," and they all showed a "strong interest in holistic medicine." New Age spirituality drew fresh attention to the esoteric sects of traditional religions such as Jewish Cabala, Christian Hermeticism, and other secretive mystery schools that not only opposed the desacralizing of the body but more radically often refused to participate in what Nasr with breathtaking iconoclasm called the "surrender . . . to the quantitative science of matter and motion and . . . evolutionist biology."

Of course, from the vantage of the secular rationalist, such resistance appears benighted and its unapologetically nonrational exponents seem, well—how to put this delicately—I guess the word is "bonkers." Exhibits A through Z in the case against religion. Chauvinists of the rational road have long decried faith as the projection of a primitive infantile state, a borderline psychosis, even a temporal-lobe dysfunction. While surveys show that a surprisingly large percentage of scientists believe in God, as a class they are the least inclined to faith. In the U.S., more than half of all scientists call themselves agnostic or atheistic as compared to approximately five percent of the population. Where the religious person sees spirit infusing matter, singing in stones, milk cartons, shoes, peppermills, teapots, trumpets, textbooks, knee joints, spleens, and hands, the scientist sees imaginations running wild, "self-deluded individuals acting out their revelatory fantasies," as one skeptic put it.

No surprise then that scientists are more likely to be dismayed by campaigns to insinuate religion back into medicine. Or that they have a keener appreciation of the struggle to despiritualize disease and to anchor treatments in principles shorn of goddish superstitions. In any field of knowledge—but in medicine especially—they reason that claims ought to be based on evidence, not intuition or wishful thinking. "What nonsense all this supposed intuitional truth is," the prolific science writer Isaac Asimov scoffed in an essay collected in a 1986 book *Science Confronts the Paranormal*, "and how comic is the sight of the genuflections made to it by rational minds who lost their nerve. No, it isn't really comic; it's tragic. There has been at least one other such occasion in history, when Greek secular and rational thought bowed to the mystical aspects of Christianity, and what followed was a dark age. We can't afford another."

In December 1997, thinking of my science-minded father's stark pronouncement on spirituality, I arranged to go to Boston to attend the fourth Spirituality and Healing in Medicine conference sponsored by Harvard University and the Mind/Body Medical Institute at the Beth Israel Deaconess Medical Center. I could hear my guides talking anxiously among themselves.

He's had a skepticism relapse!

But he seemed to be making such progress! What happened?

It started with that Asimov quote, and then one thing led to another. He's just registered for another conference.

Oh God, not more scientists!

Look, I had been wrestling with the relation of spirituality and healing long enough to know that Wile E. Coyote wasn't going to be conked on the head by the anvil of revelation at Harvard. But it still seemed important to attend. A decade ago, no one could have imagined a three-day, Harvard-sanctioned jamboree devoted to spirituality and healing. The time wasn't far gone when chaplains had been barred from psychiatric in-patient wards. And when heard from in 1984, the National Academy of Sciences was of the opinion that "religion and science are mutually exclusive realms of thought whose presentation in the same context leads to misunderstanding of both scientific theory and religious belief."

Then, almost overnight, the culture shifted. Faith, and by implication

God, had secured a new beachhead, and in medicine of all places! When I began my chakra travels in 1994, only three medical schools in the country offered courses in spirituality and medicine; by the fall of 1997, there were thirty. An emerging field was focused on the "epidemiology of religion." Heretical ideas that once looked as outlandish as Vegas showgirls were getting the intellectual equivalent of a Park Avenue makeover. Who could pass up the scene at this new confluence of mainstream and fringe?

Part of a series of courses for physicians and lay healers, the Harvard conference had been started in 1995 by Dr. Herbert Benson, an associate professor at Harvard Medical School and the chief of the Division of Behavioral Medicine at Beth Israel Deaconess Medical Center. One of the more famous researchers in mind-body medicine, Benson had been careful to keep his medical reputation off the reefs that had wrecked the careers of many of his adventurous predecessors. As a young cardiologist in the late 1960s, he had noticed that the act of wrapping a cuff around patients' biceps during office visits affected their blood pressure. Despite the work of Walter Cannon and other pioneers of stress physiology, Benson couldn't find data in the medical literature that said stress could actually hike blood pressure. So in 1967 he began a series of experiments with monkeys. He was able to train the lab animals to raise or lower their blood pressure. Two years later, he began working with practitioners of Transcendental Meditation who claimed they could regulate aspects of their physiology that medical science believed were off-limits to conscious control.

Predictably, some of Benson's colleagues advised him against investigating such farfetched and controversial topics, but the cardiologist's curiosity had been piqued, and he was nothing if not stubborn. He did much of the work in the evenings on his own time. He found that meditation lowered oxygen consumption and blood pressure; it slowed brain waves and decreased levels of blood lactate. The evidence was compelling that meditators could change their consciousness *and* their chemistry. It confirmed to Benson what yogis had been saying for thousands of years, and it suggested that cherished scientific assumptions about the division of mind and body were wrong. Benson was astonished by some of the data. In most people, six hours of sleep will lower the body's oxygen consumption by eight percent; after one hour of TM meditation, subjects reduced their oxygen consumption by thirteen percent.

In sum, it seemed meditating elicited a physiological state opposite the pop-eyed, ball-fisted, adrenal-tweaked mobilization Walter Cannon had described as the "fight or flight response." Benson dubbed it the "relaxation response," and made that the title of his best-selling book on the subject. Subsequent work proved that evoking the relaxation response could be deft therapy for any disease that was triggered or exacerbated by stress.

From the start, Benson could see the implications of his work. Evoking the relaxation response, many of his patients reported feeling a presence or an energy that they attributed to God or some other divine force. In asking patients to close their eyes, take a deep breath, go inside themselves, and focus on a phrase or word while letting go of any stray thoughts, Benson realized he was adapting processes of prayer and contemplation common to almost all spiritual traditions from shamanism to Buddhism to the great monotheisms of the West. "As the mind-body work was progressing, the spirituality theme always came back because the relaxation response was evoked by prayer," he recalled.

The question hung there: Is spirituality good for health? Unfortunately, at the time the issue was nothing science could digest. God had been squeezed out of medicine and no tenure-minded researcher was going to invite Him back in. In the early 1970s at Hampshire College I heard Benson speak about his work, and toward the end of the lecture someone in the hall asked if the doctor had been persuaded to start reaping the benefits of meditation himself. He shook his head and said, "I don't want to become the Timothy Leary of TM." I was struck by his reluctance to take advantage of what ought to have been his due as a stress-prone physician, the concern it expressed for keeping up appearances and avoiding the label of "believer." Benson epitomized the rigor and perhaps some of the schizophrenia of modern scientists whose commitment to the methods and perspectives of objective research are often at odds with their lives, undermining the credence they put in feelings and beliefs (except beliefs about objective data). There's a revealing scene in physician David Eisenberg's book on Chinese medicine, *Encounters with Qi*, in which Eisenberg describes Benson's response to a treatment from

a *chi gong* master named Dr. Zhou during their visit to the Shanghai First
Medical College in the early 1980s:

> Benson stood in the middle of a large room . . . closed his
> eyes, and performed his own relaxation exercise. Zhou
> approached him cautiously, then aimed his arm at the Harvard
> professor's midsection. Benson appeared very relaxed, almost
> in a trance. Then he began to move. He swayed a bit from side
> to side, lost his footing, and tripped. He did not fall, but he was
> clearly off balance. Zhou's arm tracked Benson's every move-
> ment . . . it was impossible to know who was leading whom.
> Benson then began to twist his hips, first to the right, then to
> the left. He swiveled 180 degrees with awkward jerks. Benson
> smiled an uninterpretable smile. Zhou smiled in response, but
> Benson, whose eyes were closed, could not see this. . . . In the
> end the demonstration did little to shake Benson's profound
> skepticism of man's ability to emit external energy. "It was all
> too subjective," said Benson. "Judgments cannot be made on
> the basis of subjective feelings alone. What we need is objec-
> tive, reproducible data."

In the case of the relaxation response, Benson had objective evidence
of the technique's efficacy. Nevertheless, wary of losing his objectivity, he
let more than a decade pass before he availed himself of its proven health
benefits. "I was starting to get old," he recalled, "and I thought, 'This is
ridiculous.' "

Now, on a December morning in Boston, it was a lifetime later.
Thicker in the midsection, hair gone gray, the cardiologist was standing
on a podium in the ballroom of the Westin Hotel at Copley Square, smiling an easily interpreted smile to the thousand or so people who had
enrolled in his course. What a crowd! A person for every petal on the
reigning lotus of religion: surgeons, anesthesiologists, psychiatrists, physicians in family practice; Catholic nuns, rabbis, Buddhists; social workers
interested in shamanism, HMO officials, chiropractors, lawyers, cancer
survivors, energy healers; and scattered here and there, those phosphor-
eyed seekers who looked as if they would walk a thousand miles in the
rain for another glimpse of the angel they'd once seen.

One of the main goals of the conference was to reorient physicians who had been schooled in the strict church–and–state protocols of despiritualized medicine and for whom the "epidemiology of religion" might be a strange idea. As Dr. Dale Mathews, an assistant professor of medicine at Georgetown University, put it in his talk that morning, religious and spiritual beliefs constituted the "Forgotten Factor" in healing. The Forgotten Factor advocates were not asking their colleagues to take the health effects of faith on faith. The distinguished American physician William Osler had noted the importance of faith in medicine in 1910 but added that faith was "the one great moving force which we can neither weigh in the balance nor test in the crucible." Osler, the son of an Anglican missionary, was wrong: Faith *had* been weighed in the balance and tested in the crucible of more than two hundred published studies, and some compelling conclusions had emerged.

Among them: Patients with religious faith were three times more likely to survive open-heart surgery. They were discharged more quickly from the hospital than nonreligious patients by a factor of twenty percent. Those recovering from hip fractures could walk farther and were less depressed when they got out of the hospital than their nonreligious peers. Hospital stays for all illnesses were nearly two and a half times longer for elderly patients without religious affiliations. People who attended church or synagogue services once a week had stronger immune systems, lower diastolic blood pressures, lower overall mortality rates. Mormons in America had half the cancer rate of the general public. Seventh Day Adventists in the Netherlands lived seven years longer than their fellow citizens. Church attendance was strongly correlated with levels of the biological agent interleukin 6. A lack of religious affiliation is one of the key predictors for alcoholism. And so on and so forth. As Jeffrey Levin noted in the February 1997 issue of *The Journal of the American Medical Association*: "Systematic reviews and meta-analyses quantitatively confirm that religious involvement is an epidemiologically protective factor."

But did these health benefits being attributed to spiritual and religious values have anything to do with the reality of God, spirit, or soul? Did improvements in health mean that God, spirit, and soul were actual objective entities like Mont Blanc or Jupiter and not constructs of the imagination? The distinction seemed important, given that negative emotions have been correlated with increased heart disease, diminished immune function, and premature death, and thus it stood to reason that *any* source of positive emotions, whether it was the joy of Jesus' personal attention or the antics of a clown, would be a boon to health. There was a subtle line between religion and social life in general. For example, some studies had shown that people with fewer social ties were twice as likely to come down with a cold—more of a vote, it would seem, for the healing power of congregations than for the deities they gathered in the name of. If it wasn't necessary to equate the negative health effects of negative emotions with the Devil, why equate the positive effects of positive emotions with God?

Over the years, Benson himself had pointed out the universal, not to say ecumenical, nature of the relaxation response. That people could evoke it with a prayer didn't mean the literal reality of God was the key aspect. The key aspect was the person's belief in what they were saying. The response activated the "biology of belief." You had to separate the fact of having beliefs in something from the substance of the beliefs. Catholics who used the Lord's Prayer to evoke beneficial changes in their blood pressure, heart rate, and brain waves might actually believe in a Heaven and an omnipotent Father, but diehard atheists didn't need the supernatural characters to evoke the same beneficial changes. They could simply count backwards or repeat the number "one" or possibly even, it seemed, chant the names of the five highest-yielding, lowest-priced stocks in the Dow Jones Industrial Average. (Or, if they were tech investors, perhaps mumble to themselves *Micron Technology, Micron Technology . . .*) Because the relaxation response worked as well for atheists as for believers, religion had no exclusive claim on spirituality; where health was concerned, a religious creed could not assert it was the one true way. No practical difference existed between one person's faith in a prayer to God and another's faith in a white-coated doctor. So why all the fuss? Why was the science of belief even obliged to evaluate religious frameworks and interpretations?

The opening morning of the Harvard conference, John C. Pierrakos, the well-known psychiatrist, refined this question with one of his own. The Forgotten Factor panel had finished plying the audience with data on the epidemiology of faith, and Pierrakos went to one of the audience microphones.

"What is the vital energy that makes the faith alive?" he said. "I would like to ask the panelists, would they please define this energy."

"Oh no, that's not on the agenda!" Herbert Benson broke in, adroitly deflecting the 2,500-year-old philosophical quandary. The crowd laughed, but the perennially unsettled issue haunted the agenda of the conference. What *was* the nature of the spirit that scientists were now daring to allude to? Set aside the question of how spirit might actually work—nobody even knew how to define it except in such vague, cloud-of-unknowing terms as "a power," "a force," "an energy," or, my favorite, "God, if you will." The conference had drawn people from diverse backgrounds, but they could be sorted into two camps by whether they were comfortable saying the word "God" and leaving it at that, or whether they twitched and had to add an "if you will" whenever they mentioned His name.

(And oh what perverse fun it was to watch the if-you-willers twitch. Having been on journalism watch-lists as some kind of closeted believer for the preceding three years, I found my user illusion relishing the spectacle of other people flailing around in the epistemological quagmire: schadenfreude, straight up.)

There was no break in the cloud-of-unknowing overcast the next day, when a parade of scholars and clerics marched to the podium to detail various healing practices in African, Buddhist, Jewish, Catholic, Islamic, Pentecostal, and Christian Science spiritual traditions. They had been invited for their spiritual and anthropological insight into religious traditions, and their talks were long on philosophy and short on science. So short I would have welcomed a few unrepentant atheists just to keep the presentations in perspective. I suppose I'd been over this ground too many times and was no longer listening with an open mind. I don't know; it just seemed that given the epidemics of infectious disease plaguing Africa, scholar Dr. Charles Cudjoe's enthusiasm for witch doctors and herbalists seemed more than a little naive. Rheumatism treatments made from the clay of anthills and *kma* leaves were fine, but so what? Weren't millions of Africans dying from AIDS, hepatitis, malaria—dying for lack of Western scientific medicine, and because of the inadequacies of traditional, spiritually based tribal medicine? Or was I still so obtuse, so steeped in the bias of materialism, that I had it backwards and didn't grasp that it was *because* Africans were in such spiritual disarray that their physical health was suffering?

I had much the same reaction to the other speakers that morning, who all seemed, for the most part, to be proposing remedies for what materialists would deride as hypochondria. Rabbi Simkha Y. Weintraub described the healing practices of ritual baths and psalm-reading and taught the crowd to sing a Jewish prayer. The Catholic priest Joseph J. Driscoll had something to say about the healing power of the Catholic sacraments. And the Buddhist scholar Tulku Thondup, the author of *The Healing Power of Mind*, praised the panacea-like power of cultivating peace and love in one's consciousness. The formidable Seyyed Nasr explained the holistic view of healing in the Islamic tradition, and denounced the mindset of Western science, which, in his view, had despiritualized medicine, desacralized the body, and now was shredding Mother Nature herself. He didn't get any argument from the vanguard of the Forgotten Factor. Could the Devil's advocate have mustered a critical word in this monastery, if only for the sake of pro forma opposition? Were the if-you-willers, not to say the devotees of God Unlimited, so disenchanted with modern medicine and the antispiritual philosophy of medical science, that they were ready to junk the cures of one and the methodology of the other?

Finally someone got up to speak whose views were too extreme even for the home-team crowd. Virginia S. Harris, the president of the American branch of the Church of Christ, Scientist, laid out the so-called science of spiritual healing developed more than a century ago by Mary Baker Eddy (and currently being taught in Christian Science churches in some seventy countries). "The physical world is a product or an effect of the mind," Harris explained. "To follow the healing example of Jesus, one reverses the relationship of mind and body. Instead of seeing thought as a phenomenon of matter, it is essential to see matter as a phenomenon of thought." The Christian Science concept of healing hinges on seeing "thought as primary and the body as derivative."

To be sure, such radical idealism has a lot in common with Hindu theology and the chakra doctrine of yoga masters and energy healers; in principle, it wouldn't alienate very devout believers in any number of Western religious faiths. But at a conference dedicated to fostering co-operation between modes of scientific and religious healing, Harris was adamant that the spiritual approach could not be compromised, and that medical doctors and Christian Science practitioners should not work together. That was too much for many people in the audience, some of whom were evidently wrestling with clown-monk dialectics of their own. When the time came for questions, the pendulum, which had been swinging toward spirituality all day, headed back the other way. A man who identified himself as a retired anesthesiologist and a Christian said, "A number of Christian Science patients have come to me with tumors the size of grapefruits, and it seems to me they're in denial about their condition. Their faith isn't working. When do you recommend that a Christian Scientist should see a doctor? Are there any conditions? Compound fractures? Balloon aneurysms?"

Harris refused to rule out conditions for which Christian Science treatment might not be appropriate. And she did not want to comment on specific cases. "We have one hundred twenty-five years of successful case histories," she said blandly.

Other members of the audience raised equally pointed and even hostile questions, and her answers were just as maddeningly unresponsive. Harris's fidelity to the theory of the supremacy of mind over body was so breathtakingly rigorous, so unreasonably inflexible, she made my visualization teacher, Dr. Gerald Epstein, seem the paragon of pragmatic moderation. Harris was like a character from beyond the looking glass, where up is down, good is evil, and where, since illness is health, people suffering from a burst aorta or a tibia sticking out of their shin need only change how they feel about the problem. After all, "Thought is the arena where change must take place for healing to take place."

It seemed to me that Harris's upside-down cake left such a sour taste in the mouths of the audience that for the first time they began to wonder if factoring God back into the medical equation was a good thing. One of the suggestions had been that doctors ought to pray with their patients. Was that really going to add something worthwhile to medicine? The premise of the conference was that religion was good; religion was healthy; religion brought out the best in people. Never mind that a classic study by sociologists Bateson and Bentis, cited the last day of the conference by Larry Dossey (the physician who'd introduced Oprah Winfrey to the bacteria-prayer studies), had concluded that religious affiliation was linked to greater intolerance and bigotry. Never mind that one of the more infamous statistics in the epidemiology of faith is the poll result which found that some five percent of Americans who pray do not petition for relief from suffering or the betterment of mankind but rather for harm to befall their fellow men. Maybe it wasn't all bad that medicine had disengaged Spirit and the spirits. Maybe we could not go back to the animism of premodern times and would not benefit from the resurrection of an intractable, shopworn deity, a mythic construct that over the centuries has arguably inspired as much anguish and hatred as it has eased, and that even now as it brings comfort and joy to some parts of the world is busy making pain and trouble in other places.

Proponents of respiritualized medicine made compelling arguments that we had turned ourselves into machines, and that only the return of the soul, or the Spirit, or whatever it was that rained down from the Cloud of Unknowing, could save us from the mindless purgatory of unsacred lives—lives that lack not only faith but also the ballast of value and meaning. Medicine could transplant hearts almost as readily as carburetors, but the heart had gone out of modern life, in their view, and had left us in the position of being no more than the sum of our parts, androidlike machines; robots, if you will. Given such bleak prospects, the idea of reclaiming God had an irresistible nostalgia. And yet, Virginia Harris notwithstanding, was there a single person in the Westin ballroom who would trade an operating table for an altar, if faced with certain medical emergencies? Perhaps medicine did not need to be re-Godded; perhaps it needed to be de-robotized. Or simply re-humanized. Was a supernatural being necessary to persuade doctors to approach anesthetized patients with reverence and respect? To convince them to maintain some feeling for the mystery of life, and perhaps even whisper a prayer before the procedure because they knew the ultimate outcome was not in their hands alone? More to the point, was emphasizing the religious aspects of healing more important than figuring out the right voltage for the defibrillator paddles or the ideal dose of morphine? Only an exceedingly mean view of spirituality would exclude science as one of its achievements.

And as for faith, for that matter, I wondered if the conference had really even gotten to the core of it, the palpable energetic reality of it— of God, or faith, or belief as a force, not a sentiment. For a gathering devoted to spirituality and healing, the pageant at the Westin seemed very removed from the experience of Sahasrara, which of course could not be reduced to ten million words, much less a half-hour presentation with five minutes for follow-up questions. Only the Pentecostal speaker, Samuel Solivan—who was born two months premature on the altar of a church in the Bronx and was thought to be retarded but bootstrapped himself into a Ph.D. and became a minister—only he brought the charismatic energy of faith into the hotel ballroom. He brought the energy of his beliefs to life, and a thousand people jumped to their feet to give him a standing ovation. It was as if the sun had suddenly burst out and spurred a thousand-petaled lotus into bloom. And yet even Solivan's triumph had more to do with the power of good theater than with the truth of his doctrine.

I suppose on a deeper level my disquiet owed to the sense that it seemed absurd, and even, well, sacrilegious, to reduce the shattering epiphanies of the Mystic Way to "health outcomes" and strategies for HMO cost containment. If you'd never had an epiphany, you didn't know what you were butchering when you started chopping the visions and transcendent experiences of religious ecstasy into bite-sized bits, making them useful as stress-management techniques or, even worse, making them seem reasonable—little rationalized trinkets to put on the shelves of reason's clubhouse, that "grubby hutch for schoolboys" as the poet Theodore Roethke disdainfully called it. The schoolboys had grown up, of course. They had degrees. They sat on panels for expenses, honorariums, and the greater glory of their scientific careers, but in their dowdy tweeds they seemed irredeemably part of old Harvard and its ilk, more comfortable talking about the "faith factor" than faith itself, more comfortable meeting Spirit as a concept than a feeling. Oh, I'm probably not being fair. Most of the presenters seemed like academics who'd worked out a compromise between science and religion . . . It was just the nature of academic show-and-tell, perhaps, that the scales tipped more toward tell than show. During those three days in Boston I ran into a few healers I knew, and as one of them put it, the eggheads on the podium "were running a lot of yellow." Yellow being the color of most philosophy departments, the vibe of the mind, of ego, of thinking.

Toward the last day, I found myself wondering about a distinction between faith and belief I'd read in V. S. Naipaul's *A Bend in the River*, the gist of it being that beliefs were ideas that could be shaken, but faith was different, faith was the result of having been shaken. Could you envy someone with the conviction of faith and yet not take them seriously? In a way, having faith disqualified you from the opera of modern life, whose leitmotif was instability and whose emblematic figures were Beckett's clowns. And yet it was starting to seem as if the great to-do about healing in our time was nothing but a roundabout way of wrestling with the absence of faith. I still had no faith to speak of, but I did realize in the course of the conference that I was vacillating wildly. Not between matter and spirit, or mind and body, but between head and heart. Those old standbys. I was unreasonably vexed one minute by a seemingly reasonless mind (and wanting to indulge the temptations of judgment), and irrationally irked the next by a fresh outbreak of mindless reason. This ongoing discord seemed to signify more double folly, not the single wisdom of the Fool, and I wondered if I was ever meant to find anything that I actively looked for and if perhaps the true discoveries were to be found only when you gave up, when you sank to your knees exhausted from searching. I was tired from all the two steps forward and the three steps back. And yet here was the thing: It was beginning to dawn on me that some truths could be perceived only in the throes of illness, heart truths, if you will, and some truths could be learned only from petri dishes and meta-analyses, truths of the head, and that in the broadest sense of the word, in this age of the half believer we were bound to take them both on faith.

3. LADY LAMA

The Harvard conference was hardly lacking in *think-think*. Running yellow all day, the brigade of eggheads had established a kind of community, but it was a community doomed to disappoint anyone wanting to delve into the instrumental nature of belief—belief as a living experience, not an abstraction. For all their earnest intentions, the eggheads could not transcend the limits of their method, and it seemed to me that in their determination to reason their way toward faith, they were missing the forest for the trees. When you were starving for weather—for the taste of rain, the smell of lightning, the crack of thunder—what did the reductionist's approach offer? A package of anemometer readouts and satellite photographs. There were no mysteries of communion in the Harvard tabernacle, just journal reprints and buttons that said "Get Well Sooner with God, If You Will."

A line from Wallace Stevens kept running through my head: "We keep coming back and coming back / To the real: to the hotel instead of the hymns / That fall upon it out of the wind." Which is not to say in the case of the Harvard conference that the meretricious Westin at Copley Square was more compelling than the psalms of data being chanted by academics. Hotel and hymns alike seemed only to *refer* to something authentic, something out of reach, something I imagined to be like the world beyond the bars that Shin the snow leopard saw before she died. Wasn't it Stevens's point that we all were caged in conceptions and fettered by our methods? (As it had been Blake's point with his "mind forged manacles.") Didn't we all keep coming back and coming back to the edge to put our whiskers through the wire mesh in hopes of sensing the truth of what lay where we could not go, the reality beyond our idea of reality? Given that hymns nowadays were not appreciably less authentic than corporate hotels, you could take issue with the poet's metaphor but not with his larger point. Everything we made, everything we thought or said was a human construct and as such was fatally imbued with our user illusion's longing for life ever after, for wholeness, for redemption, for irrefutable truth—for whatever it was that we needed to voice when we cried out together in prayer from the cage of the Sabbath.

And yet I kept coming back to those hymns as if they were as real and essential as a great river. I kept coming back to the intricate and as yet unmastered trick of negative capability, and to the portents of the wise Fool that promised the union of human and divine realms. I kept coming back to the baited hook of faith itself, which promised that something sacred and irreducible would emerge from wherever two or three were met; and to the lure of community, which dangled the prospects of revelation, of transcendent energies and Tomberg's "supra-individual" states of being that could be attained only in the context of other people.

It was the depth of these last attractions, the beautiful seductions of faith, that made me realize my passage up the chakras had accomplished at least one thing: I was thoroughly disenchanted with scientific weather reports and Harvard-style presentations about the faith factor. In a heart-before-head way, I was eager to return to the empiricists, who were standing out in the rain of the inner world, those self-revelatory fools who had attuned their user illusions to the nuances of energy and dared omit the "if you will" from their idea of God. And so, even as I was finishing this book, I went back again, returning as I had been returning over the years to the community of people who were gathered around the renowned healer Rosalyn Bruyere.

Let me go back to the beginning, when I first encountered Bruyere. This was in December 1994, when she was booked into the Barbizon Hotel in New York City for a weekend seminar in what she called the "Egyptian Mysteries." A crowd of about two hundred turned out, many of them healers who had been studying with her a long time. They were familiar with her shrewd monk-and-clown mix of solemnity and hijinks and her way of what she called "teaching on a circle," which meant that tyros and experts were mixed in with each other. She wasn't afraid to belabor material, repeating stories and lessons on the theory that you couldn't get smart as a healer until you got a little stupid. Running yellow was no good. The goal of her training program was to produce not graduates but ordained ministers for the church she'd founded in Glendale, California, the Healing Light Center. I liked the way she punctured sanctimony and joked around. Her lectures were a trove of odd facts, ranging discursively from the energetic aspects of chocolate and stained-glass windows to indigenous Cree healing traditions, Bedouin joint manipulation, and the Nazi-profaned geometry of the swastika. Hotels and graveyards are doorways to the astral plane, she said. If you come to a door in a dream, go through it—doors are symbols of the soul's progress. Can't remember your dreams? Try curling your right toes. When you increase your vibration rate—your psychophysical clock speed, as it were—your head becomes less compact and you can enter the microscopic precincts of your body, including the space between your synapses. At the time, I confess, it sounded like a recipe for creating airheads, but maybe it was possible. In her view, increasing the vibration rate was part of human potential. In her view, our limitations, especially in the West, were reflected in our curtailed, numbed-out nervous systems. "Stories, not facts, strengthen the immune system," she said. "Quantification helps the intellect, but paradox helps the soul." Who was I to argue?

Two months later, I went up to Boston to attend her weekend course in "Body Symbology." Bruyere presented some of her ideas about the chakras. They were not just a model of the whole body's energy system; they offered a way of looking at individual organs and levels within the body. To move from the marrow of the thigh bone to the surface of the skin was to run the ladder from red to orange to yellow to green to blue to purple to white. The same rainbow spectrum could be detected in the lungs, the liver; each frequency was as distinct (dare one say scientific?) as the isobars on a weather map. What applied to the body as a whole applied to its parts: The essence of healing was the flow of energy that righted and reset the organism. The chakras promoted and organized the flow. Each had a function.

"You are supposed to know a concept in one," she said, "have a feeling about it in two, form an opinion of it in three, have a second feeling in four that ameliorates the initial feeling in two, speak about the feeling in five, gain some insight or understanding about it in six, and release it to God in seven."

Releasing it to God, that was the tricky part.

Each chakra was also associated with an element and an age, and marked a stage in the growth of one's personality. The first chakra glowed with life's foundational fire and was fully developed by the time you were four years old. The second was linked to water and the emotions, and was fully developed by age seven. The third chakra matured at around twelve; its element was air. If you were stuck in orange, you might be prone to lachrymose sentimentality, but overemphasizing yellow could turn you into an emotional desert and you might desiccate your heart in the chakra above with an excess of dry wit. Or worse, dry witlessness. In Bruyere's experience, people who used the third chakra to do the work of the first chakra often made themselves sick because they were relying on their intellect and their opinions for their power. In chakra-speak, they were like the Harvard eggheads running yellow in lieu of red. Their likely exhaustion and depletion of spirit stemmed from drawing on the comparatively limited energy of the adrenal glands when they should have been drinking from the ground-of-being energies of the bone marrow and the Earth itself.

Above the solar plexus, one reached the heart chakra, whose opening was indicated in the rapturous agonies of teenage love, love which could later be turned into a first novel when the speak-your-heart throat chakra was consolidated, in the early twenties. And then, later still, when real insight supposedly emerged, in the thirties, with the opening of the sixth chakra, you would be ready to repent all that youthful folly in an Augustinian memoir.

Bruyere even had commentary to hang on the ineffable Sahasrara, the crown chakra, which she said was at least eighteen thousand years old and, given its seat in the dense nerve plexus of the neocortex, was by far the most complex of the seven. The purpose of a king's crown was to amplify the crown chakra. The crown held the monarch half in, half out of his body, and thus enabled him to function as a spiritual bridge between Heaven and Earth. (Wasn't that the fool's job too?) The bishop's miter, the dunce's cap, the wizard's Matterhorn-like headgear all had the same energetic purpose of fortifying or awakening the connection with higher energies. There were various ways to open the crown chakra, some of them profoundly mundane. Pets could coax it open. So could humor.

Humor! At the time, I wondered: Maybe a more suitable name for Sahasrara was the Clown Chakra.

In both Boston and New York, Bruyere's students insisted it was as important to mind what she was doing energetically as to listen to what she was saying—something disciples typically say of their gurus. And though Bruyere was clearly a teacher and a healer, she did seek to impart something that only her presence could convey. As she said on a later occasion: "I cheat. When I talk to people, I've usually got my hands on them, and I'm running my worldview through their body."

From her appearances in New York and Boston, I would not have guessed Bruyere was a grandmother. She was forty-eight that winter, with a broad, youthful face and cascade of auburn hair. She was battling her weight and tended to wear long dresses or pants and loose tops. But her stamina was formidable. She practiced karate with her second husband, Ken, a sixth-degree black belt. "You have to be in shape to be a healer," she said. "The same energy people use to break boards with in karate, healers use to dissolve gallstones." She had a virtuosic command of her own energy, but she had to be careful about keeping it reined in. A few minutes of meditation could quickly expand the circumference of her aura, which usually attracted her cats and provoked her green parrot, Amigo. Once when she was rushing for a flight at London's Heathrow airport, she set off the metal detector, and when the security officers couldn't find any metal on her, they asked if she had a pacemaker. It was easier to lie than to serenade them about the chakras and the strength of her field. Yes, governor, a pacemaker.

One of the more boggling anecdotes in her quiver came from an incident in 1994 in Phoenix, on the Fourth of July. She and Ken and some other people were being driven to a concert in a limousine when the engine quit. The driver was unable to start it back up, and concluded the limo's two batteries had died. What the hell, Bruyere thought, maybe we can do something. She got out. "The batteries are dead, lady," the driver said. Ken got out too. They stood on either side of the limo and held their hands about six inches over the hood. They began a Native American healing chant and ran energy at the batteries. "I felt one of those healing releases," Bruyere recalled, "a sort of whoosh, the same feeling you get in karate during a good brick break. I told the driver to give it a try, and when he turned the ignition, the engine started. I don't know if I believe we had anything to do with it, I only know that I cared that it started. The most fantastic thing was the look on the driver's face."

At those first weekend seminars in New York and Boston, the idea that someone could set off a metal detector with their energy field, or maybe jump-start a battery with their hands, was as intriguing to me as any Egyptian mystery. Newcomers were always more impressed by effects than theories. It would not have occurred to me to say that what Bruyere was doing as she spoke was opening her crown chakra and mobilizing the secondary chakras in her feet and making herself into one of those pontifical bridges between Heaven and Earth. I was not familiar enough with energy to know that when it served her purpose she shifted her energy from her solar plexus to her heart or her third eye, changing the locus and frequency of her being as easily as a pianist changes key. But even without any special sensitivity to energy, anyone could grasp the overall effect, which was of a charismatic, stage-savvy actress relishing her time in the limelight. Initially I wondered: Was she doing anything a good performer didn't do? What actors would credit to natural ability and good technique, she framed in energetic terms and insisted was a function of chakra mastery and auric know-how. Only the shop talk, the idiom, was different. Bruyere was catching and playing and communing with the energy coming at her from the crowd. What mattered was managing the flow and knowing how to shape the interchange. That was the lesson inside the lectures.

All this was nearly four years ago. I'm not prepared now to say that if I had to drive somewhere with Bruyere I'd ditch the jumper cables and vest my die-hard faith in the charging power of her hands. But over years of seeing her at various venues, I suppose I have grown used to . . . what? Not to outlandishness per se, but to some elasticity in the boundaries of the possible. Is this just a case of habituation, similar to what afflicts souvenir vendors at Virgin Mary manifestation sites who hardly bother looking up when pilgrims shout that the sun is spinning backwards? Well, maybe. Repeated exposure to bizarre phenomena can go a long way toward helping even a negatively incapable rationalist relinquish his desire to reach irritably after fact and reason. But I think more was involved than simply the numbness of custom setting in.

I once watched a healing where Bruyere worked on a young woman named Jennifer Halls. Halls was studying healing herself and earning a living as an assistant curator at a South Carolina museum. She had developed a serious inflammation in her eyes and had been advised by her doctor that her sight was in jeopardy. Bruyere called on four healers in the audience to assist. She had one stand at Halls's feet and run red, two others go to Halls's hips and run green, and the fourth one hold Halls's shoulders and run blue. Bruyere laid her own hands on Halls's face and edged her fingers up around the eyes. As she worked, she spoke to the hundred or so people in the room.

"All I'm going to do at first is begin to fill the eye area with gold and white light."

She glanced at the other healers, who were standing with their knees slightly bent and their eyes half closed.

"Now I can feel the field doubling."

There was a sense of unity about them that reminded me of a jazz quintet.

"I'm being very slow and careful, because I didn't trim my fingernails," Bruyere said, to the surprise of those students who thought the reason for her deliberate manner might be more profound. "Now I'm going through the eyeball to the back. I'm making one curved line and one straight line. I want to close a fissure in the energy."

Halls was lying motionless with her eyes closed, quiet as a corpse.

"Rosalyn, can you tell us what you feel in your body?" someone asked.

"I have a soft feeling in my heels. The arch of my right foot is pulsing. The ball of the foot is pressing down harder." Bruyere had been talking earlier about being able to articulate varying frequencies of energy just by changing where she applied pressure to the soles of her feet. "There's an odd tingle around my knees, thighs, and spine."

More time passed. "Jennifer's left eye is cool and soft, the right eye has a sparky red sensation."

"Wow!" Halls said suddenly. "I felt that!"

"I'm running gold now, because you've got to get a level of energy going that is twice as fast as the tissue in the brain. The frequencies in this part of the body are so high. I don't want to put energy into her eye. The eye tissues are much too delicate. I want her body to pull the energy off my finger and into the eye."

"Are you using any particular finger?" someone asked.

"You can use any finger except the ring finger. The ring finger doesn't give *chi*; it sucks *chi*. It's like a little pipette. That's why we wear rings on it."

Bruyere had her hands on Halls's face for about half an hour, first on the right side, then on the left. She said that the problem in the left eye was in a different spot than the problem in the right eye, and that she was trying to loosen the connection of the muscles and the nerves—to get some play and suppleness into what had become rigid with inflammation. The air in the room seemed as delicate as the tissue she was treating. We were all like tuning forks that had begun to resonate at the high pitch Bruyere was sustaining in her hands. I know that someone who was not there might dismiss the effect as another example of the "power of suggestion." I can say only that I felt the alignment of healer and client. I felt it in my eyes, of all places, in my right eye mainly, the eye that had seemed to be enveloped in that weird cloud of unknowing, the eye tagged or implanted with some bit of something ostensibly from a far-faraway place.

At long last, Bruyere dropped her hands from Halls's face, disengaging with a bittersweet reluctance. It was as if she were withdrawing from the keys of a piano on which she had just played one of Eric Satie's melancholy studies—and leaving all of us to listen with her to the echo of the last notes dying away in a deserted ballroom, late at night, all the dancers and the gaiety gone . . .

"Has the eye changed in there?" someone asked, breaking in on the reverie like a beer vendor at the opera.

Halls looked spellbound and could only nod.

"How?"

"It doesn't prickle anymore," she murmured.

Months later, I got a note from Halls. The trouble in her eyes had defied medical predictions. She'd lost none of her vision, and the retinas had stabilized; what's more, she had pinpointed what she thought was the source of her problem—her fear about quitting her museum job to pursue a career as a clairvoyant and healer. One of the many repercussions of her session with Bruyere was that she'd seen her way into the leap. She'd gone out on her own. She had a new sole proprietorship now. "Insight," she was calling it.

I picked up the details of Bruyere's life story as many of the healers in her community did, in bits and pieces gleaned in the course of her lectures. She often used the twists of her own history to convey the processes of the subtle world. She was the oldest of three children. Her father worked as a telephone installer, and her mother had a job in a soap factory. They eventually divorced. Bruyere spent some time in a Catholic orphanage and was raised mainly by her grandparents and her clairvoyant great-grandmother, Nana, who taught her to see the energy around plants and pets and people. At age five, conducting experiments with Nana, Bruyere discovered bulbs with auras produced healthier gladioli and dahlias than bulbs without auras. The light around plants moved more slowly than the light around animals; and animal light was slower than the light around people.

Nana was eventually hospitalized for what the family called a nervous breakdown, and Bruyere's caretakers made it plain that trafficking in the auric realm was dangerous. By seven, she'd been weaned from second sight. At Pacific Grove High School, Bruyere cut her rhetorical teeth as the captain of debating team. She enrolled in college in 1965 and hoped to pursue studies in engineering, but she dropped out after a year, married her first husband, and gave birth to two sons. When her boys were about three years old, they began to mention "the fuzzy light" around plants. Bruyere was inspired to find every bit of information available on chakras, auras, and illimitable whirlwinds. She devoured the occult literature section at the L.A. County Public Library, riffling through several hundred books, no two of which agreed, it seemed to her. She read Alice Bailey and the turn-of-the-century Theosophists, who popularized chakras in the West. A book critic in *The New Yorker* disparaged the "intolerable woolliness . . . of addlepated theosophist enthusiasts," but Bruyere wasn't bothered by it. The theories weren't so woolly when the rocking chair in your house moved by itself for seven minutes every day at 2:12 P.M., and the lights switched on and off, and the water faucets opened and closed. Friends started declining invitations to stop by for coffee.

Bruyere went to see Pat Allison, an elderly medium and healer in the spiritualist tradition. When Bruyere walked in, Allison said, "We've been waiting for you." Bruyere looked around, but there was nobody else in the room. Allison seemed to know Bruyere's family history, the intimate details of her life; she insisted Bruyere's exceptional psychic abilities would someday lead her to teach. It was all too incredible—Bruyere was twenty-three years old with two rambunctious kids and a job checking groceries in a local Safeway. But she started studying with Allison and a group of Los Angeles spiritualists at night. Dormant since childhood, her clairvoyant abilities returned. One night in Los Angeles her younger son, Mark, fell against a heater and suffered second-degree burns from his waist to his knees. Driving him to Children's Hospital, Bruyere stopped by Allison's house. The healer laid Mark facedown on her lap and said to Bruyere, "I want you to watch this." Then over the burns she made what looked to Bruyere like an icy blue light. She blew air across the boy's knees, making nine or ten passes in one direction and three in another. That was it. At the hospital the burns were confirmed as second degree; forty-eight hours later, the doctors were astonished to discover they were gone, and the skin had healed.

The discoveries, the miracles—whatever they were—kept coming. Bruyere apprenticed herself to the master healer Bill Gray. She learned to flex her psoas muscles to draw energy up from the ground. Current hummed through her like water through a hose. The Theosophists *were* a little addlepated, she realized. They had cut off the lower body. You couldn't pull divine energy down from the sky as reliably and safely as you could reach up toward it from a solid footing on the Earth. As she would later say to her students: "Your hands can't feel what your feet don't provide."

In 1974, Bruyere participated in landmark research conducted by Valerie Hunt at UCLA. A professor of physiology, Hunt had gotten interested in studying energy-field phenomena after a visit from a shamanic healer named Emilie Conrad Da'oud, who had been able to exert a beneficial influence on a disturbed patient's brain waves simply by chanting and performing ritualistic movements. (Da'oud went on to invent the

well-known breathing therapy called Continuum.) Hunt commenced
what would eventually become six hundred hours of electromyograph
recordings of muscle and tissue frequencies emanating from the chakras.
Using Bruyere as the "aura reader," Hunt correlated verbal descriptions
of fluctuating colors in a person's energy field with various wave patterns
recorded on the chakra points. Hunt described her work in her 1996
book *Infinite Mind*, but she never published her results in a peer-reviewed
journal—she was drawn away from science and into a healership of her
own—and consequently the experiments were not replicated or taken
as seriously as they might have been.

That same year, 1974, Bruyere founded the Healing Light Center
Church in Glendale, California, and began to develop its training program, and with it her reputation. Within a decade, she was considered
one of the world's foremost practitioners and teachers of hands-on healing. She had been accepted as an honorary medicine woman in six Native
American tribes; people twice her age addressed her as "grandmother."
She was traveling to teach healing in Germany, England, Norway, Ireland,
South Africa, and all over the U.S. and Canada. She was on the road
thirty-six weeks a year and spending so much time on airplanes her dogs
didn't recognize her when she returned because her clothes reeked of jet
fuel. ("My body thinks jet fuel is a food group," she said.) When I first
encountered her, Bruyere had scaled her practice back to three healings
a month, but when she wanted to demonstrate a technique, she would
often pick someone whom she knew was sick from the audience. And
she could draw on the experience of having treated some ten thousand
people since the start of her hands-on career.

Bruyere's only book, *Wheels of Light*, was published in 1989. It outlined the ideas she had synthesized from Hindu chakra theory, ancient
Egyptian theology, and Native American spiritual traditions. She had
superimposed a bit of Egyptian temple architecture onto the chakra system, specifically the idea that reality has four levels: literal, symbolic, paradoxical (or irrational as it is sometimes called), and divine. Each level
offered its own slant on health and disease, and as you moved up the
chakras you ascended through the four levels. The first chakra and its
related illnesses resided in the literal; the second and third chakras (feeling and opinion) belonged to the symbolic. The heart lay halfway

between the symbolic and paradoxical levels. And the third eye lay on the boundary between the paradoxical and the divine.

She illustrated these distinctions using the commandment "Honor thy father and mother." Its literal meaning was obvious: Mother's Day cards for Mom, ties for Dad. At the symbolic level, you were obliged to honor teachers and mentors who had served you in the role of father or mother. At the irrational or paradoxical level, you were bound to credit those who had opposed you, whose resistance or refusals resulted in some valuable lesson—an idea most eloquently echoed in the Native American concept of the "good enemy" who teaches you what you need to know. From the vantage of the third level, the task of parents was not to nurture and protect their children per se, but to inflict the "sacred wound" that would shape and organize their children's lives—the wound that the child's soul required for its own development and for which its parents had been selected precisely because they were equipped to deliver it. (A radical take on child abuse, to say the least.) And from the vantage of the divine, the commandment could be read as an injunction to honor your father and mother by creating on Earth what would otherwise exist only in Heaven, and dedicating that act of service to your parents' memory.

Even something as basic as light could be refracted through the four levels: Literally, light was photons; symbolically, aesthetic beauty; paradoxically, the revelation of darkness; and divinely, the cosmic illumination that blossomed in the petals of the thousand-petaled lotus. Certain diseases, in Bruyere's view, were primarily diseases of the literal. Others stemmed from distortions in symbolic thinking, as any psychologist would agree. Auto-immune diseases in Bruyere's view were the essence of the irrational—the self attacking itself. Healers had to attune themselves to the irrational level to comprehend the source of diseases that literally *didn't make sense.*

As she joined the chakras to the four levels, so she joined the four levels to the Native American medicine wheel. Found in many aboriginal cultures, the medicine wheel is a kind of map that assigns stations and duties to members of a tribe based on their age. With its eight lodges set at eight points of the compass and the Children's Fire in the center, it underscored your changing responsibilities as you progressed through your allotted time. One complete turn took twenty-four years. Then you passed back into the Children's Fire for three years and emerged for another round, beginning as always in the east, in the Men's Lodge, and moving clockwise around the circle at the rate of three years per lodge. It was not just your responsibilities that changed with each lodge but your perspective too. You were obliged to speak from the vantage of that lodge, be it the Peace Chiefs or the Warriors. Each lodge marked certain milestones and entailed certain rituals of passage; each afforded a certain way of interpreting diseases and problems.

Bruyere had combined the wheel and the four levels so that on your first circuit you took the meaning of the lodges literally. Warriors fought literal battles on their inaugural circuit; when they returned to the lodge twenty-four years later, they were still bound to fight, but the battles were symbolic. (For example, a journalist wouldn't punch his enemy, he would hit him with a nasty profile.) On their third go-round, warriors carried the standard of paradox and irrationality into the fray, and would probably piss off a lot of their friends in the community for pursuing what seemed to everybody a senseless crusade. On their last time around the wheel, assuming they lived long enough to qualify, warriors brought the vantage of the divine to their contest. They might go to war on behalf of the environment, or in some other way fight the battle for the divine outcome.

I was intrigued when I heard Bruyere lay out the structure of the wheel. My interest in healing had arisen during my tenure in the lodge of Mediums and Singers, where the duties were self-explanatory. If you wanted to serenade a hotel with hymns, you couldn't pick a more auspicious lodge. But my next stop was the Women's Lodge, where the assigned task was to keep the silence—which augured ominously for someone with a book contract. As I was on my symbolic turn through the wheel, I resolved to interpret the duty to keep the silence as an obligation to speak for the silence, to bludgeon the ineffable, if you will. (If the ineffable had to be bludgeoned, and from the evidence of the literature it did, best it were done by someone in a quasi-official capacity, no?) Apart from the qualifications of each lodge, I loved the meanings that seemed to coil up out of the wheel, the circular perspectives that brought the old times around again in a new way; without the wheel, your days would unfold one after another in a dull, straight, A to Z line, implying that life could be reduced to the dash on the tombstone between your first year and your last. Reality was deepened and enriched by the repetitions of the wheel. Once you got started seeing with lodge- and level-minded eyes, it was hard to stop. I had been literally curious about community in New York and symbolically curious about it in Boston, and my further curiosity was . . . well, irrational, paradoxical. *And that was precisely the point.* The need to participate, to experience, to understand and revel in community had nothing to do with reason. It had everything to do with what might be learned or felt outside the methods of reason.

So later that spring, after the seminars in New York and Boston that had served as introductions to the construct of a healing community, I drove my father's rattle-trap Toyota up to Epping, New Hampshire, to attend my first "intensive." Bruyere's New England community was the oldest of half a dozen groups around the country. They met for a week every May, and that year—1995—they were convening at a farm-cum-conference-center called Green Pastures.

On the road north, I found myself thinking of a previous foray into self-consciously spiritual fellowship, a grisly Baha'i pow-wow back in high school that I'd been dragged to by my then-girlfriend and her mother. It was okay at first: innocuous speeches about the universality of religious truth, friendly people, and no sense that some tense customer might burst from his chair brandishing a volume of Sartre and shriek, "See, it says right here, 'Hell is other people!' " But then as things were winding up, the Baha'is asked everybody to form a giant circle and link hands. I looked around at all the painfully sincere faces, and I realized that Hell is other people in their heart-rending earnestness, in their poignant needs. Hell is all of us in our heart-rending earnestness and poignant needs. Hell is my own poignant needs . . . One of the pleasures of being seventeen is fleeing from unbearable revelations, and hell quickly became the idea of delay. I took the first opportunity to get the hell out of there, bolting through a fire door. And I've been, let's say, a little dodgy ever since about ideas that premise the life of the soul on the interaction with others.

Green Pastures was a working farm. I found my room in the bunkhouse I was sharing with the badly outnumbered males in the New England community. My roommate Cleave was in his late forties. He used to sell mini-computers. Cleave and Peter, a ponytailed massage therapist across the hall, spent half an hour unpacking satchels of vitamins, supplements, and tinctures. One of the other guys, Christopher, used to be in the army. He'd moved on to aromatherapy; each night before bed he rubbed his face with rosewood oil and coated his feet with oil of pine and spruce. The free time of one of our other roommates was monopolized by his colon; each night he fixed a ghastly-looking cocktail of colloidal bentonite and drank it down with a grim devotion. I was the only brother in the men's dorm who'd packed a commercial deodorant in his dopp kit.

Being in community was nothing like sitting in a room alone reading about being in community. We gathered in a large meeting room that had been smudged with sage smoke. A small altar had been set up with a vase of flowers, candles, pictures, a Tibetan bell, and a wooden ark that each year was entrusted to one of the members of the community. Offerings had been made; prayers had been raised petitioning discarnate beings for guidance. After the main morning session, the community repaired for lunch, and then the members took a break in the afternoon to do healings or rest before reconvening after supper. As always, Bruyere and various elders emphasized the importance of building the *chi*. Group *energy* was the chief attraction of community. It's not easy even now for me to describe group energy, except to say that it paradoxically exhausts and innervates. I found I was revved up and bone-tired that first night. I couldn't drink enough water. Everyone was drinking gallons of water, prompting a regular exodus to the john. The fatigue I felt was almost the athletic kind you feel returning to exercise after a long lay-off, when muscles report in that you haven't heard from in ages. Only these weren't muscles reporting in; they were dimensions or aspects or parts of my being that I hadn't been conscious of. They rose into my awareness like images emerging on Polaroid film. I marked their arrival in new and oddly altered perceptions. One night at dinner, I found myself bewitched by the never-before-perceived beauty of a green bean. People's eyes began to fill with a sweet, unironic light. Naps seemed like deep-sea dives. If you imagine the combined field of a healer and client as being like a ripple on a pond, then the field of a hundred healers communing with a *sui generis* teacher was the equivalent of a tsunami.

Of course all the while the doubts that I have belabored since the beginning of this narrative were mobbing my thoughts. Who are these snowballs? Who is this Bruyere woman? What are we doing here? Not bad questions. One time Bruyere decided to demonstrate a technique for cleaning the liver. Not the literal liver but its crucial energetic analog, familiar to the community as the "etheric liver." Most of the people in the community of course perceived the etheric liver to be as real and substantive in its way as any liver laid out for autopsy.

Bruyere called for a volunteer. A woman got up. Bruyere put her hands near the woman's torso and told us that she was gently extracting the etheric liver. It wasn't something I could see, but I could see that others saw it, or thought they saw it, and that others felt it, or thought they felt it. And since it was becoming apparent to me that all knowledge about the subtle world had to include some basic suspension of disbelief, I took it on faith that Bruyere was not simply acting out her revelatory fantasies but had her hands on something real. It was a bigger assumption in 1995 than it seems now. With what seemed an air of frolic, Bruyere flung the visible/invisible liver over the heads of the community, and at least twenty pairs of eyes tracked its outbound flight, like spectators at a tennis match, and then its boomerang-like return. They saw Bruyere catch it and with one smooth motion shovel it back into the woman's body. Many of the healers grinned with delight.

If only laundry were so easy to clean!

Or so I thought at the time, ducking into the clown. The elders in the community were quick to point out that the feeling of being out of step, of not getting it, of doubting the consensus, were characteristic perturbations of a self in transition. Familiar pitfalls on the spiritual path. The value of the elders couldn't be overstated. Listening to Jim Kepner, a gestalt therapist from Cleveland who had a sharp feel for the coercive potential of groups, I remember thinking, "Here's a very smart guy and he believes this stuff . . ." And there were many other people in the community who had good educations, advanced degrees, successful careers, who were service-minded, kindhearted, who were surprisingly down-to-earth and conversant with a reality principle. If they'd been to Zork, they'd found their way back. Barbara Sorce was a registered nurse. Steven Weiss had a thriving practice as an osteopath. I found myself especially sympathizing with a radiologist named Jonathan Kramer who was struggling to hold on to his identity as a physician as the verities of his medical education were supplanted by a new model of how energy functioned in the body. Many of the elders in the community knew how they seemed to outsiders. When it was important to look conservative—say, when they were giving a healing in a hospital—they presented a conservative facade. When it didn't matter what others thought, they let their colors fly.

The influence of elders in the community notwithstanding, I'm amazed when I look back now, three years after that New Hampshire intensive, that I ever signed up for another one. I mean, the Quote Clown's absolute favorite line was Voltaire's famous dictum about the dangers of repeating certain kinds of experience: "Once a philosophy, twice a pervert." But I did sign up again. I kept coming back and coming back to the hotels and the hymns, to the unreal realities of etheric livers, to inexplicable results. I saw Bruyere take away the back pain of a Harvard graduate and extract the energetic traces of ovaries from a man. I watched her float her hands over the Kaposi's sarcoma lesions on the face of Joseph Carman, a New York writer; she ran a delicate energy back and forth across the blemishes until they visibly faded from his skin, and many months later he said, "She removed a huge lesion on my nose that radiation and chemo didn't take out. But when I look back at the work she did, the most important thing was the spiritual re-rooting of the disease. I still have HIV in my system, but she got me started on a whole new life where the disease was not applicable." I watched Bruyere channel a four-thousand-year-old Tibetan guide named Master Chang, whose disembodied voice had been authenticated by His Holiness Lungtok Tenpai Nyima, the exiled head of the Bon religion; her relationship with Master Chang and her healing work had inspired the monks in the Menri monastery in Dolanji, India, to call her the "lady lama."

So I kept coming back and coming back, and not for the fodder of miracles so much as for the possibility that there were parts of the world you could not discover by yourself. It is one of the commonplaces of spiritual healing that we cannot know ourselves apart from others. Our most inward aspect—the soul, "the within" as the Jesuit paleontologist Teilhard de Chardin once called it—can be realized only in the context of others. G. K. Chesterton said as much when he observed that a person "can acquire everything in solitude, except character." And not too long ago, I found the same idea beautifully echoed in Harvard Divinity School professor Harvey Cox's 1973 book *Seduction of the Spirit*. Cox had replaced de Chardin's "within" with the word "interiority." He wrote: "Interiority arises within us only as community emerges amidst us, and vice versa."

So bold, that proposition! *Interiority arises within us only as community emerges amidst us.* It was the essence of my midnight epiphany on the Pont des Arts. But it was complicated. Were they to be pitied, the world's hermits, the unshared souls of the lovelorn, the maiden aunts, the aging Upper West Side bachelors with only their home entertainment centers to snuggle up to? Was their isolation rapidly morphing them into zombies? Had they only warrants to a soul or an inner life, warrants that would soon expire? To hold that marriage—the community of two—and participation in the social life of larger communities could be equated with spiritual depth was nothing if not paradoxical. It implied that one of the most sacred aspects of our privacy was contingent on our capacity for interaction. Was that the paradoxical bargain tendered by communities— that it was only others who could cash the check of our innermost self? Only others who could unlock our deepest interiority, the within of all withins?

Interiority arises within us only as community emerges amidst us: By this idea, identity did not depend on the ways in which you distinguished yourself from the crowd but on the ways in which you overcame your essential differences—the ways in which you allowed those differences to be broken down. That theory opposed the old truism of meditation that it is hazardous to attempt to transcend the self before you take the trouble of developing one. Maybe Sartre was right, hell is other people. Certainly that bargain for interiority seemed hellish. Given the history of mobs and cults and political parties and religious crusades and Elks Club luncheons, a good argument could be made that the idea of interiority had been conceived and was useful only because without it there would be nothing to be breached when people were drafted into the miseries of coexistence. What drill sergeant would not be disappointed if the new snowball privates in his charge didn't have some notion of their inner lives, however tender and provisional, that he, their new master, could melt or dismantle on behalf of platoon unity? In community, wasn't it a fine line between unity and oblivion?

Small wonder that in New Hampshire my second chakra was awash with emotions and my third was tempted by the siren song of the fire exit. Community was humbling. Intensives were intense. You couldn't get away from other people. Or yourself. During the seminars in Boston and New York, people had felt free to interrupt Bruyere with questions or comments; her talks sometimes seemed more like conversations than lectures, and my mouthy clown had found it great sport to dart the dialogue with wisecracks. In New York, when Bruyere was discussing the crown chakra and the significance of ceremonial hats and making the point that part of being the Pope was assuming the power of the Pope's miter—when you put the hat on you *are* the Pope—I asked rhetorically if putting on the hat would quicken you with the desire to ban birth control. One line, and suddenly I had a reputation in the community as a joke machine! And it was completely undeserved; making jokes around and about healers is child's play. Their spirituality is often so ponderously earnest it jeopardizes the light they are generating in its name. Any clown confronted with the weight of that sincerity can see it has to be made light of, lest it tip the Earth out of orbit and send the whole caboodle crashing into the sun.

But by the latter part of the week in New Hampshire, I felt solemn and unaccountably vulnerable in community. I take this now as progress, however paltry. I had discovered how unsatisfying it was to stand off at a distance and lob jokes like a know-nothing pot-shotter, too frightened to open himself up. That was the hard part—opening up. Easy enough to do alone. But in front of others, yikes! It gave me a bad case of Baha'i-style heebie-jeebies. And then one morning I found myself raising my hand to ask a question that became a confession before the community that I envied their sensitivity, the nuanced world that they could see and feel. It seemed so out of reach.

"That's because you're living without water and earth," Bruyere said.

Water and earth, meaning chakras two and four. I had not cultivated the center of emotional energy, the energies of the heart. I was not attuned to the movement of feeling through my body, or how a passion that arrived at the heart chakra could be tempered into compassion.

"You're living half a life. It's joyless."

More than three years ago this was, and yet that sense of nakedness is still fresh. Bruyere's glib self-deprecation had always seemed a measure of her ability to present a norm-minded newspaper facade. But it was not a mask she used to hide from people; it was a way of disarming the egg-heads who blitzed her with yellow. She could run yellow stride for stride with them, but when she saw an opening, she didn't hesitate to shift the color of the conversation.

"Is it that apparent?" I asked.

"No, it's not," she said gently. "But you are unable to ask for what others can give."

I remember bowing my head, washed by waves of shame, and of unforeseen longing too. Was my distress so transparent? What had everyone else in the room figured out fifteen lifetimes ago that I hadn't?

Asking for what others can give . . .

Asking for what others can give is an excruciating idea when you have to be self-sufficient, when you are struggling to believe that what you have done on your own, or can do on your own, is well enough and good. Somewhere I had seized on the prideful-teen idea that I had to measure up on my own, without help. I had gone as far as I could on the impetus of that energy. In the context of a healing community, it was clear the momentum of self-definition had run out. It was pathetic to remember the binds it had gotten me into, and was still causing. In France I learned that I'd rather go hungry than ask for help ordering dinner in a foreign language.

And it was precisely a language problem that I had in New Hampshire too. The members of the community had fluent hands. Their eyes saw spirits. Their ears heard guides. Their hearts understood the centrality of love, the redemptive beauty of devotion and service. Their lives were anchored in the instrumentality of Sahasrara. Let mainstream priests and rabbis fret over the prospect of God as an energy source; let them drone on about the lack of moral emphasis in New Age theology; let them question relationships with God that were built on mystical experiences and patronize their little sparrows with injunctions to stick to time-tested theologies and liturgies. The members of the community were traveling abroad, voyaging down the spinal cord and into the back-beyond of the peripheral nerves, where they could hold the neural tissue open until some radiance burst from the bonds of matter itself. They had rid themselves of the need to make judgments. They didn't insist on what had to be true and what could not be true. They didn't gainsay their own perceptions. They had crossed into the enchanted world where you doubted your sanity if you *didn't* hear voices.

So now you want postcards!

No, I wanted a visa. We sleep in a matrix of assumptions until suddenly one night it collapses beneath us like a rotten hammock. In retrospect, I can see that in New Hampshire I was alarmed by the depth of the rupture in my definition of my self. I could not grasp its dimensions except as they were intimated in those symptoms that were made ineluctably visible in community: the hollowness of my clowns; the shockingly transparent unhappiness, the shame of exposure; and all that clairvoyant evidence of haywire chakras.

And there was also the unresolved business about my eye. It might seem a small problem beside the spiritual abyss of a joyless existence, but at that point the possibility that some object of unearthly origin might be lodged in or behind my right eye symbolized everything that I did not understand about the matrix that was fraying beneath me. Of course, the possible existence of an otherworldly implant made no literal sense. It still makes no sense. But now, looking back, having struggled to enlarge my idea of what I might consider *real*, the weirdness in my eye seems part of a brilliantly personalized teaching from the domain of the irrational. What more perfectly ludicrous talisman could I have received to expose the narrow base of my beliefs? In New Hampshire, though, I was ready to announce that if this bug existed, it was at the expense of everything I believed.

The truth was that I was afraid of losing what I believed in—terrified, even—and not just by the prospect of confronting the implant itself, whatever it was, but by the madness it might signify, and by the madness that might be signified in simply entertaining it as real. I was terrified of the upheaval it might create—of the abyss that might open beneath the threadbare hammock where I had been bedded down in a blissfully clueless sleep. What hotel would I turn back to when that strange hymn had fallen out of the wind?

Bruyere's words were swimming in my head that night. And the next morning, waiting for the session to get under way, I struck up a conversation with a healer named Lisa Platt, who was sitting in a nearby seat. She had dark hair and warm brown eyes; she was in her early thirties. She supported herself with her healing practice. At length, I asked if she had ever heard of implants.

"Oh, sure," she said.

"Can you get them out?"

"Sure."

She sounded so confident, so completely unfazed that I told her about my right eye and my experience with the two healers who had already grappled with it without success. She nodded sympathetically.

You are unable to ask for what others can give.

I got my nerve up—why was it so hard?—and asked her if she might take a look.

"Sure," she said. "Tomorrow afternoon. I'll get my team together."

4. A MOTH IN A MOSQUE

L isa Platt's hands looked much older than her face. They were weathered and full of stories, the sort of hands you might expect to find on a carpenter or a boatbuilder or an army cook. And, indeed, she had traveled on them. At thirty-four, she was a youngster in the community, but her prowess at tracking energy had inspired some people to call her "the queen of the etheric."

Platt had a busy healing practice in southern New Hampshire, but continued to study with Rosalyn Bruyere. That May at Green Pastures was her sixth intensive. She had discovered her sensitivity to energy in her early twenties. She had dropped out of college and was working as a cook, and one night she had a great run playing pool in a bar. She attributed it to what seemed a weird perceptual insight that could have been chalked up to tequila—if she'd been drinking tequila. "I could see what looked like lines of light between the balls," she said. "If I hit along the lines of light, the balls would go in. I hadn't played much pool, but the balls seemed connected. I practically ran the table. I was playing against guys who had played for a long time, and I won."

On the appointed afternoon, I helped Platt set up her healing table in a room in one of the bunkhouses. Her team arrived: Ticia, a Rolfer in her early fifties; Candace, who was about the same age, with a head of white hair; and Dawn, who, like Lisa, was in her early thirties and, also like Lisa, was wearing a sweater of the same royal purple that routinely surfaced on my visual field when I shut my eyes to meditate. I took off my shoes and lay down on the table. Dawn stood at my feet. Ticia and Candace stationed themselves at my hips. Lisa stood behind my head: an eight-handed healing! I was nervous. Ticia had beautiful unveiled blue eyes and smiled at me—moved, she told me later, by some transparent sign of longing in my gaze.

Lisa asked Ticia and Dawn and Candace to run red and orange— first and second chakra energies. Particularly orange. My emotional body was cracking and drying out, she said, and it was obvious to her that I was in sore need of the water of the second chakra. She said she wanted to see my overall field enlivened. If it was flush and dynamic, changes would be easier to effect. It was easier to work clay when it had been warmed in the hand.

"Okay," Lisa said, "which eye is it?"

And suddenly I didn't know, I couldn't say, I didn't remember. It felt as if both eyes had the mysterious affliction, the irritating feeling of a bug caught behind the lids. I was aghast. Suddenly not to know what I had been so specifically aware of for months was profoundly disturbing. For months it had been my right eye, but now it seemed as if I could feel the same unidentified floating object in my left eye too.

"Well, let me tune in," Lisa said. Her hands floated down to my temples. She closed her eyes and concentrated.

"There are two of them," she said.

The first came out easily. The way she worked was familiar to me, but what she was doing was so specific that it seemed extraordinary. All the while, the four of them just stood there, running their current into mine, filling my field.

"I'm in behind the brainstem," Lisa said, speaking not so much to me as to her team. Though the other healers were older, they were not as experienced, and they were following her intently. One of them asked a question.

"When I put my hands on somebody," Lisa replied, "sometimes I can feel where the blocks are, but it's not like I can draw a picture. I just know the area is blocked. Once I touch them, I can see the block in my mind's eye."

"Do you ever doubt your perception?" Ticia asked.

"I doubted it all the time at first. I wasn't sure what I was seeing and feeling. But then I would get feedback. I'd find a block at the throat, and the client would say, 'My throat's getting tight.' "

My legs began to heat up.

"There, I've got it," she said.

I couldn't feel the link she'd made.

"I'm going to bring it out through a secondary chakra at the side of the head. There's a secondary chakra at the temple."

"Why are you doing that?" asked Ticia.

"It's less disruptive when you can use an existing trail."

Her hand was at my right temple, and I felt something passing over my right eye. As it passed, I wondered how I might describe it, limited as I was to five senses. It was as if . . . what? As if I had swallowed a spoonful of ice cream mixed with sand, and some of it had gotten behind my eye. As if my eye were wriggling out of a scratchy old pair of long johns. There was the coolness of an irritant absenting itself.

"Okay, the first one's out," Lisa said. She held up her hand. "It's very small, and it seems like it's made of some nonterrestrial metal. I'm going to let it dissolve in the light . . ."

If there was something real in her hand, it was nothing I could see when I opened my eyes to peek at what she was doing. She was offering her hand up to the air above her head. She was holding what she had rather serenely described as the energy of a small nonterrestrial object. My legs felt kindled and tremulous with the current of the extra hands.

"There it goes," Lisa said.

"Wow," said Ticia.

"Did you hear the *pffttt* sound it made?" Lisa asked.

Dawn and Ticia and Candace seemed to be following along without difficulty.

"Okay," Lisa said. "I'm going to get the other one."

Many minutes passed in silence.

"Keep the energy up," Lisa entreated. It was as if Candace and Dawn and Ticia were holding a long, shaky ladder, and Lisa had to climb up it to reach the frequency of the thing she was seeking. The implant.

"It's deep down there," she said. "At the base of the sixth chakra . . . Oh, wow, it's moving, it's like it doesn't want to come out."

I could feel it moving. Wow. More startling was the fact that it *could* move. *These freaking things have locomotion? Energy? The will to evade? They're defending their purchase on my real estate?* They had the properties of any number of parasites. But it wasn't the parasite properties that were upsetting. It was the fact that the operation was proving trickier than even Lisa had expected. Lisa, the master, making the third attempt. If Lisa couldn't pluck the bugs out . . . And at that moment, the reality of the bugs seemed inarguable. It occurred to me that the parameters of some old and happily conventional world were gone, or lay far off, as at the wrong end of a telescope. How unutterably strange it was to accept the reality of these things, whatever they were. And yet there was a serenity in yielding, too. Yielding to practical matters. I didn't care what they were: I just wanted them out. Later, I would wrestle with what they were, and cancel my subscription to the *The Skeptical Inquirer* if necessary. Later, perhaps, I would scrape some rationalizations together. Maybe implants, bugs, entities, whatever, were no different from the millions of viruses and bacteria that were holed up in my interiority. Hell, wasn't the "self" an implant of sorts? A self believed it could move. A self had energy and volition and the desire to defend its turf. Truth be told, I hardly felt a self at that moment, but rather some kind of arena, half petri dish, half parliament, teeming with various life-forms and their conflicting interests. An image loomed up of a mosque full of moths. Was I the mosque or one of the moths?

"I need you guys to keep running *chi*," Lisa said.

She fell silent.

"A guide is working?" one of the team asked.

"My guide Philippe," she said. "He's a French surgeon."

"Fill" and "leap," I thought.

Lisa's effort had not slackened, but the quality of it had changed. She seemed to be concentrating on holding still, holding some tone in her being, holding the space where the work was being done—done through her, not by her: her hands, her focus, but not her will . . . She held the space patiently, like a doorman holding an umbrella over a socialite getting out of a cab.

"It's in so deep, and there's no nearby chakra to take it out through. He's working the implant through the tissue."

I could feel that Lisa, or Philippe, or Lisa-Philippe, had a hold of . . . something. It was as if she or he or they had hooked a tiny larval salmon on the finest thread, or had thrown a lariat made of spiderwebbing around the one black moth that was fluttering in the chiaroscuro of the mosque. And they were delicately leading this captured thing to some exit. Reeling it along, guiding and gently tugging it. I was worried that Lisa might not get it all the way out. That the connection would break and the fish slip away, or the moth wriggle free of the gossamer line. I could feel a ripping sensation in my brain, the brain, which isn't supposed to be able to register pain, which doesn't feel the surgeon's knife. I could feel the progress of this little hulk of perplexity as it was being dragged through the gray matter.

"It's almost there, keep the *chi* up," Lisa exhorted her team. Then she said, "Oh, cool. Did you see that? He dissolved the implant—vaporized it."

"Wow," Ticia said.

"What did it look like?" I asked.

"It was a strange metal."

Lisa set her hands on my temples and then behind my ears. I felt another sharp pain and the onset of a headache.

"I'm going to reset the etheric matrix so it's not displaced. It was askew."

She worked for about ten more minutes, essentially, as I understood it, trying to realign my physical body proper with the energy body pitched one level above it. I felt very calm and peaceful, drifting in a shallow sea of blissfulness. The irritation and pressure were gone from my eyes.

And when I opened them again and gazed through the window, I found myself drinking in the pageant of the virgin green leaves and the gray bark of the maple trunks. I found myself following along the trace of the brown farm paths, and the tan painterly panels of the clapboard buildings, and the yellow splash of daffodils under a blue delirium of sky, and, oh, those azaleas blazing like a succulent purple fire—colors and textures and patterns so ravishing I could almost taste them. Who could get enough of the world in his eyes?

Lisa was smiling at me.

"Welcome home," she said.

5. WILD PRAYERS OF LONGING

Home. *Home.* But where was that? Where was home if you were not grounded in your body—if it were truly the case, as the metaphysicians of healing said, that you weren't in your body, your body was in you? Somewhere between everywhere and nowhere . . .

Not long ago, a connoisseur of irony asked me what sort of "genius" I thought I'd become after four years in the swim of the subtle world. Oh, that was easy: a genius of the highest disorder, who in the course of devolving into fooldom had picked up the equivalent of tourist French in the language of energy, and now lived more acutely in the debt of his assumptions, and found that sometimes he would lose track of his body, that the ground of his being would suddenly shift out from under him and for a moment he would be unable to tell himself apart from some kinship with Nature, the community of ducks and azaleas and the livelong configurations of matter that were all braided together like an ensemble of voices in a great Sahasrara hymn; and his guides chiming in, too, caroling sweetly as he crossed the park: "You could learn something from that elm, buddy boy."

It was not faith I got the hang of so much as the Keatsian knack of suspending disbelief, of hovering in a sort of useful irresolution. I said "Enough already!" to some things. Enough with the irritable reaching after fact and reason. Enough getting *verklemmt* about the provenance of the Zorkian energy in my eyes. I didn't understand the provenance of energy, period, so I might as well lump the specific mystery of one in with the general mystery of the other. Put the puzzle piece in the box with everything else I didn't understand about the subtle world, everything that would never fit through reason's sieve or add up to a pretty picture for the yellow-breasted eggheads who looked askance at second sight, chakras, guides, subtle bodies, healing hands. On good days, when the method of inner empiricism was cooking, who could doubt the results, who'd bother getting lathered up about self-revelatory delusions? Some days during meditation, I could feel the air between my hands grow as pliant and tacky as a ball of cotton candy; I could send the purple cursor gadding around my ground of being, feel myself extended beyond my skin . . .

But suspended disbelief should not be mistaken for faith, or for the conquest of skepticism. Soon after I started into the chakras, I decided to revisit the Reverend of the Lilies. This was in August 1994, nearly ten years after my first eventful psychic reading. Reverend Diane lived in the same house in Washington, D.C. And she looked scarcely a day older, either, even though in the long interim between my visits, her husband, Henry, had died—"graduated" was how she had put it in a letter to her clients. It had been, as I remembered, a touching note: For all her professed insight into the future, her faith that someday she and Henry would be reunited, she'd confessed that "one is never quite prepared for the death of a loved one."

Anyway, when I showed up on her doorstep again, she had moved on in her no-nonsense fashion. As before, we climbed the stairs to her consulting room. She made the familiar invocations. It was nice to hear the word "hast" again. I wish I could say the reading moved me as it had before. The second time, her second sight seemed off. She told me a lot of stuff that was just plain wrong. I would be making a brief research trip to New York, she said—New York, where I had been living for nine years already. I would be picking up a companion at the Baltimore Washington

International Airport and wearing safari clothes. Prospects for my love life were so bleak I ought to consider getting a dog; she could see me "sitting in a chair, eating cereal, all alone" and skulking around like a "lone wolf" with only the comforts of work. Oh, all right, at the time she wasn't *that* wrong about the love-life stuff, or my cereal habits. And some minor predictions were on the money (as if anyone needs a psychic to forecast out-of-state travel), but egad, safari clothes? And a lone wolf cuddling up to a dog? Barely a year later, when I assessed her psychic gifts from the vantage of the Pont des Arts, they seemed deeply un-Delphic.

I suppose a defender of the faith could argue that her bleak forecast of my future as a lupine professional trolling for company at BWI Airport helped precipitate my resolve to make some fast adjustments. Who knows. At the time, the reading left me with the queasy feeling that I'd mythologized our initial flower-of-the-dead encounter and, like Wile E. Coyote, had boldly headed out across the deep water of the mind-body problem on a bridge of woo-woo lily pads, which would give way the moment I realized they were not the stones I took them for.

I find now from the aerie of the seventh chakra that I am still divided and equivocating: skeptical sometimes of my own enthusiasm, and yet drawn again and again to the hymns, to the longing to believe. Just this last spring I went back for another week-long intensive with Rosalyn Bruyere's New England community, now gathering in a monastery in West Hartford, Connecticut. My book was virtually finished; I had no good "reason" to be there. But I'd formed bonds with people; in a way, I had become a part of the community. The attachments of the subtle world are not easily broken when intellectual or professional interest is satisfied. Traveling up the chakras is not like zipping down to the Caribbean for a week. You just don't switch them off when the trip's over, and you can't condense the experiences into a few delicious anecdotes to amuse guests at dinner parties. (Then again, if you get far enough into the subtle world, dinner party invitations start to dry up, so maybe it's not an issue.)

At the intensive in West Hartford I felt once again that strange sense of a rootless, free-floating home. But some of the old qualms that dated back to New Hampshire were still around. I still didn't know what to make of the material Bruyere channeled from the four-thousand-year-old Tibetan entity Master Chang. Extraordinary as Chang's provenance was—the current abbott of the monastery in Menri believed that he knew Chang in an ancient incarnation, and had apologized for once striking him with a bell—it was the content of what Chang said that troubled me.

For the newcomers to the community, Bruyere explained again how she had developed a relationship with Chang; how he personified an energy of almost unendurable majesty and sweetness; how his advice and willingness to make himself available were great gifts intended for our benefit, to help all of us in the community on our spiritual paths. When she channeled Chang, Bruyere left her body, taking some of her chakras with her, but usually leaving the throat chakra in so Chang could speak. Serving as a channel required a tremendous amount of energy; she had learned to make her exit by reciting the Lord's Prayer. The first night, as was customary, we all joined in as the prayer was said—a prayer I hadn't recited since my boyhood at St. Clement's, where I remembered it mainly for the oil-on-a-hot-skillet hiss of the word "trespasses" when the congregation said "Forgive us our trespasses." Around "Hallowed be thy name," Bruyere's head nodded forward, and then she was gone, out, whisked up through the crown chakra like a genie through the neck of a bottle. (When she was out, she said, she often hovered near the back of the room, but she had to be careful moving around because thoughts were speeded up, and what you intended happened much faster; if she intended to move herself toward a chair, she might sail right through it.)

And here was Chang in Bruyere's body, saying, "Good evening."

"Good evening, Master Chang," replied the members of the community.

Many of the veterans doted on Master Chang's visitations, and after his preliminary talk, they plied him with questions about their lives, or issues of interest to the entire group.

It was hard for me to get past the Ti'nglish voice Chang spoke in. It sounded like a parody of an Asian accent. Even harder—and I hope Chang and his devotees will forgive me if I am trespassing—was what seemed the lack of substance in what the entity had to say. While genial enough, with plenty of references to dragons, his advice tended toward pseudoprofundities on the order of "buy low and sell high." Bruyere always struck me as being more interesting when she spoke as herself. The caliber of Chang's remarks, along with the spectacle of some one hundred people hanging on his every word, always created a certain amount of cognitive dissonance. What was I missing that these bright and thoughtful people found so fascinating? It was as if they were parsing song lyrics from the Monkees' Greatest Hits under the illusion that the words were verses from one of Shakespeare's lost plays.

But then again, as was said time and again, it was not the words that mattered so much; it was the vibe in the room, the grain of the air. And the feeling when Master Chang had the floor was completely different. It was often said if you didn't have the antenna to pick up his frequencies, his energy would put you out faster than a turkey dinner. I had gone down hard the first few times I heard him, but was sure it was my own invincible drowsiness in the face of boredom, not high frequencies of spiritual energy. In time, witnessing repeated channeling sessions at a series of intensives, I learned to stay awake, and, even more important, I learned to stop minding the words and to attend instead the quality of the silence between them, to the energy they were riding on. It was an astonishing discovery, that energy: like being borne up on a giant wave, or on the recoil of a bungee cord. You felt half the Earth's gravity had been revoked and you were light enough to walk across a cloud.

This last time, in Hartford, it wasn't my Chang qualms that preoccupied my thoughts, but more of that shyness in the context of others, the continuing demonstration of what we can learn about ourselves alone versus what we can discover only in the setting of a group. I had asked a question, to which Bruyere replied, "Come on up and let me demonstrate something." People in the audience were dying for her to demonstrate any sort of technique on them, under the belief—a belief I subscribe to—that when she got her hands on you, she could do a lot of energetic work in a short amount of time. But for some reason, I was suddenly freaked out by the prospect of having to expose myself, of being up there on stage, so I shook my head and said in a jocular way that there was no way I was going up there, not realizing at the time what I was turning down, or how strange it was to say no. That "no" haunted me the rest of the week. I wanted to undo it, but what was done was done, and there it sat, defining me as shuttered-up, a refusenik, a chicken. My beliefs were shaken. I did not think of myself as someone who was so full of resistance and judgment that he would decline a public encounter with a healer he had been seeking out and studying with for four years . . .

Ticia, who had assisted Lisa Platt with my eye surgery in 1995 in New Hampshire, sat next to me at dinner a few days later. She told me that she didn't know what it was but that she felt as if I were her brother or something. And then she said, "You're not sure you belong here, are you?"

She was right. It seemed the bind you'd be in if you were caught up in the endless counterpoint of doubt and faith, or doubt and the longing for faith. It was hard to explain the vacillation to believers. I reread a passage of prose that I'd been brooding over in W. H. Auden's beautiful long poem *For the Time Being: A Christmas Oratorio*, a monologue in the voice of Herod, who is lamenting his failure to convince the citizens to live by the dictates of reason and to resist the lure of faith:

> I have tried everything. I have prohibited the sale of crystals and ouija-boards; I have slapped a heavy tax on playing cards; the courts are empowered to sentence alchemists to hard labor in the mines; it is a statutory offence to turn table or feel bumps. But nothing is really effective . . . Legislation is helpless against the wild prayer of longing that rises, day in day out, from all these households under my protection: "O God, put away justice and truth for we cannot understand them and do not want them. Eternity would bore us dreadfully. Leave Thy heavens and come down to our earth of waterclocks and hedges. Become our uncle. Look after Baby, amuse Grandfather, escort Madam to the Opera, help Willy with his homework, introduce Muriel to a handsome naval officer. Be interesting and weak like us, and we will love you as we love ourselves."

When reason is replaced by revelation, Auden warns, knowledge "will degenerate into a riot of subjective visions—feelings in the solar plexus induced by undernourishment, angelic images generated by fevers or drugs, dream warnings inspired by the sound of falling water." *Beliefs can be shaken.* Including religious beliefs. Surely no second sight is required to foresee the dangers of saviors or to anticipate the explosive potential of summoning heavenly forces to govern earthly business. The dementias of religion challenge the wisdom of the Fool, who tries to marry heaven and earth.

And Herod's indictment of unscientific knowledge neatly mirrors the criticism of spiritual medicine made by professional skeptics—the hierophantic quantifiers of the National Science Foundation, the white-coats at the National Institutes of Mental Health, and those self-appointed quack-busters and op-ed warriors who are always deploring homeopathy or "touch therapy" or "psychic healing" on the grounds that it can't be true because it doesn't make sense, it's not rational.

I thought I had gotten their voices out of my head, but this past April, as I was concluding my four-year odyssey through the chakras, virtually persuaded that healers could sense a field of energy around the human body and that sometimes I could too, the *Journal of the American Medical Association*, which has seldom printed anything about "energy medicine," published a study finding that twenty-one practitioners of "energy healing" were unable to detect energy fields at rates better than chance. It was amazing that the powerful voice of the medical mainstream had anything at all to say about energy medicine; even more amazing was that the study—published on April Fool's Day, of all days!—was based on data gathered by a fourth-grade girl named Emily Rosa, from Loveland, Colorado. The fact that a child had obtained results that undermined the foundations of a popular alternative therapy was irresistible to the news-media. Emily's picture appeared on the front page of the *New York Times* and she made the nightly news.

In her first experiment, which was a project for a science fair, Emily recruited nineteen female and two male practitioners of Therapeutic Touch, the form of energy healing pioneered by Dolores Krieger and one of the mostly widely practiced types of energy healing in the country. The healers put their hands through a screen, palms up, about a foot apart; Emily flipped a coin to determine which of their hands she would target and then held her own hand a few inches above the healer's hand. The healers were to report which of their hands Emily's was hovering above. They had, of course, a fifty-percent chance of guessing which hand she was targeting, but they did worse than chance. Each healer was tested ten times, and in two averaged sets of trials they called the correct hand forty-four percent of the time.

Told of their poor results, the healers offered excuses. Their hands had gotten hot. They could have been misled by the different energy profiles of the hands—the left hand typically received energy; the right one transmitted it. Or maybe they had been confused by the energetic traces of Emily's hand from the previous trial. Some wondered if they'd been thrown off by the kid's "experimenter bias." Emily's "intention" might have been disposed toward a negative result, given that her mother, registered nurse Linda Rosa, was a well-known critic of Therapeutic Touch.

The *JAMA* paper was written by Linda Rosa, Larry Saner, and the noted quack-buster physician Stephen Barrett. The assumption of the study was that if the premise of TT was faulty then it didn't matter what studies had concluded about TT's efficacy. In a note accompanying the article, the editors of *JAMA* apparently accepted this proposition and, on the basis of this one article, rendered the lordly judgment that "further professional use of Therapeutic Touch is unjustified."

It seemed to many healers that the publication in *JAMA* and the subsequent media coverage had less to do with science or the reality of the human energy field and its potential to be sensed and harnessed by healers than it did with the politics of alternative medicine. Why was that the healing study published in *JAMA* and not the experiment Mehmet Oz had recently done, which showed a healer could slow the growth rate of breast-cancer cells? Alternative-medicine partisans wanted to blast the study, but it was hard to rip into the work of a clever child. Was now a time for faith? Maybe somewhere out in the heartland a third-grader would emerge bearing data that proved the energy field did exist . . .

So it goes, skeptics, believers; critics, advocates. I followed the debate for a while until the whole back-and-forth began to make me feel like one of April's fools. I have to say there is something unappealingly grim about professional skeptics who set themselves up as quack-busters. They are the science police, and often seem less interested in discovery than enforcement. For sure, they do great good public service at times, especially in medicine, but their adamancy is sometimes no more subtle than the certitude of believers. Enough with inflexibly fixed positions! Skepticism in the end can't work as a way of life. Logic requires you to turn your skepticism on itself, which is to say skepticism in the end is bound to devour itself. And at that point you are left with your metaphysics and your faith.

Beliefs can be shaken, but faith is the result of being shaken. Perhaps there are a million moments that I might point to, but the one that has stayed with me was a time from my first year in college. I had gone rock climbing in New Hampshire on a cliff called Cathedral Ledges. Cathedral Ledges specialized in creating spiritual epiphanies. I was roped to an older student whose name I have forgotten. We were set on a route known as Standard, which was one of the easier climbs on the cliff, but was very exposed, and scary for the greenhorn climber I was. The route went up a crack in the massive gray face and then traversed out a long way to the right.

My partner was an experienced climber, a few years older. He led out and climbed up to a ledge about 120 feet off the ground. He anchored himself to the rock and then belayed me up the pitch, which I managed without too much trouble. The view was beautiful; I could see over the treetops fired in the colors of a New England fall. I could also see across the thin footing of the next pitch, the traverse where the cliff sheared away below. My partner took the lead again, edging across faint nubbins of rock. He wore a sling of aluminum nuts and carabiners that jingled as he moved. Ordinarily, the leader places a nut in a crack and attaches it to the rope with a carabiner, but on the traverse, spots to put in the protection were hard to find. And the pitch didn't look too hard. From my stance on the ledge, I watched him edge his way to a bulge in the cliff face about forty feet out. He paused a moment and then with some effort crabbed around the bulge, and continued smoothly across the traverse, gaining another forty or fifty feet of height. He called out "Off belay," which meant that he was no longer depending on me to hold the rope tight if he slipped. He began hauling in the slack.

Now it was my turn to climb. I edged onto the traverse. The going wasn't hard, but it was fearsomely exposed—the abyss of air beneath me reached ever greater depths as I moved right, along the crack. I came to the bulge that had detained my partner. It was inclined almost to the vertical. I tried to step out around it, but I had to retrace my steps immediately. It was harder than it looked. Anxiety was weakening my arms; my hands were damp. I tried again. There seemed to be no spot for my feet, nothing for my hands. My partner shouted something I couldn't hear. "I'm stuck," I shouted back. My legs began to tremble—shaking violently. Sewing machine leg, they called it. Sweat ran into my eyes. The rope trailed off to my right, not directly above me; if I fell, I wouldn't slide a foot or two, I would pendulum across the cliff, spinning and careening off the rock, and I would be in even worse circumstances, stranded in a blank section with nothing to grab on to . . . I had to move past the bulge even though I didn't know what holds might lie around the bend. I had to move with only the hope something would be there. My hands were soaked, my breath shallow. I crouched at the side of the outcrop and then levered myself up onto the bulge. No turning back now. But I saw with panic that my prayers were not answered. There was nothing to hold on to. I couldn't go forward or back, I could only hold on where I was, and within seconds I felt the last of my strength ebbing.

I was lost. God was deaf. I had nothing to summon. No energy. No will. Nothing that could deliver me from this impasse high on a plunging wall in the mountains of New Hampshire. It was only the terror of falling—of still greater calamity—that kept me hanging on . . .

And then the strangest thing happened: I saw myself move. On the strength of some unknown initiative, I watched as I moved—as I was moved. Watched as if from above my body. One trembling leg flailed out to the right and found a purchase. And then my exhausted fingers crept across the rock face to some hitherto-unseen fleck of stone and grasped it, and then I saw my clown bulk miraculously shifting to the right, around the burl of rock. I was not the conscious agent of these actions. I was beside myself and being moved, like a zombie possessed by some other sort of agency, some hidden force or will that had drawn on reserves I could not invoke but could only bear witness to—could only hail in a chorus of hallelujahs issuing from my throat at the instant of my extrication. Here was Fate's Pawn ready to shout praise to . . . something! Something had delivered me! Something had spared me from the abyss. But what, exactly? What had happened? Whose bidding had I done? There was something I should believe in, and to this day I'm not sure what it is.

When was it ever faith in and of itself that the faithful wanted? We wanted deliverance. We wanted lily pads to hold us up. Rescue from dire straits. Most of all, we wanted meaning. A sense of purpose, the possibility that events had some larger order, and the motions and the shapes of matter were part of a design.

This was the paradise where healing ended: that nothing happened just by chance, that some lesson or design was imbued in the calamity of an accident, some reason or purpose vested in the misfortune of disease. This renunciation of chance was the ultimate revelation, the final enlightenment, what exponents will dare say was the healing of healings. As Nietzsche wrote in a letter in December 1888 to the playwright August Strindberg, alluding to one of the signal epiphanies of his life: ". . . there is no longer any element of chance in my life."

And in a chanceless realm, no event is too trivial to convey a message from the divine order. Once during a break in a Rosalyn Bruyere seminar in New York, I went to get a sandwich with a healer named Susan, whom I had been badgering with questions. She was constantly alluding to Spirit. Spirit this, Spirit that. Her enthusiasm for divine signs and portents was positively Mesopotamian. We found a place to sit on a bench in Central Park. What was Spirit, anyway? I asked. Where was it? What did it have to do with anything? Suddenly, as if to answer, a pigeon on the elm branch overhead dumped a load of guano that sailed down and splattered the lapel of my camel-hair Dolce & Gabbana jacket. Susan practically ruptured an artery laughing. "That's Spirit," she gasped when she got her voice back. The intersection of my lapel and the waste of a defecating pigeon was not chance; it was Spirit rushing to parry my belligerent thrust. And if Spirit had taken it into its mind to make the point with a tree limb or debris from a disintegrating communications satellite, well that would have had nothing to do with chance either.

I had a hard time believing that Spirit, the force that made the universe, could even hear a critic, much less be bothered enough to transmit a rebuttal in the semaphore of pigeon shit. I wondered later: Is it "chance" our minds can't stand? Is "chance" the true Cloud of Unknowing? There is a beautiful passage in Brian Friel's play *Faith Healer*. All his life, the protagonist, Francis Hardy, has suffered the doubt of not knowing whether he would have the power to command a miracle of healing on any given night. In his final moments, he walks toward a man in a wheelchair; he knows he cannot heal the man. He knows the man's friends will beat him to death when he fails. And it is precisely this fatal, ineluctable certainty that exalts him: "For the first time, I had a simple and genuine sense of homecoming," he says. "For the first time there was no atrophying sense of terror; and the maddening questions were silent. At long last I was renouncing chance."

As Nietzsche had, when he emancipated himself from the horrifying arbitrariness of fate. Of course, Nietzsche's fate is nothing if not a caution. It was not long after his letter to Strindberg proclaiming the conquest of chance that he encountered a horse being whipped to death in Turin, and went mad. Mad he remained for the last eleven years of his life.

Mad in a chanceless world. Was it syphilis that drove him out of his senses? Or perhaps was it that he shouldered responsibility for the entirety of his fate? Having declared himself the author of his destiny, he could not escape its dire turns. In randomness there is the element of luck. Good or bad, luck as an idea helps relieve the burden of complete responsibility. Nietzsche assumed responsibilities normally vested with God or Fate or Nature, and refused to cast himself as a pawn beholden to the power of superior forces. No Twelve Step capitulation for him. Having announced the death of God, he struggled to assume divine duties. He had no recourse in faith, even the mundane faith embraced by the baldest atheist—faith that the branch won't break, the plane won't crash, the heart will not, in the words of the Swedish poet Tomas Transtromer, be stopped by "the sudden axe-blow from within."

I have learned not to clutch too tightly this idea that there is an intrinsic meaning in all events. At times it seems contemptibly nuts, a screwball decree with all the inhuman harshness of any fundamentalist edict. People create their own reality? Give that lecture on the train tracks and see who scatters when the whistle blows. Let's talk about the reality of idealism outside in the tornado or up there in the plane with four engines out. Almost any tragedy will test the proposition that everything happens for a reason. People who, invite leukemia patients to take responsibility for their disease by getting in touch with their anger can't say they didn't ask for it when they get punched in the nose. When the sister of a friend was killed in a freakish car crash not long ago, the randomness and senselessness of her death was inescapable. There were no lessons to draw, no meanings to glean. It was a bolt from the blue and to suggest otherwise seemed monstrously absurd. To intimate that the soul had made a choice seemed almost a form of cruelty. If nothing else, the tragedy defined the limits of personal intention. Why should illness be different? Fate is what befalls us.

And yet the idea of intrinsic meaningfulness is central to the metaphysics of healing. At times nothing seems more powerful than the willful disavowing of chance precisely because it does turn every misfortune into a lesson; it does render meaning; it does ask you to search the flux of events for your complicity. Maybe the very effort to live by such a code creates its own meaning. You learn to pretend that everything happens for a reason and you are astonished to find that meaning appears, like magic, out of nothing. You lack belief? Well then, why not make believe? In the midst of accidents and setbacks, what is faith if not the call to rededicate yourself to a hard-won vision of ultimate purpose? What is faith but the strength not to yield to the pointlessness of life? To espouse faith is to practice some kind of knowingly lunatic alchemy by which the lead of randomness is converted to the gold of meaning. I am not saying the idea is not entirely paradoxical or nuts. Maybe it is. But maybe it is fox crazy. Maybe there is also real magic in magical thinking. Maybe the alchemy of faith is like the loom that weaves itself into being, or the artist's hand that draws itself into the world.

Consider a dream it sketched for me. After great effort, I was granted an audience with a famous oracle and apprised that I could ask one question.

"Who are the two greatest philosophers of healing?"

The answer came back right away.

"Mr. Stephen Aeger, and C. Fred Wynn."

"Who are they?"

"No more questions," the oracle said.

But just then two figures came up the road, apparently the fellows in question. One was a man, dressed in robes. I knew him instantly to be my monk. The other was a chimpanzee in a party hat—a clown, of course, but not the one I knew. They stopped. They asked me where I was going.

"I'm going home," I said.

"You'd better come with us," said the monk, putting the chimp's hand in mine.

"Why?" I said.

He nodded to C. Fred.

"Because he knows the way."

NOTES

CHAPTER ONE

page

3   *"The gods have become diseases."* C. G. Jung quoted in "Commentary on the Secret of the Golden Flower" in *Psyche and Symbol* (New York: Anchor Books, 1958), 331. The complete thought does not flatter the Fourth Estate: "The gods have become diseases; not Zeus but the solar plexus now rules Olympus and causes the curious symptoms of the physician's consulting room, or disturbs the brains of the politicians and journalists who then unwittingly release mental epidemics."

5   *. . . fallible god . . .* "To fall in love is to create a religion that has a fallible God," quoted in Jon Winokur, *A Curmudgeon's Garden of Love* (New York: New American Library, 1989).

5   *. . . whiff of charlatanism . . . not half as ripe as it seems now . . .* Telephone psychics are a $300-million-a-year business according to figures quoted in Joanne D. S. McMahon and Anna M. Lascurain, *Shopping for Miracles: A Guide to Psychics and Psychic Powers* (Los Angeles: Lowell House, 1997). For a history of psychic charlatanism, see Ruth Brandon, *The Spiritualists* (New York: Knopf, 1983). For a review of the use of psychics by law enforcement agencies, see Arthur Lyons and Marcello Truzzi, *The Blue Sense* (New York: Warner Books, 1991), which reports that the California Dept. of Justice officially recommends using psychics in certain dead-end cases. Also see the note to page 129, on Remote Viewing referencing.

8   *. . . the flower of the dead . . .* And thus, also, Christianity being what it is, the symbol of resurrection.

9   *. . . had her colon periodically flushed . . .* Colonic irrigation, which was practiced by the ancient Egyptians and is part of the ayurvedic regimen known as *panchakarma,* has gone in and out of fashion in the West. See Paul Beeson, "Fashions in Pathogenic Concepts During the Present Century," *Perspectives in Biology and Medicine,* 36, 1 (Autumn 1992): 13. Beeson quotes A. F. Hurst, "The Sins and Sorrows of the Colon," *British Medical Journal* 1 (1922): 941–43, that the fad for intestinal douching reached its apex in France during the reign of Louis XIV, who underwent colonic lavage, as the procedure was called, "several thousand" times.

10   "She Started to Do Better" is based on an interview with Nancy Chan of the San Francisco Zoological Society and press accounts by Karen Commings, *Catfancy,* January 1996. And Larry D. Hatfield in the *San Francisco Examiner* (June 13, 1995).

12   *. . . In Ireland in the seventeenth century . . .* Quoted in Richard Gordon, *The Alarming History of Medicine* (New York: St. Martin's Press, 1993). Many of the other bizarre therapies presented are detailed in Benjamin Walker, *Encyclopedia of Metaphysical Medicine* (London: Routledge & Kegan Paul, 1978).

12   *. . . a horse chestnut . . . for relief from rheumatism . . .* Quoted in Joseph C. Aub and Ruth K. Hapgood, *Pioneer in Modern Medicine: David Linn Edsall of Harvard* (Cambridge, MA: Harvard Alumni Medical Association Books, 1970).

13   *. . . "someone of worthless estate" . . .* Walker, *Encyclopedia of Metaphysical Medicine.*

13   *. . . mail-order panaceas . . .* Warren E. Schaller and Charles R. Carroll, *Health, Quackery and the Consumer* (Philadelphia: W. B. Saunders, 1976).

14   W. Haggard, *Devils, Drugs and Doctors* (New York: Harper & Brothers, 1929).

page

15 . . . *Charles was a practitioner.* . . . Marc Bloch, *The Royal Touch: Sacred Monarch & Scrofula in England and France* (London: Routledge & Kegan Paul, 1973). Bloch notes that Charles usually gave hands-on treatments on Fridays except if the weather was unusually hot. The patients received a gold or silver coin, but when the royal treasury was strapped for funds, they were given a token bearing the impress of St. Michael slaying a dragon. For information about the life of the king, see also Tony Palmer, *Charles II: Portrait of an Age* (London: Cassell, 1979).

15 . . . *crowds were so large* . . . cited in Haggard, *Devils, Drugs and Doctors.*

15 Harry Clements, *Magic, Myth and Medicine* (London: Health for All Publishing, 1952).

16 Among the sources for "A Deplorable Story": Henry E. Sigerist, *The History of Medicine: Primitive and Archaic Medicine* (New York: Oxford University Press, 1951), vol. 1; Henry E. Sigerist, *On the Sociology of Medicine* (New York: MD Publications, 1960); Charles M. Leslie, *Asian Medical Systems* (Berkeley: University of California Press, 1976); Ari Kiev, ed., *Magic, Faith and Healing: Studies in Primitive Psychiatry* (Glencoe, NY: Free Press of Glencoe, 1964); David J. Weatherall, *Science and the Quiet Art: The Role of Medical Research in Health Care* (New York: Norton, 1995); Byron Good, *Medicine, Rationality, and Experience* (New York and Cambridge: Cambridge University Press, 1990); Ted Kaptchuk and Michael Croucher, *The Healing Arts* (London: BBC, 1986); Bernard Lown, *The Lost Art of Healing* (Boston: Houghton Mifflin, 1996); Guido Majno, *The Healing Hand: Man and Wound in the Ancient World* (Cambridge, MA: Harvard University Press, n.d.)

17 Virgil J. Vogel, *American Indian Medicine* (Norman: University of Oklahoma Press, 1970).

17 . . . *epilepsy could be explained* . . . For an interesting discussion of epilepsy see G.E.R. Lloyd, *Magic, Reason and Experience* (New York and Cambridge: Cambridge University Press, 1979).

18 Majno, *The Healing Hand.* This is a beautifully illustrated and endlessly interesting book that ranges across the history of early medicine.

20 . . . *"the arrival of a good clown"* . . . Thomas Sydenham quoted in *Familiar Medical Quotations,* ed. Maurice B. Strauss (Boston: Little, Brown, 1968).

20 . . . *Galen attained such cult authority* . . . Daniel J. Boorstin, *The Discoverers* (New York: Random House, 1983).

22 Albert B. Sabin, *Perspectives in Biology and Medicine* 25, 2 (1983): 188–97.

28 Henri F. Ellenberger, *The Discovery of the Unconscious* (New York: Basic Books, 1970).

28 . . . *the age of the "half-believer"* . . . Richard L. Gregory, ed., *The Oxford Companion to the Mind* (New York and Oxford: Oxford University Press 1987), 677.

29 The details of Abraham Flexner's life are drawn from *I Remember: The Autobiography of Abraham Flexner* (New York: Simon & Schuster, 1940); *Medical Education in the United States and Canada,* Bulletin no. 4 (1910), Carnegie Foundation for the Advancement of Teaching. I also drew on Howard S. Berliner, *A System of Scientific Medicine* (New York: Tavistock Publications, 1985); Barbara Barzansky and Norman Gevitz, eds., *Beyond Flexner: Medical Education in the Twentieth Century* (New York: Greenwood Press, 1992); Charles Vevier, ed., *Flexner: 75 Years Later: A Current Commentary on Medical Education* (Lanham, MD: University Press of America, 1987).

33 Leo Galland, *The Four Pillars of Healing* (New York: Random House, 1997), 20–21.

page

34   Paul Starr, *The Social Transformation of American Medicine* (New York: Basic Books, 1984).

34   E. Richard Brown, *Rockefeller Medicine Men* (Berkeley: University of California Press, 1979).

36   . . . *adverse reactions to medication* . . . Jason Lazarou, Bruce Pomeranz, Paul N. Corey, "Incidence of Adverse Drug Reactions in Hospitalized Patients: A Meta-analysis of Prospective Studies," *Journal of the American Medical Association* 279, 15: 1200–1205. An account by Denise Grady can be found in *The New York Times,* April 15, 1998.

36   . . . *no more free of dogmas than any other cultural activity* . . . For a ringing indictment of scientific dogmas see Morris Berman, *The Reenchantment of the World* (Ithaca: Cornell University Press, 1981), 232–33: "At the level of the dominant culture we are supposed to believe that scientific knowledge is the only knowledge real or worth having; that analogue knowledge [i.e., intuitive, tacit, poetic] is nonexistent or inferior; and that fact and value have nothing to do with each other. None of this is true, but we are all required to live by these rules. . . . [W]e now live in a world turned upside down, a systemic double bind that has resulted in a kind of collective madness. The only way out of this double bind, it would seem, lies in rising to a new level of holistic consciousness which will facilitate new and healthy modes of behavior."

38   Mary Hesse, *Miracles: Cambridge Studies in their Philosophy and History,* ed. C. F. D. Moule, quoted in Dan Wakefield, *Expect a Miracle* (San Francisco: HarperSanFrancisco, 1995).

38   Elliot S. Dacher, *Whole Healing* (New York: Dutton, 1996).

40   Paul B. Beeson, "Changes in Medical Therapy During the Past Half Century," *Medicine* 59, 2: 79–86.

41   . . . *Flexner himself began to have some qualms* . . . Quoted in Pellegrino, *Flexner: 75 Years Later.* Pellegrino chides Flexner not for "apotheosizing science" but for his failure to "be more specific about how humanism and compassion could be taught." In Flexner's defense, he notes that Flexner "is not the prophet who led us into the desert of narrow fact-packed anti-humanistic medical curricula. If we are there now it is because we have taken to heart only half of his educational legacy."

42   "The Mantra of No" draws on a number of sources including: Carol E. McMahon, *Where Medicine Fails* (Owerri, NY: Trado-Medic Books, 1986); Robert S. Mendelsohn, *Confessions of a Medical Heretic* (Chicago: Contemporary Books, 1979); Oscar Janiger and Philip Goldberg, *A Different Kind of Healing* (New York: Putnam, 1993); Andrew Stanway, *Complementary Medicine* (New York: Arkana Penguin Books, 1994); Edward Parker Luongo, *American Medicine in Crisis* (New York: Philosophical Library, 1971); Kristine Beyerman Alster, *The Holistic Health Movement* (Tuscaloosa: The University of Alabama Press, 1989); Robert C. Fuller, *Alternative Medicine and American Religious Life* (New York and Oxford: Oxford University Press, 1989); Marc S. Micozzi, ed., *Fundamentals of Alternative and Complementary Medicine* (New York: Churchill Livingstone, 1996); Stanley Joel Reiser, "The Era of the Patient," *Journal of the American Medical Association* 29, 8 (February 24, 1993): 1012–17.

42   . . . "*rabid dogs*" . . . The chiropractors' case against the American Medical Association is told in Howard Wolinsky and Tom Brune, *The Serpent on the Staff* (New York: Tarcher/Putnam, 1994).

page

43   . . . *"The credulous believe"* . . . For more on what the credulous believe, quackery, and quack-busting, see Stephen Barrett and William T. Jarvis, *The Health Robbers* (Buffalo: Prometheus Books, 1993); Jack Raso, *"Alternative" Healthcare: A Comprehensive Guide* (Buffalo: Prometheus Books, 1994). Robert Buckman and Karl Sabbagh, *Magic or Medicine: An Investigation of Healing and Healers* (New York: Prometheus Books, 1995), tries to avoid "taking sides." An interesting skeptical introduction to paranormal phenomena such as clairvoyance can be found in Theodore Schick Jr. and Lewis Vaughn, *How to Think About Weird Things: Critical Thinking for a New Age* (Mountain View, CA: Mayfield Publishing, 1995).

43   René Dubos, *The Mirage of Health* (New York: Harper, 1959).

44   . . . *the word "holism"* . . . was coined by the former prime minister of South Africa and biologist Jan Christiaan Smuts, *Holism and Evolution* (New York: Macmillan, 1926).

44   Anne Harrington, *Reenchanted Science* (Princeton, NJ: Princeton University Press, 1996).

44   Harry Schwartz, "A Half Century of Health Progress," *The Ohio State Medical Journal* 71, 1 (January 1975): 58–59.

44   Ivan Illich, *Medical Nemesis: The Expropriation of Health* (New York: Pantheon, 1976).

45   . . . *2.2 million nonfatal adverse reactions to medications, up from 1.5 million* . . . Ralph Greene, *Medical Overkill* (Philadelphia: George Stickley, 1983). Other statistics are from the National Center for Health Statistics.

46   . . . *From 1990 to 1994, health-care spending in the U.S. doubled* . . . Joseph W. Duncan and Andrew C. Gross, *Statistics for the 21st Century* (New York: Dun & Bradstreet, 1993). Health-care spending was six percent of the gross domestic product in 1990 and twelve percent by 1993.

46   . . . *physicians who asked patients* . . . It's worse than I remembered: Physicians would interrupt after an average of eighteen seconds. H. Beckman and R. Frankel in "The effect of physician behavior on the collection of data, *Annals of Internal Medicine* 101, 5 (November 1981): 692–96.

47   Harris L. Coulter, *Divided Legacy: A History of the Schism in Medical Thought*: vol. 3, *The Conflict Between Homeopathy and the American Medical Association* (Berkeley: North Atlantic Books, 1973); vol. 4, *Twentieth Century Medicine: The Bacteriological Era* (Berkeley: North Atlantic Books, 1994).

47   David Eisenberg, et al., "Unconventional Medicine in the United States: Prevalence, Costs and Patterns of Use." *New England Journal of Medicine* 328 (1993): 245–52.

CHAPTER TWO

51   *If I aspire to a metaphysical career* . . . E. M. Cioran, *The Temptation to Exist* (London: Quartet Books, 1987), 33–34.

53   . . . *Joel B. Wallach* . . . Joel B. Wallach was at pains to include his middle initial on his card in order to distinguish himself from Joel D. Wallach, a veterinarian who has gained notoriety in alternative medicine circles for his controversial taped lecture "Dead Doctors Don't Lie."

page

54   Joseph Campbell, *The Inner Reaches of Outer Space: Metaphor as Myth and as Religion* (New York: Harper & Row, 1988), 110.

54   Bill Moyers, *Healing and the Mind* (New York: Doubleday, 1993).

58   *"What lies in that space"* . . . Upanishads, translated by W. B. Yeats, in F. C. Happold, *Mysticism: A Study and an Anthology* (New York: Penguin, 1963).

60   *"Force, Force, everywhere Force"* . . . Thomas Carlyle, quoted in Eric R. Bentley, *A Century of Hero Worship* (Philadelphia: Lippincott, 1944).

60   . . . *detect a ridge of glass* . . . Quoted in Paul W. Brand and Anne Hollister, *Clinical Mechanics of the Hand* (St. Louis: Mosby Year Book,1993).

61   Freeman Dyson, *Infinite in All Directions* (New York: HarperCollins, 1988).

62   . . . *the doctrine of vitalism* . . . Discussed in Rainer Shubert-Soldern, *Mechanism & Vitalism: Philosophical Aspects of Biology* (South Bend, IN: University of Notre Dame Press, 1962).

64   . . . *adaptation energy* . . . Hans Selye, *The Stress of Life* (New York: McGraw Hill, 1956), 209.

64   . . . *variety of pulses in the Nei Ching* . . . Summarized in Majno, *The Healing Hand,* and in Masoshing Ni, trans., *Neijing Suwen: The Yellow Emperor's Classic of Medicine* (Boston: Shambhala, 1995). For a Western perspective, see *Harper's,* January 1976, in which the noted surgeon and author Richard Seltzer describes watching Yeshi Donden, physician to the Dalai Lama, do a pulse diagnosis of a female patient: "For the next half hour, he remains thus, suspended above the patient like some exotic golden bird with folded wings, holding the pulse of the woman beneath his fingers, cradling her hand in his. All the power of the man seems to have been drawn down into this one purpose. . . . And I know that I, who have palpated a hundred thousand pulses, have not truly felt a single one."

66   John Mann and Lar Short, *The Body of Light* (Boston: Charles E. Tuttle, 1990).

66   . . . *detect a strand of hair* . . . Quoted in Robert C. Fulford, *Dr. Fulford's Touch of Life* (New York: Pocket Books, 1996).

67   . . . *kundalini* . . . *that aspect of the life force coiled in the sacrum* . . . Eliade, *Yoga: Immortality and Freedom,* pp. 241–45, reports that kundalini is "coiled eight times like a serpent around [the root chakra], as brilliant as lightning."

67   Werner Bohm, *Chakras: Roots of Power* (York Beach, ME: Samuel Weiser, 1991). The discussion of the chakras through the book draws heavily on Arthur Avalon, Sir John Woodroffe, *The Serpent Power: The Secrets of Tantric Yoga and Shaktic Yoga* (New York: Dover Publications, 1974); Mircea Eliade, *Yoga: Immortality and Freedom* (Princeton: Princeton University Press, 1958). Also I relied on Shafica Karagulla and Dora van Gelder Kunz, *The Chakras and the Human Energy Fields* (Wheaton, IL: The Theosophical Publishing House, 1989); Zachary F. Lansdowne, *The Chakras and Esoteric Healing* (York Beach, ME: Samuel Weiser, 1986): Carolyn Myss, *The Anatomy of the Spirit* (New York: Harmony Books, 1996); Hiroshi Motoyama, *Theories of the Chakras* (Wheaton, IL: The Theosophical Publishing House, 1981); Klansbernd Vollmar, *Journey Through the Chakras* (Bath, ME: Gateway Books, 1987); Harish Johari, *Chakras: Energy Centers of Transformation* (Rochester, VT: Destiny Books, 1987).

68   . . . *and only four mentioned in Buddhist tantras* . . . Eliade, p. 243: "four chakras situated

page

respectively in the umbilical, cardiac, and laryngeal regions and the cerebral plexus." In other words, numbers two, four, five, and seven.

68   *... one could just as easily substitute the days of the week* ... A number of commentators have remarked on the symbolic correspondence between the chakras and the endocrine glands. Physician William A. McGarey, *In Search of Healing* (New York: Perigee, 1996), also suggests a symbolic correspondence between the chakras and—clown alert!—the seven dwarfs. The first chakra belongs to Dopey, the second to Bashful, and then Grumpy, Sneezy, Happy, Sleepy, and finally, Doc. "The unconscious is much more knowledgeable than the conscious mind in many regards," McGarey writes. "If we dig deeply into these areas, as the Seven Dwarfs did while searching for gold in the earth, then we must expect something valuable to be brought to light."

68   *... chakras seemed more like metaphysical speculations* ... Eliade, *Yoga: Immortality and Freedom,* p. 234, notes: "[C]areful reading of the texts suffices to show that ... these 'centers' [chakras] represent yogic states—that is, states that are inaccessible without preliminary spiritual *ascesis.* Purely psychophysical mortifications and disciplines are not enough to 'awaken' the chakras or to penetrate them; the essential and indispensable factor remains meditation, spiritual 'realization.' Thus, it is safer to regard 'mystical physiology' as the result and the conceptulization of experiments undertaken from very remote times by ascetics and yogins. Now we must not forget that the yogins performed their experiments on a 'subtle body' (that is, by making use of sensations, tensions, and transconscious states inaccessible to the uninitiate), that they became masters of a zone infinitely greater than the 'normal' psychic zone, that they penetrated into depths of the unconscious and were able to 'awaken' the archaic strata of primordial consciousness, which, in other human beings, are fossilized."

69   Barbara Brennan, *Hands of Light: A Guide to Healing Through the Human Energy Field* (New York: Bantam Books, 1988).

73   Barbara Brennan, *Light Emerging* (New York: Bantam Books, 1993).

78   *... like Robert Benchley doing his immortal parody* ... Robert Benchley, *The Treasurer's Report and Other Aspects of Community Singing* (New York: Harper & Brothers, 1930).

78   *... Socrates frequently heard ... the voice of a semidivine being* ... In Plato, *Theagetes,* quoted in Jeffery Mishlove, *The Roots of Consciousness* (Tulsa: Council Oaks Books, 1975, rev. 1993).

83   *... astonishingly narcissistic* ... For a more skeptical (and psychologically conservative) view of what healers are doing, see Stephen A. Appelbaum, "The laying on of health: personality patterns of psychic healers," in *Bulletin of the Menninger Clinic* 53, 1 (Winter 1993): 33–40. "A case can be made for healing as an expression of the kind of love that predominates early in life, based on the wish and expectation of mother and child that mother will 'make it right,' " Appelbaum notes. He takes the position that "the typical healer basically tests reality accurately, but nonetheless is open to self-delusion through being less interested in checking ideas with reality than in having wishes supported by like-minded people. Made anxious by the hemming in of rules and structure, healers are typically committed to finding their own path and rejecting that of others. Healers are aided in this pursuit by sublime self-confidence, however cloaked in humility, and are drawn, in fact or fantasy, to center stage." And he goes on to say, for what it's worth: "Healing stems from an infantile layer of the mind that includes

page

such oral traits as eating and garrulousness and a merging givingness modeled on the relationship between mother and child."

85 Diane Goldner, "High Energy Healer," *New Age Journal,* January/February 1996.

92 . . . *a set of intriguing studies* . . . See Valerie V. Hunt, *Infinite Mind: Science of Human Vibrations of Consciousness,* (Malibu, CA: Malibu Publishing, 1996); also Valerie V. Hunt, "Electromyographic High Frequency Recording of Human Informational Fields," in *Energy Fields in Medicine* (Kalamazoo, MI: The John E. Fetzer Foundation, 1989).

C H A P T E R   T H R E E

103 Charles W. Leadbeater, *Man Visible and Invisible* (Wheaton, IL: The Theosophical Publishing House, 1925).

105 . . .*Viki Buchanan* . . . That would be Victoria Lord Riley Burke Buchanan Buchanan Carpenter, "The First Lady of Llanview."

105 Kim Heron letter, personal correspondence.

106 . . . *"Oprah: OK. Now what is the bo—"* . . . Transcript, *Oprah,* April 6, 1994, Harpo Productions.

110 "This Mad Glory of Hands" draws on a number of books including Daniel J. Benor's two-volume summaries of healing research, *Healing Research: Holistic Energy Medicine and Spirituality:* vol. 1, *Research in Healing* (Munich: Helix Editions, 1993), and vol. 2, *Holistic Energy Medicine and the Energy Body* (Munich: Helix Editions, 1994). There is also a comprehensive overview of "mental healing" in Jerry Solfvin, "Mental Healing, *Advances in Parapsychological Research,* ed. Stanley Krippner, vol. 4 (New York: Plenum Press, 1974), 31–63; I also relied on Richard Gerber, *Vibrational Medicine* (Sante Fe: Bear & Company, 1988); Dean Kraft, *Portrait of a Psychic Healer* (New York: Putnam, 1981); and Malcolm S. Southwood, *The Healing Experience: Remarkable Cases from a Professional Healer* (London, Piatkus, 1994). See also Lori J. Zefron, "The History of the Laying-on of Hands in Nursing," *Nursing Forum* 14, 4 (1975): 350–63.

110 . . . *described in the Ebers papyrus* . . . Stanley Krippner, "Energy Medicine in Indigenous Healing Systems," in *Energy Medicine Around the World,* ed. T. M. Srinivasan (Phoenix: Gabriel Press, 1988).

111 Finbarr Nolan, *Seventh Son of a Seventh Son* (Edinburgh: Mainstream Publishing, 1992).

111 . . . *starting with the Synod of Ancyra* . . . Lilla Bek and Philippa Pullar, *The Seven Levels of Healing* (London: Rider, 1986), 35.

112 *Alternative Medicine: Expanding Medical Horizons, A Report to the National Institutes of Health on Alternative Medical Systems and Practices in the United States,* NIH Publication No. 94-066, December 1994, U.S. Government Printing Office.

112 . . . *ten to twelve watts of bioelectricity* . . . *The Incredible Machine* (Washington, D.C.: National Geographic Society, 1986). See also Elmer and Alyce Green, *Beyond Biofeedback* (Fort Wayne, IN: Knoll, 1977), and Robert O. Becker, *The Body Electric* (New York: William Morrow, 1985).

113 . . . *decapitated torpedo fish* . . . Quoted in *Bulletin of Historical Medicine* 20 (1946): 112–37. According to Krippner in "Energy Medicine in Indigenous Healing Systems," the

page

Roman physician Scribonius Largus used electric fish to cure headaches, and the Abyssinians used electric catfish to drive out harmful spirits.

113   . . . *Some bioenergy that healers can generate* . . . On just the question of healing and energy there are some strange findings. For example, researcher Elmer Green found that electrostatic fields of meditating healers were marked by mysterious voltage surges lasting an average of three and a half seconds. See "Anomalous electrostatic phenomena in exceptional subjects," *Subtle Energies* 2, 3 (1991): 64–94. What these phenomena mean, nobody knows. Energy, as science understands it, may not even be required for healing, given the studies of William Brande and Marilyn Schlitz, which suggest that healers and psychics can influence autonomic activity in people at a distant location. These so-called distant-intentionality studies raise the possibility that energy is an outmoded metaphor and the transaction between healers and patients occurs in some other form or domain. See Schlitz, M. and Brande, W., "Distant Intentionality and Healing: Assessing the Evidence," *Alternative Therapies* 3, 6 (November 1997).

114   "Chain of Thumbs" draws on two irresistible books: Alan Gauld, *A History of Hypnotism* (New York and Cambridge: Cambridge University Press, 1992); and Adam Crabtree, *From Freud to Mesmer: Magnetic Sleep and the Roots of Psychological Healing* (New Haven: Yale University Press, 1993). Also: Frank Podmore, *From Mesmer to Christian Science* (New Hyde Park, NY: University Books, 1963).

118   . . . *the commission's now classic report*: Jean Bailly, et al., *Report on Animal Magnetism by the Royal Commissioners,* trans. Charles and Danielle Salas, published in *Skeptic* 4, 3 (1996): 68–83.

121   . . . *attach a secret report* . . . Translated and discussed in Alfred Binet and Charles Fere, *Animal Magnetism* (London: 1887).

121   . . . *eight thousand people* . . . Podmore, *From Mesmer to Christian Science.*

121   Ellenberger, *The Discovery of the Unconscious.*

123   . . . *one arm, one breast, and two penises* . . . James Esdaile, *Mesmerism in India and Its Practical Application in Surgery and Medicine* (London: Longman, Brown, Green and Longmans, 1846; reprinted by Arno Press, 1975).

125   Stefan Zweig, *Mental Healers* (New York: Frederick Ungar Publishing, 1932).

126   Karl von Reichenbach, *The Odic Force* (New Hyde Park, NY: University Books, 1968).

128   J. Gordon Melton, ed., *Encyclopedia of Occultism and Parapsychology* (Detroit: Gale Research Inc., 1996).

129   Walter J. Kilner, *The Human Aura* (New Hyde Park, NY: University Books, 1965).

129   Arthur J. Ellison, "Some Recent Experiments in Psychic Perception," *Journal of the Society for Psychical Research* 41, 713 (1962): 355–65.

130   . . . *the formidable Wilhelm Reich* . . . W. Edward Mann, *Orgone, Reich & Eros* (New York: Simon & Schuster, 1973).

134   . . . *a Canadian biologist* . . . Biographical material on Bernard Grad is based on author interviews with the biologist.

138   . . . *Oskar Estebany* . . . See David M. Rorvik, "The Healing Hand of Mr. E.," *Esquire,* February 1974.

139   . . . *"I wanted to create some unfavorable conditions that healers could overcome"* . . . Among Grad's many publications are: Bernard Grad et al., "An Unorthodox Method

page

of Treatment on Wound Healing in Mice," *International Journal of Parapsychology* 2, 3 (1961): 5–19; Bernard Grad, "Some Biological Effects of the Laying On of Hands," *Journal of the American Society for Psychical Research* 59 (1967): 95–129. Bernard Grad, "The Laying On of Hands: Implications for Psychotherapy, Gentling and the Placebo Effect," *Journal of the American Society of Psychical Research* 61: 286–305. See also "An Anatomy of Healing, *ASPR Newsletter* 18, 1, published by the American Society of Psychical Research.

144 ... *a speech [Grad] had delivered* ... Bernard Grad, "Invited Address," *Research in Parapsychology 1988* (Metuchen, NJ: Scarecrow Press, 1989).

146 Sister M. Justa Smith, "Paranormal Effects on Enzyme Activity," *Human Dimensions* 1, 2, (1972), The Human Dimensions Institute; Dolores Krieger, "The Response of In-Vivo Human Hemoglobin to an Active Healing Therapy by Direct Laying on of Hands," *Human Dimensions* 1, 3 (1972), The Human Dimensions Institute.

146 Dolores Krieger, *Accepting Your Power to Heal: The Personal Practice of Therapeutic Touch* (Sante Fe: Bear & Company, 1993). See also Janet Quinn, "Building a Body of Knowledge: Research on Therapeutic Touch 1974–1986," *Journal of Holistic Nursing* 6, 1 (1988): 37–45.

CHAPTER FOUR

151 "*In this body, in this town of Spirit*" ... Book VIII, The Doctrine of the Chhāndôgyas, translated by W. B. Yeats and Shree Purohit Swami, *The Ten Principal Upanishads* (New York: Macmillan, 1937).

153 "Valentine/Pump." I drew on books by Daniel E. Schneider, *The Image of the Heart* (New York: International Universities Press, 1956); Julius Comroe, *Exploring the Heart* (New York: Norton, 1983). The origins of the shape of the valentine heart are addressed in Gordon Bendersky, "The Olmec Heart Effigy: The Earliest Image of the Human Heart," *Perspectives in Biology and Medicine* 40, 2 (Spring 1997). "In ancient Greco-Roman and Etruscan times, the heart acquired a conventionalized form which may be the prototype of the traditional valentine card symbol; however the actual origins of this symbol may lie in a botanical form, fashioned from the vine leaf."

153 ... *young ascetic Dayānand Sarasvatī* ... Quoted in John Nicol Farquhar, *Modern Religious Movements in India* (New York: Macmillan, 1919, reprinted by Garland Publishing, New York, 1980), 106: "His books on Yoga contained anatomical accounts of the human body. Reading in these volumes long and intricate accounts of nerve-circles and nerve-centers which he could not understand, he was suddenly filled with suspicion. As it happened a dead body was floating down the river on the banks of which he was walking. He drew the corpse to the shore, cut it open, satisfied himself that the books were false, and in consequence consigned them to the river along with the corpse. From this time his faith in many works on Yoga gradually dwindled."

154 *Galen's "Prince of all Bowels"* ... Quoted in Robert A. Erickson, *The Language of the Heart* (Philadelphia: University of Pennsylvania Press, 1997).

157 C. Richard Conti, *Clinical Cardiology,* March 1997.

page

167 *. . . five quarts of blood a minute . . .* James J. Lynch, *The Broken Heart* (New York: Basic Books, 1977), 234.

178 *. . . CIA had spent $20 million . . .* Mainstream press accounts include: R. Jeffrey Smith, "Pentagon Has Spent Millions on Tips from Trio of Psychics," *The Washington Post,* November 29, 1995; Douglas Waller, "The Vision Thing," *Time,* December 11, 1995. Headline-writing clowns on the copy desks of many American newspapers had a good laugh lampooning this story: "Pentagon Peepers"; "It's Shaped Like a Nut. Coincidence?" "Hey, Agent 000 has another hunch!" For more sober accounts of the government-funded remote viewing work, see H. E. Puthoff, "CIA-Initiated Remote Viewing Program at Stanford Research Institute," *Journal of Scientific Exploration,* 10, 1 (1996): 63–76, and Edwin C. May, "The American Institutes for Research Review of the Department of Defense's STAR GATE Program: A Commentary," *Journal of Scientific Exploration* 10, 1 (1996): 89–107.

182 *. . . one of the few replications . . .* Daniel P. Wirth, "The Effect of Non-contact Therapeutic Touch on the Healing Rate of Full Thickness Dermal Wounds," *Subtle Energies* 1, 1 (1990): 1–20.

194 *He was from a small rural town in New England . . .* At his request I have withheld Steve's last name and presented only a general description of his background.

196 *. . . kundalini awakenings sometimes entailed discharges of energy . . .* See Bonnie Greenwell, *Energies of Transformation* (Saratoga, CA: Shakti River Press, 1990), also B. S. Goel, *Third Eye and Kundalini* (Kurukshetra, Haryana, India: Third Eye Foundation of India, 1985), especially Chapter VII, "The Divine Process of Kundalini and Its Understanding."

CHAPTER FIVE

211 *Healer and patient are destined actors . . .* Edward C. Whitmont, *The Alchemy of Healing* (Berkeley: North Atlantic Books, 1993), 195.

213 Rachel is a pseudonymn.

215 W. Brugh Joy, *Joy's Way* (New York: Jeremy P. Tarcher, 1979).

224 Henry Miller, *The Smile at the Foot of the Ladder* (New York: New Directions, 1958).

225 Stephen E. Braude, *First Person Plural: Multiple Personality and the Philosophy of Mind* (Lanham, MD: Rowman and Littlefield, 1995).

227 *. . . further elaborated by Alexander Lowan and John Pierrakos . . .* See John C. Pierrakos, *The Core Energetic Process in Group Therapy* (monograph), Institute for the New Age, 1975.

242 *"One always perishes" . . .* Cioran, *The Temptation to Exist.*

CHAPTER SIX

261 Daniel Dennett, *Consciousness Explained* (Boston: Little, Brown, 1991).

264 *. . . a third eyeball . . .* Some clairvoyants claim Ajna is depicted in the Christian/

page

      Masonic image of the eye that peers out from atop the pyramid on the back of the American dollar bill.

265 G. A. Gaskell, *Dictionary of All Myths and Scriptures* (New York: The Julian Press, 1960).

266 . . . *in the words of Hiroshi Motoyama* . . . Motoyama, *Theories of the Chakras.*

266 . . . *"one establishes himself in the place"* . . . Johari, *Chakras: Energy Centers of Transformation.*

267 St. Augustine, quoted in Happold, *Mysticism.*

267 Leadbeater, *Man Visible and Invisible.*

270 Ludwig Wittgenstein, from *Tractatus-Philosophicas,* 1922, quoted in *The Healing Arts: An Oxford Illustrated Anthology,* ed. R. S. Downie (New York and Oxford: Oxford University Press, 1995).

270 "The Consciousness Bazaar" draws on material in Owen Flanagan, *The Science of the Mind* (Cambridge, MA: MIT Press, second edition, Cambridge MA, 1991); David J. Chalmers, *The Conscious Mind* (New York: Oxford University Press, 1996); Antonio R. Damasio, *Descartes' Error* (New York, G. P. Putnam's Sons, 1994); John Searle, *The Rediscovery of the Mind* (Cambridge, MA: MIT Press, 1992).

275 . . . *famous research by neuroscientist Benjamin Libet* . . . is well summarized in Nicholas Herbert, *Elemental Mind* (New York: Plume/Penguin, 1993); Benjamin Libet, "subjective Antedating of a Sensory Experience and Mind-Brain Theories," *Journal of Theoretical Biology* 114 (1985): 563–70.

278 *"As for the point about my not being a zombie"* . . . For clarity's sake I have interpolated Dennett's definition of a zimbo, which is drawn from *Consciousness Explained,* p. 310.

279 . . . *an eloquent Sub* . . . See David Hodgson, *The Mind Matters* (Oxford: Clarendon Press, 1991).

284 Dr. Philip West's account of "Mr. Wright" is included in Bruno Klopfer, Psychological Variables in Human Cancer," *Journal of Projective Techniques* 21, 4 (December 1957).

284 . . . *Krebiozen* . . . *produced by injecting horses* . . . *Report on Krebiozen,* pamphlet, Krebiozen Research Foundation, 1962.

285 Daniel E. Moerman, "Physiology and Symbols: The Anthropological Implications of the Placebo Effect," in *The Anthropology of Medicine,* eds., Lola Romanucci-Ross, Daniel E. Moerman, Laurence R. Tancredi (New York: Bergin & Garvey, 1991).

286 Anthony Campbell, "Cartesian Dualism and the Concept of Medical Placebos," *Journal of Consciousness Studies* 1, 2 (1994): 230–33.

287 I drew on three books by Gerald Epstein: *Waking Dream Therapy* (East Hampton, New York: ACMI Press, 1981); *Healing Visualizations* (New York: Bantam Books, 1989): *Healing into Immortality* (New York: Bantam Books, 1994). Also: Leon Eisenberg, "The Subjective in Medicine," *Perspectives in Biology and Medicine* 27, 1 (Autumn 1983).

292 Susan Sontag, *Illness as Metaphor* (New York: Farrar, Straus & Giroux, 1978).

295 Richard S. Broughton, *Parapsychology: The Controversial Science* (New York: Ballantine Books, 1991).

296 . . . *postmodern critics who insist that reality is a social construction* . . . See Walter Truett Anderson, ed., *The Truth About the Truth: Deconfusing and Reconstructing the Postmodern World* (New York: Tarcher/Putnam, 1995).

page

296 James Randi, *Flim Flam: ESP, Unicorns and Other Delusions* (Buffalo: Prometheus Books, 1982).

297 . . . *the most withering dismissal* . . . The National Research Council report: D. Druckman and J. A. Swets, eds., *Enhancing Human Performance* (Washington, D.C.: National Academy Press, 1988).

297 . . . *the benefits of aspirin* . . . Quoted by Jessica Utts at the 1996 Parapsychological Association annual meeting.

298 Radin's work discussed in "Afterwards, You're a Genius" has recently been summarized in: Dean Radin, *The Conscious Universe* (New York: HarperCollins, 1997).

298 . . . *Radin had coauthored a paper* . . . Dean Radin and Roger Nelson, "Evidence for Consciousness-Related Anomalies in Random Physical Systems, *Foundations of Physics* 19 (1989): 1499.

298 . . . *the Princeton Engineering Anomalies Research Lab* . . . The work of the PEAR lab is summarized in Robert G. Jahn and Brenda J. Dunne, *Margins of Reality: The Role of Consciousness in the Physical World* (New York: Harcourt Brace Jovanovich, 1979).

299 . . . *the article from which her talk was drawn* . . . Susan Blackmore, "Do You Believe in Psychic Phenomena? Are they likely to be able to explain consciousness?" *The Times Higher Education Supplement,* April 5, 1996, p. v.

306 . . . *moon-behavior correlations, which are controversial* . . . See "Seventeen Red." Gravitational effects of the moon are addressed in George O. Abell, "Moon Madness," in *Science and the Paranormal,* ed. George O. Abell and Barry Singer (New York: Scribner's, 1981). George O. Abell's "Moon Madness" piece is not to be confused with E. L. Abel's book *Moon Madness* (Greenwich, CT: Fawcett, 1976). Abell writes that the gravitational force exerted on a two-hundred-pound man by the moon will increase his weight by an amount approximately equal to the weight of a mosquito landing on his shoulder.

307 C.E.M. Hansel, *ESP: A Scientific Evaluation* (New York: Scribner's, 1966).

308 Dean I. Radin, "A Possible Proximity Effect on Human Grip Strength," *Perceptual and Motor Skills* 58 (1984): 887–88.

310 *One was . . . Jessica Utts. . . . The other was Ray Hyman* . . . Their positions are summarized in UCNewsWire, University of California Davis News, November 28, 1995. Utts's review in full can be found at http://www-stat.ucdavis.edu/users/utts. See also: Jessica Utts, "An Assessment of the Evidence for Psychic Functioning," *Journal of Scientific Exploration* 10, 1 (1996): 3–30. Hyman's "Evaluation of Program on Anomalous Mental Phenomena" can be found at http://darkwing.uoregon.edu/~uocomm/newsrel/Hyman.html.

CHAPTER SEVEN

319 Anonymous (Valentin Tomberg), *Meditations on the Tarot* (Rockport, MA: Element, 1993).

327 Woodroffe, *The Serpent Power.*

327 . . . *temporal lobe is the wellspring of religious visual imagery* . . . See Michael Winkelman, "Physiological and Therapeutic Aspects of Shamanistic Healing," *Subtle Energies* 1, 2

page

(1990): "Some temporal lobe seizures are primarily subjective experiences such as visual, auditory, tactile or olfactory hallucinations, a distorted sense of time, or feelings of intense emotion such as fear or ecstasy, while others are associated with sensory experiences or personality changes." He cites a long list of references.

327   Rudolf Otto, *The Idea of the Holy* (Oxford and New York: Oxford University Press, 1923).

328   . . . *a spiritual healer in the Christian tradition* . . . See, for example, Agnes Sanford, *The Healing Light* (Shakopee, MN: Macalester Park Publishing, 1947, rev. 1972), 97, 85. "I found that those who came to me for help received at first a tremendous inflowing of power." And: "[T]hat power of God . . . works through the being of one person for the healing of another. . . . It is only the channeling of a flow of energy from God's being through man's being. It is the entering in of the Holy Spirit of God through the spirit of man, via the conscious and subconscious mind of that man, via the nerves of his body, via the center and thence to his mind and spirit. . . . Thus he makes of his whole being, spirit, mind and body, a receiving and transmitting center for the power of God."

331   . . . *new forms of spirituality* . . . See Jacob Needleman, *The New Religions* (New York: Crossroad Publishing, 1970). See also David G. Bromley and Anson D. Shupe, *Strange Gods* (Boston: Beacon Press, 1981).

331   Robert C. Fuller, *Mesmerism and the American Cure for Souls* (Philadelphia: University of Pennsylvania Press, 1982).

332   Damian Thompson, *The End of Time: Faith and Fear in the Shadow of the Millennium* (Hanover, NH: University Press of New England, 1996).

332   Seyyed Nasr, *Religion and the Order of Nature* (Oxford and New York: Oxford University Press, 1994).

333   Isaac Asimov, "Science and the Mountain Peak," in *Science Confronts the Paranormal,* ed. Kendrick Frazier (Buffalo, NY: Prometheus, 1986).

335   Herbert Benson, *The Relaxation Response* (New York: William Morrow, 1975).

335   David Eisenberg, *Encounters with Qi* (New York: Norton, 1985).

337   William Osler, "The Faith That Heals," *British Medical Journal,* 18 (1910): 1470–72.

337   . . . *some compelling conclusions* . . . Jeffrey Levin, "Religious and Spirituality in Medicine: Research and Education," *The Journal of the American Medical Association* 298 (September 3, 1997): 792–893.

341   . . . *Harris's fidelity* . . . *was so breathtakingly rigorous* . . . A view of Christian Science less pissy than mine can be found in Robert Peel, *Spiritual Healing in a Scientific Age* (San Francisco: Harper & Row, 1987).

345   "*We keep coming back and coming back*" . . . Wallace Stevens, "An Ordinary Evening in New Haven," *The Collected Poems of Wallace Stevens* (New York: Knopf, 1971), 471.

355   Hunt, *Infinite Mind.*

355   Rosalyn Bruyere, *Wheels of Light* (New York: Simon & Schuster, 1989).

361   . . . *lesions on the face of Joseph Carman* . . . Personal correspondence and an unpublished eleven-page account by Joseph Carman: *Miracles Are Hard Work: Five Days of Healing with Rosalyn Bruyere.*

361   Teilhard de Chardin, *The Phenomenon of Man* (New York: Harper & Row, 1959).

page

362 Harvey Cox, *Seduction of the Spirit* (New York: Simon & Schuster, 1973).

366 For more on Lisa Platt, see Chip Brown, "When You Need a Miracle," *Mademoiselle,* April 1996.

373 . . . *dinner party invitations start to dry up* . . . A good illustration of the social costs of espousing an interest in, and a gift for, healing can be found in the example of the Earl of Sandwich. According to Haggard, in *Devils, Drugs and Doctors*, "The Earl of Sandwich believed he had a gift for healing, and practiced on his servants and others. His friends were skeptical. 'Old friends so disliked the idea,' he said, 'that they began by shunning all allusions to the subject and now avoid my society.' " Haggard notes rather tartly that "it is probable that his enthusiasm in his new acquisition made the earl something of a bore."

376 W. H. Auden, "For the Time Being: A Christmas Oratorio," in *Collected Longer Poems* (New York: Random House, 1969).

377 . . . *based on data gathered by a fourth-grade girl* . . . Linda Rosa, Emily Rosa, Larry Sarner, Stephen Barrett, "A Close Look at Therapeutic Touch," *Journal of the American Medical Association,* 279 (April 1, 1998): 1005–1010. An account of the experiment by Gina Kolata was published on the front page of the *The New York Times,* April 1, 1998. A report on the same experiment appeared in 1996 in *Skeptic,* 4, 4.

381 . . . *Nietzsche's letter to Strindberg* . . . Quoted in Richard Elliot Friedman, *The Disappearance of God* (Boston: Little, Brown, 1995). Nietzsche commented on the standardization of people and medicine in *The Joyful Science*: "[T]he more we put aside the dogma of the 'equality of men,' the more must the concept of a normal health, along with a normal diet and the normal course of an illness be abandoned by our physicians. Only then would the time have come to reflect on the health and sicknesses of the *soul,* and to find the peculiar virtue of each man in the health of his soul: in one person's case this health could, of course, look like the opposite of health in another person." Quoted by Kaptchuk and Croucher, *The Healing Arts,* p. 254.

381 Brian Friel, *Faith Healer* (New York: Samuel French, 1980).

ACKNOWLEDGMENTS

This book has had a long advent, and I want to thank some of the people who if they didn't directly contribute to the preparation of its pages nevertheless contributed to the preparation of the author. Foremost is Howard Simons, who died of pancreatic cancer in 1989. As the managing editor of the *Washington Post,* he brought me to the fairgrounds of a great metropolitan daily from a small weekly newspaper in Homer, Alaska, and I doubt I would have ever qualified for a checking account much less a book contract without his visionary faith in a far-fetched protégé. It pains me he's not around to read this opus and, no doubt, to confide in his affectionately hard-boiled way that yes, mentors have to range far afield to find new talent, but in my case he'd probably beaten the bushes too hard.

Also from the *Post* days, thanks to David Maraniss, who urged his then-young writers to follow Lorca and search for the drop of duck's blood under the statistics; and to Bob Woodward, who made me curator of his "nut file," which contained all the bizarre stuff mailed to him by the lunatics of Washington, D.C., and which piqued my curiosity about the possibilities of altered states in a hidebound capital. For life lessons, long-standing guidance, and friendship from the *Post* days on, I thank Mary Battiata, Lloyd Grove, Bill Hamilton, Blaine Harden, Elsa Walsh, and Diane Martinelli Weeks.

As the body of the text makes plain, I'm much indebted to the blessed lapse that allowed Tina Brown to send me off to a healing school on a *New Yorker* assignment. Thanks also to senior editors Robert Vare and Kim Heron for close readings and guidance. Jack Rosenthal, Adam Moss, Stephen Dubner, and Alan Burdick gave me the chance to explore some medical and scientific topics under the aegis of *The New York Times Magazine.* I am grateful to a number of other editors who underwrote my travels in the subtle world and helped shape some of the material: Mary Murray and Karen Marta at *Vogue,* Laurie Abraham at *Mirabella,* Valerie Frankel at *Mademoiselle,* Kim Brown at *Travel & Leisure,* Kurt Andersen and Michael Hirschorn at *New York,* and Terry McDonell, David Hirshey, and Will Blythe at *Esquire.* It's a measure of how long this project took that hardly any of these people are still employed at the same magazines.

For professional interviews, conversations, and guidance, I thank: Stephen Barrett, Daryl J. Bem, Daniel Benor, Susan Blackmore, Stephen E. Braude, Deepak Chopra, Larry Dossey, Gerald Epstein, James S. Gordon, Bernard Grad, Keith Harary, Ruth-Inge Heinze, Valerie Hunt, Alex Imich, Patrice Keane, Stanley Krippner, Jeffrey S. Levin, Richard J. Levinson, Bill Lovallo, Ed May, Woody Merrell, Daniel Moerman, Reed Moskowitz, Mehmet Oz, Herbert Pardes,

Janet Quinn, Dean Radin, Jack Raso, Jannine Rebman, Ruth Reinsel, Beverly A. Rubik, Richard P. Sloan, James Spottiswoode, Nancy Sondow, Marilyn Schlitz, Tony Schwartz, Elisabeth Targ, Eric Rose, Dana Ullman, Rhea White.

Thanks especially to the resourceful Joanne MacMahon, director of the Eileen J. Garrett Library at the Parapsychology Foundation, and to the librarians and staff at the New York Academy of Medicine, and to Andrew Kolonos at the library of the American Society of Psychical Research.

Thanks to practitioners of energy healing who showed me what was in their hands: Karen Aarons, Ticia Agri, Barbara Brennan, Susan Brown, Rosalyn Bruyere, Joseph Carman, Yuliya Cohen, Carol DeSanto, Virginia Dutton, Howie Golde, Marcia Gunsberg, Jennifer Halls, Shelby Hammitt, Alix Harden, Susan Jameson, Catherine Karas, James Kepner, Theo Kyrkostas, Joan Luly, Michael Mamas, Philip Marden, Julie Motz, Diana Muenz, Nancy Needham, Eileen F. Oster, Lisa Platt, Jason Shulman, Traci Slatton, Barbara Sorce, Rolf Steiner, Elizabeth K. Stratton, Susan Traill, Bonnie Vancelette, Marjorie Valeri, Joel Bruce Wallach, Steven Weiss, Susan Weiley, Kathleen Joy Woeber.

From outside the subject matter, I thank Geraldine Baum; my in-laws, Hobart Betts and Glynne Robinson Betts; Mark Bryant; Molly Castelloe; Chris and Stephanie Clark; Joel Gay; John and Stephanie Golfinos; Barbara Greenburg; Miriam Horn; Trea Hoving; Linda Keslar; Bill Kimball; Tom Kizzia; Michael and Sydney McDonnell; Will McGreal; Jeff Maguire; Ann Marsh; Terry Monmaney; Anton Mueller; Carlo Orth-Pallavicini; David Roberts; Kim Shelton; and Ethan and Andrea Topper.

Elizabeth Betts found the photo illustration for the cover; thank you, Liz. Pamela Hanson took the photophobic author's picture; thank you, Pamela. Thanks to the Riverhead angels, past and present: Nicky Weinstock, Nicole Wan, and Hanya Yanagihara.

If in this list of tributes I fail to mention my parents, there will be hell to pay on the holidays. Thank you, Mom and Dad, for love, humor, and support over the years. Long live the Bears!

I come now to the four women who more than any others brought this book into being. My deepest thanks: to my agent, Kris Dahl, who sold the thing on a wing and a prayer; to the publisher, Susan Petersen, who bought the thing on a wing and a prayer. (Look Ma, no book proposal!) To my editor, Julie Grau, who had a vision of what it all might add up to, and whose brilliance helped me find the shape of a story within the sprawl of a subject. (To the degree that this book has a spirit guide of its own, it's Julie.) And finally, to my wife, Kate Betts, who singlehandedly solved my mind-body problem and, with her great unstinted flow of love, helped me through the most difficult days of this long adventure: She walks on water. *Namaste.*

ABOUT THE AUTHOR

C hip Brown, a former staff writer for the *Washington Post,* has written for *The New York Times Magazine, The New Yorker, Harper's, Esquire, Outside, Vanity Fair, Vogue, Condé Nast Traveler,* and more than twenty other national magazines. He has won numerous honors for his journalism, including a National Magazine Award for feature writing. He lives in New York City with his wife, Kate Betts.